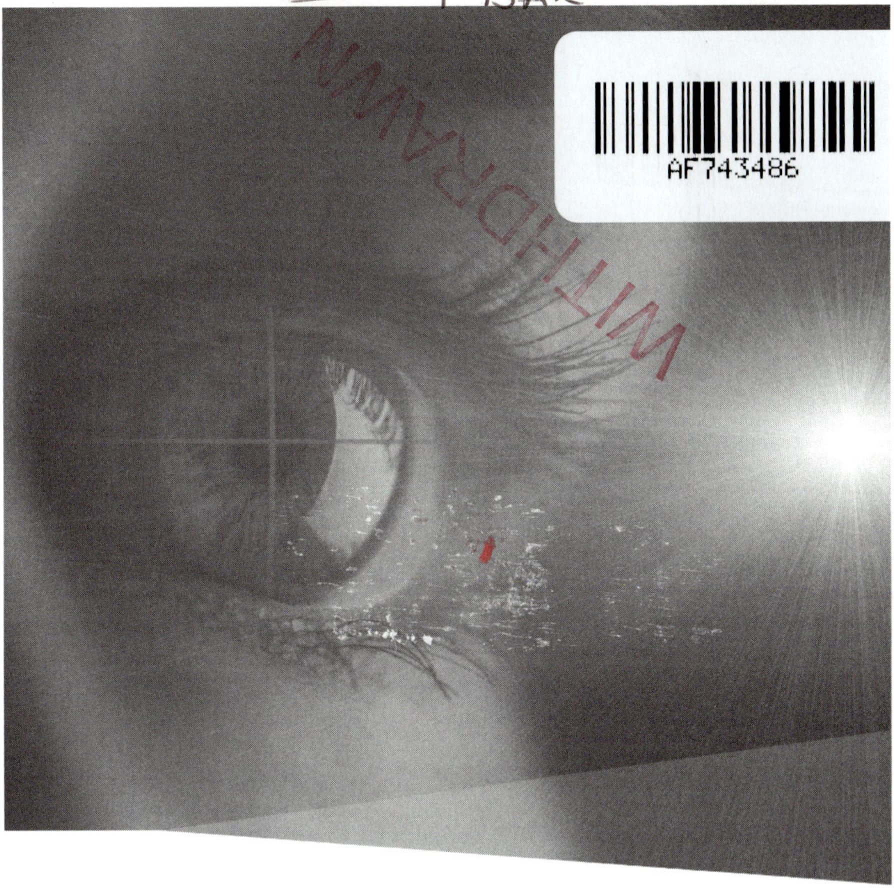

Ophthalmic Drug Facts

19th Edition

Wolters Kluwer Health | Facts & Comparisons

Ophthalmic Drug Facts®

Manuscript indexed by Graves Editorial Service, Colorado Springs, Colorado.

Adapted from *Drug Facts and Comparisons®* loose-leaf drug information service.

ISBN-10: 1-57439-275-1
ISBN-13: 978-1-57439-275-3

Printed in the United States of America

Wolters Kluwer Health
77 Westport Plaza, Suite 450
St. Louis, Missouri 63146-3125
Phone 314/216-2100 • 800/223-0554
Fax 314/878-5563
www.factsandcomparisons.com

Ophthalmic Drug Facts®

Editor

Jimmy D. Bartlett, OD, DOS, DSc (Hon)
Professor of Optometry,
School of Optometry
Professor of Pharmacology,
School of Medicine
University of Alabama at Birmingham
Birmingham, Alabama

Ophthalmic Drug Facts® Editorial Panel

Edward S. Bennett, OD, MSEd
Associate Professor
Co-Chief, Contact Lens Service
School of Optometry
University of Missouri – St. Louis
St. Louis, Missouri

Richard G. Fiscella, RPh, MPH
Clinical Professor
Department of Pharmacy Practice
University of Illinois at Chicago
Chicago, Illinois

Siret D. Jaanus, PhD, LHD (Hon)
Professor of Pharmacology
Southern California College of Optometry
Fullerton, California

Thom J. Zimmerman, MD, PhD
Emeritus Professor and Chairman
Department of Ophthalmology and Visual Sciences
Emeritus Professor of Pharmacology and Toxicology
University of Louisville
School of Medicine
Louisville, Kentucky

Global Ophthalmic Medical Director
Global Medical Affairs
Pfizer Ophthalmics

Table of Contents

Editor's Preface

The mission of *Ophthalmic Drug Facts* is to provide reliable and objective ophthalmic drug information to facilitate therapeutic decision making. This book is intended to promote efficient, quality eye health care. Although general information is available for ophthalmic drugs, there are very few sources that provide comparative drug and drug product information in a concise format; none is as comprehensive.

Ophthalmic Drug Facts was conceived and developed through a team approach and will be of value to both the student and eyecare practitioner. Ophthalmologists, optometrists, and pharmacists should find this text particularly valuable in their daily practices.

Ophthalmic Drug Facts provides a broad range of information including pharmacologic and pharmacokinetic information on drug entities, commercial product information, and specific formulation availability. The text is arranged in a pharmacotherapeutic format, with emphasis on drug action and current product availability rather than on pathophysiology of disease states.

Ophthalmic Drug Facts is a comprehensive ophthalmic drug information resource. Detailed information on specific entities is included as well as many drug combinations. There is also a comprehensive section of contact lens products and extemporaneous preparations. Selected bibliographies are provided for all chapters. In addition, *Ophthalmic Drug Facts* includes valuable information on:

- Systemic medications for ocular conditions
- Systemic drugs affecting the eye
- Off-label uses for FDA-approved drugs
- Orphan ophthalmic agents and investigational drugs
- Ophthalmic product manufacturer index
- Extemporaneous preparations

We hope the reader finds this a valuable guide in ophthalmic drug product selection and use. As any practitioner is aware, ophthalmic practice is constantly adapting to incorporate the latest information. We intend to continue the effort with future editions; therefore, your comments, criticisms, and suggestions are always welcome.

Jimmy D. Bartlett, OD, DOS, DSc (Hon)
Edward S. Bennett, OD, MSEd
Richard G. Fiscella, RPh, MPH
Siret D. Jaanus, PhD, LHD (Hon)
Thom J. Zimmerman, MD, PhD

Introduction

Ophthalmic Drug Facts is a comprehensive ophthalmic drug information compendium. The unique format is designed to facilitate comparisons between drugs. To enable the reader to quickly locate needed information, it has been organized by:

- Therapeutic drug class
- Table of contents
- Chapter summary tables
- Comprehensive alphabetical index
- Extensive cross-referencing

The following pages explain the organization and contents of *Ophthalmic Drug Facts* in detail. All readers are urged to review this information to ensure efficient and effective use of *Ophthalmic Drug Facts.*

♦ Editorial Policy

Accurate, unbiased information; concise, standardized presentation; comparative, objective format; and timely delivery are the principal editorial guidelines governing *Ophthalmic Drug Facts*. Review of FDA-approved product labeling, hundreds of journal articles, textbooks, policies, and recommendations from many authoritative and official groups form the base of evaluation of information for *Ophthalmic Drug Facts.* FDA-approved indications and dosage recommendations are included. In addition, other established or potential uses are discussed and are designated as *"Off-label Uses."*

Most of the products listed are protected by letters of patent and their names are trademarked and registered by the firm whose name appears with the product. Identification of the product distributor is given in parentheses next to the brand name. The distributor may or may not be the actual manufacturer or fabricator of the final dosage form. Listing of specific products is an indication only of availability on the market and does not constitute an endorsement or recommendation.

Products that contain identical amounts of active ingredients are listed together for comparison as an aid in product selection. Drug product interchange is regulated by state laws; listing of products together does not imply that they are therapeutically equivalent or legally interchangeable. Caution is particularly advised when comparing sustained release, timed release, or repeat action dosage forms.

♦ Editorial Panel

The Editorial Panel for *Ophthalmic Drug Facts* is an interdisciplinary group of established, respected, and renowned clinicians and researchers. The panel includes recognized experts in the fields of ocular pharmacology, therapeutics, and drug information. These experts contribute the introductory material, review monographs, and provide direction for *Ophthalmic Drug Facts.*

The Facts and Comparisons® Editorial Advisory Panel consists of a very distinguished group of physicians, pharmacologists, and pharmacists. This panel reviews monographs and provides editorial direction for the entire Facts and Comparisons® database.

♦ Organization

Information in *Ophthalmic Drug Facts* is organized by therapeutic use. Twelve chapters are divided into groups and subgroups to facilitate comparisons of drugs and drug products with similar uses. The remaining chapters provide information on chapter summary tables, ophthalmic dosage forms and routes of administration, miscellaneous products, contact lens care, systemic drugs affecting the eye, extemporaneous preparations, systemic medications used for ocular conditions, and investigational and orphan drugs.

Products most similar in content or use are listed together. This format of presenting the facts makes it easy to make comparisons of identical, similar, or related products. Because drugs are listed by use, some drugs may be listed in more than one section of the book.

♦ Index

The alphabetical index includes page references for drugs by their generic name, brand or trade name (in italics), and therapeutic group names. Additionally, many synonyms, pharmacological actions, and therapeutic uses for agents are included.

♦ Chapter Introductions

The chapter introductions provide information about the drugs in each therapeutic class, including general treatment guidelines. A selected bibliography located at the end of each chapter introduction provides additional sources of information.

♦ Drug Monographs

Prescribing information is presented in comprehensive drug monographs. General information on a group of closely related drugs may be presented in a group monograph. Specific information relating to a particular drug is presented in an individual monograph under the generic name of the drug. All monographs are divided into sections identified with bold titles for ease in locating the desired information.

Actions: Provides a brief summary of the known pharmacologic and pharmacokinetic properties.

Indications: All FDA-approved indications or uses are listed. When available, drug monographs also include "Off-label Uses." These include investigational uses for drugs and uses not yet approved by the FDA.

Contraindications: Specifies those conditions in which the drug should NOT be used.

Warnings and Precautions: Lists conditions in which use of the drug may be hazardous, precautions to observe, and parameters to monitor during therapy.

Drug Interactions: A brief summary of documented, clinically significant drug-drug, drug-food, and drug-lab test interactions is provided.

Adverse Reactions: Reported adverse reactions are presented. Incidence data on adverse effects are included when available.

Overdosage: Clinical manifestations of toxicity and treatment of overdosage are given for most agents.

Patient Information: Provides the essential information to be communicated to the patient by the health professional to allow the patient to safely and effectively administer the medication.

Administration and Dosage: Dosage ranges and administration methods are presented.

♦ Charts and Tables

Charts and tables are included in many monographs to make drug-drug comparisons easier. Examples of tables include: Pharmacokinetics (onset, peak and duration of action), routes of administration, dosage ranges, and adverse reactions.

♦ Special Features

Contact Lens Care: Chapter 13 provides guidelines and product information for soft and rigid gas permeable contact lens care.

Extemporaneous Preparations: Chapter 15 provides guidelines for the use and preparation of extemporaneous compounding of ophthalmic solutions.

Systemic Drugs Affecting the Eye: Chapter 16 discusses the effects systemic drugs have on ocular structures and functions.

Systemic Medications Used for Ocular Conditions: Chapter 17 discusses systemic medications and their uses and dosing in ocular conditions.

Orphan Drugs: The Orphan Drugs section of the Appendix briefly describes Orphan Drug legislation and includes a table that provides generic name, trade name, indication, and manufacturer information on Orphan Drugs for ophthalmic conditions.

Manufacturer Index: This index provides the unique manufacturer/labeler codes found in the National Drug Code (NDC) numbers, as well as the addresses and phone numbers of the manufacturers and distributors of ophthalmic products listed in *Ophthalmic Drug Facts.*

♦ Product Listings

Individual products are listed following each monograph. The format and components of the product listings are discussed below and illustrated on the following page.

1. **Chapter title** is located at the top of the right-hand page.
2. **Generic titles** appear at the beginning of general drug monographs and individual drug monographs.
3. **Cross references** to the appropriate drug monograph appear for complete prescribing information.
4. **Distribution status** of products is indicated as *Rx* or *otc.*
5. **Identical brand name products** are listed in alphabetical order. Combination products are listed in tables to facilitate comparisons. Products most similar in formulation are listed next to each other.
6. **Products are grouped** by dosage form or strength.
7. **Package sizes** are given for all dosage forms and strengths of each product.
8. **Products available by their generic name** from multiple sources are indicated as available from (Various) distributors. Selected multiple-source distributors and manufacturers are provided. The list of distributors and manufacturers is intended to provide an example and is not an attempt to be comprehensive.
9. **Distributor's name** is given in parentheses next to the product name.

ATROPINE SULFATE ——②

For complete prescribing information, refer to the Cycloplegic Mydriatrics group monograph. ——③

Indications:

Mydriasis/Cycloplegia: For cycloplegic refraction or pupil dilation in acute inflammatory conditions of iris and uveal tract.

Administration and Dosage:

Solution:

Adults - Uveitis – Instill 1 or 2 drops into the eye(s) up to 4 times daily.

Children - Uveitis – Instill 1 or 2 drops of 0.5% solution into the eye(s) up to 3 times daily.

Refraction – Instill 1 or 2 drops of 0.5% solution into the eye(s) twice daily for 1 to 3 days before examination.

Ointment: Apply a small amount in the conjunctival sac up to 3 times daily.

Compress the lacrimal sac by digital pressure during and for 2 to 3 minutes after instillation.

Individuals with heavily pigmented irides may require larger doses.

Storage/Stability: Keep away from heat.

④ ⑤

Rx	**Atropine Sulfate Ophthalmic** (Various, eg, Bausch & Lomb)	⑥ **Ointment:** 1%	In 3.5.
Rx ⑧	**Atropine Sulfate** (Various, eg, Alcon, Bausch & Lomb, Fougera) ⑨	**Solution:** 1%	⑦ In 2, 5, and 15 mL.

Monographs

Dosage Forms and Routes of Administration

For ophthalmic drugs to be effective, they must reach ocular tissues in relatively high concentrations. Depending on the specific diagnostic or therapeutic objective, ophthalmic drugs may be delivered to the eye through various routes of administration, including the following:

- Topical
- Oral
- Parenteral
- Periocular
- Intracameral
- Intravitreal

TOPICAL ADMINISTRATION

Topical application is the most common route of administration for ophthalmic drugs. Advantages of topical application are convenience, simplicity, noninvasive nature, and the ability of the patient to self-administer. Except for some nonsteroidal anti-inflammatory drugs, most topical medications do not typically penetrate in useful concentrations to posterior ocular structures and usually are of no therapeutic benefit for diseases of the retina, optic nerve, and other posterior segment structures.

Inactive Ingredients

The following inactive agents may be present in ophthalmic products:

Preservatives: Destroy or inhibit multiplication of microorganisms introduced into the product by accident. Each preservative can cause epithelial toxicity, especially with excessive or prolonged use.

benzalkonium chloride
benzethonium chloride
benzododecinium bromide
cetylpyridinium chloride
chlorobutanol
EDTA
mercurial preservatives (eg, phenylmercuric nitrate, phenylmercuric acetate, thimerosal)
methyl/propylparabens
phenylethyl alcohol
polyquaternium
sodium benzoate
sodium propionate
sorbic acid

Less Toxic Preservatives:

Purite
sodium perborate

Viscosity-Increasing Agents: Slow drainage of the product from the eye, increasing retention time of the active drug. Increased bioavailability may result.

carbopol gels
carboxymethylcellulose sodium
dextran 70
gelatin
glycerin
hydroxyethyl cellulose
hydroxypropyl methylcellulose
methylcellulose
PEG
poloxamer 407
polysorbate 80
propylene glycol
polyvinyl alcohol
polyvinylpyrrolidone (povidone)

Antioxidants: Prevent or delay deterioration of products by oxygen in the air.

EDTA
sodium bisulfite
sodium metabisulfite
sodium thiosulfate
thiourea

Wetting Agents: Reduce surface tension, allowing the drug solution to spread across ocular surface.

polysorbate 20 and 80
poloxamer 282
tyloxapol

Buffers: Help maintain ophthalmic products in the range of pH 6 to 8, which is the comfortable range for ophthalmic instillation.

acetic acid
boric acid
hydrochloric acid
phosphoric acid
potassium bicarbonate
potassium borate
potassium carbonate
potassium citrate
potassium phosphate
potassium tetraborate
sodium acetate
sodium bicarbonate
sodium biphosphate
sodium borate
sodium carbonate
sodium citrate
sodium hydroxide
sodium phosphate

Tonicity Agents: These agents help ophthalmic solutions to be isotonic with the pre-ocular tear film. Products in the sodium chloride equivalence range of 0.9% ± 0.2% are considered isotonic and will help prevent ocular irritation and tissue damage. A range of 0.6% to 1.8% is usually comfortable for ophthalmic use.

buffers
dextran 40 and 70
dextrose
glycerin
potassium chloride
propylene glycol
sodium chloride

Packaging Standards

To help reduce confusion in labeling and identification of various topical ocular medications, drug packaging standards have been generally adopted. The standard colors for drug labels or bottle caps include the following:

Topical Ophthalmic Drug Packaging Standards

Therapeutic class	Color
Beta blockers	Yellow, blue, or both
Mydriatics and cycloplegics	Red
Miotics	Green
Nonsteroidal anti-inflammatory drugs	Grey
Anti-infectives	Brown, tan
Carbonic anhydrase inhibitors	Orange
Prostaglandin analogs	Teal

Medications

Solutions and Suspensions: Most topical ocular preparations are commercially available as solutions or suspensions that are applied directly to the eye from the bottle, which serves as the eye dropper. Avoid touching the dropper tip to the eye because this can lead to contamination of the medication and may cause ocular injury. Resuspend suspensions by shaking to provide an accurate dosage of drug.

Betaxolol 0.25% (*Betoptic S*) and rimexolone (*Vexol*) are classified by the FDA as suspensions but are much less viscous products suspended in carbopol gels than is pilocarpine gel (*Pilopine HS*). A drop can be administered with less concern for prolonged blurred vision. Although *Betoptic S* and *Vexol* are classified technically as suspensions, little shaking is required to suspend or resuspend these agents.

RECOMMENDED PROCEDURES FOR ADMINISTRATION OF SOLUTIONS AND SUSPENSIONS
1. Wash hands thoroughly before administration. 2. Tilt head backward or lie down and gaze upward. 3. Gently grasp lower eyelid below eyelashes and pull the eyelid away from the eye to form a pouch. 4. Place dropper directly over eye. Avoid contact of the dropper with the eye, finger, or any surface. Keep the tip 1 inch from the eye to avoid contact. 5. Look upward just before applying a drop. 6. Release the lid slowly and close eyes gently. 7. With eyes closed, apply gentle pressure with fingers to the inside corner of the eye for 2 to 3 minutes (see Figure 1). This retards drainage of the solution from the intended area. 8. Do not rinse the dropper. 9. Do not use eye drops that have changed color or contain a precipitate. 10. If > 1 type of ophthalmic drop is used, wait ≥ 5 minutes before administering the second agent.

Solutions, Suspensions, and Emulsions – Drops

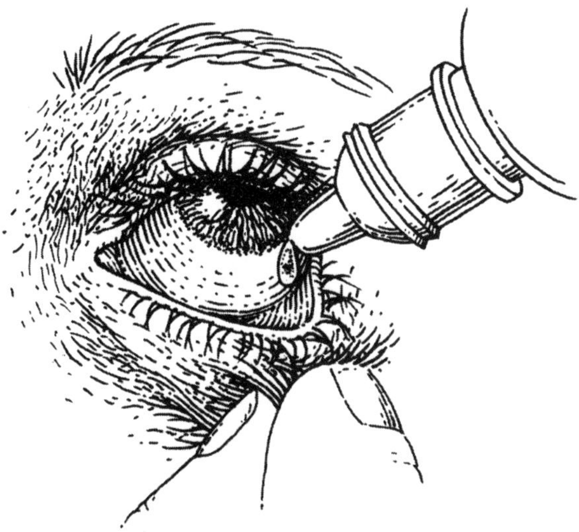

Emulsions: Emulsions are oil-water mixtures that behave clinically like solutions and suspensions. Unlike suspensions, the commercial formulation does not require shaking to resuspend the product. Available emulsions are mixtures of glycerin, polysorbate 80, and caster oil. *Refresh, Endura,* and *Restasis* each contain such an emulsion vehicle.

Nasolacrimal Occlusion

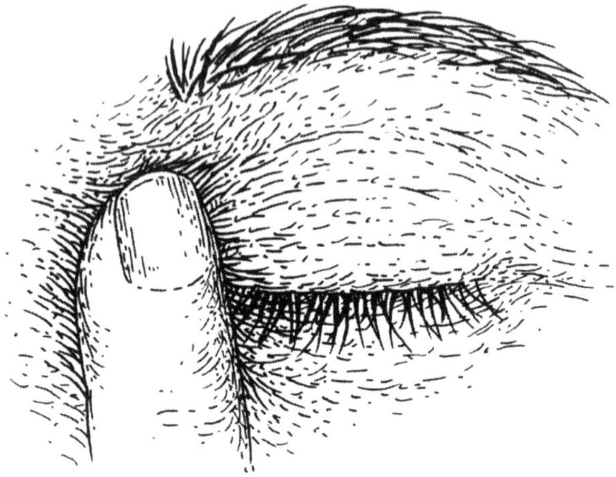

Ointments: The primary purpose for an ophthalmic ointment vehicle is to prolong drug contact time with the external ocular surface. This is particularly useful for treating children, who may "cry out" topically applied solutions, and for medicating ocular injuries, such as corneal abrasions, when the eye is to be patched. Administer solutions before ointments. Ointments may prevent entry of subsequent drops.

RECOMMENDED PROCEDURES FOR ADMINISTRATION OF OINTMENTS
1. Wash hands thoroughly before administration.
2. Tilt head backward or lie down and gaze upward.
3. Gently pull down the lower lid to form a pouch.
4. Place 0.25 to 0.5 inch of ointment with a sweeping motion inside the lower lid by squeezing the tube gently, and slowly release the eyelid.
5. Close the eye for 1 to 2 minutes.
6. Temporary blurring of vision may occur. Avoid activities requiring visual acuity until blurring clears.
7. Remove excessive ointment around the eye or ointment tube tip with a tissue.
8. If using > 1 kind of ointment, wait ≈ 10 minutes before applying the second agent.

Ointments/Semi-Solid Gels

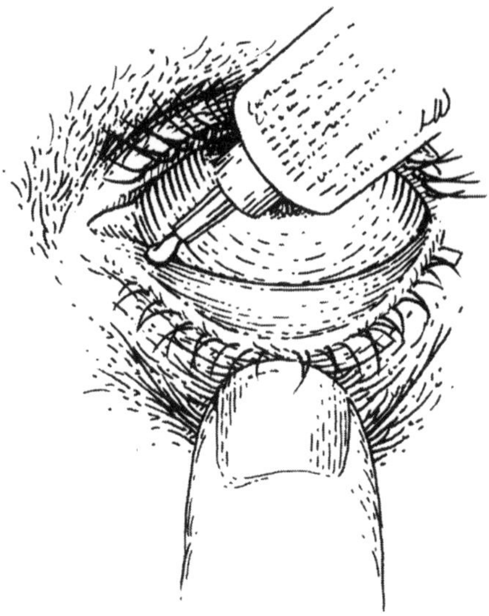

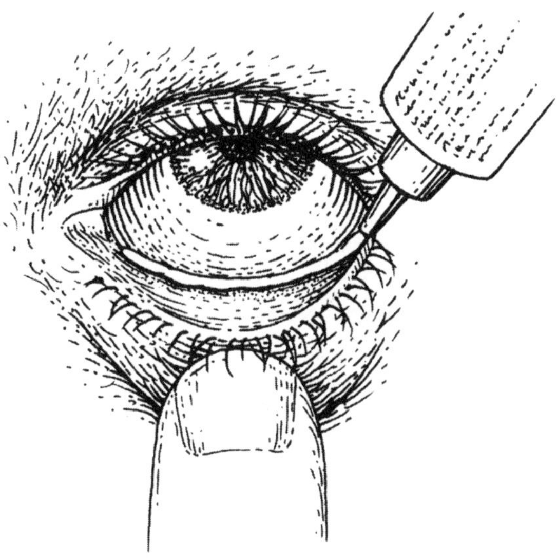

Gels: Ophthalmic gels are similar in viscosity and clinical usage to ophthalmic ointments. Pilocarpine (*Pilopine HS*) is formulated in carbopol gel. *Pilopine HS* is more viscous than a traditional gel and is applied at bedtime to avoid blurred vision. Timolol maleate (*Timoptic XE*) is a slightly viscous solution that forms a gel when it makes contact with the cations in the preocular tear fluid. This formulation provides a prolonged contact time for the timolol within the precorneal tear film. A limited number of gels are available as artificial tear products for treatment of dry eye. These products (eg, *GenTeal Gel*) make treatment more convenient by reducing required dosing frequency.

Sprays: Some practitioners use mydriatics or cycloplegics, alone or in combination, administered as a spray to the eye to dilate the pupil or for cycloplegic examination. This is most often used for pediatric patients, and the solution is administered using a sterile perfume atomizer or plastic spray bottle. *Nature's Tears* and *Tears Again Liposome Spray* also are available for treatment of dry eye.

Lid Scrubs: Commercially available eyelid cleansers, antibiotic solutions, or ointments can be applied directly to the lid margin for treatment of blepharitis. This is best accomplished by applying the medication to the end of a cotton-tipped applicator and then scrubbing the eyelid margin several times daily. The gauze pads supplied with commercially available eyelid cleansers are also convenient.

Lid Scrub – Cotton-Tipped Applicator

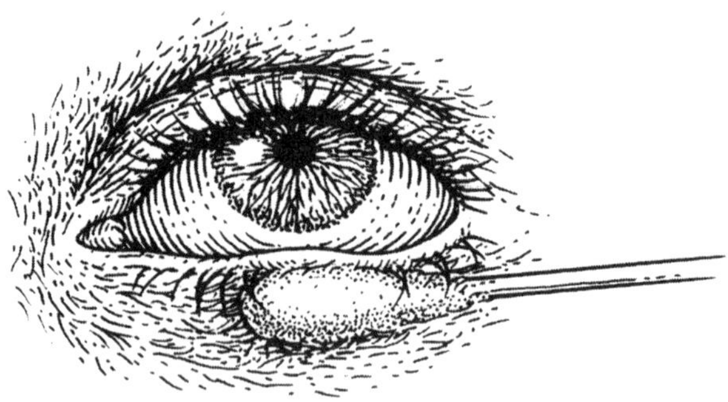

Lid Scrub – Gauze

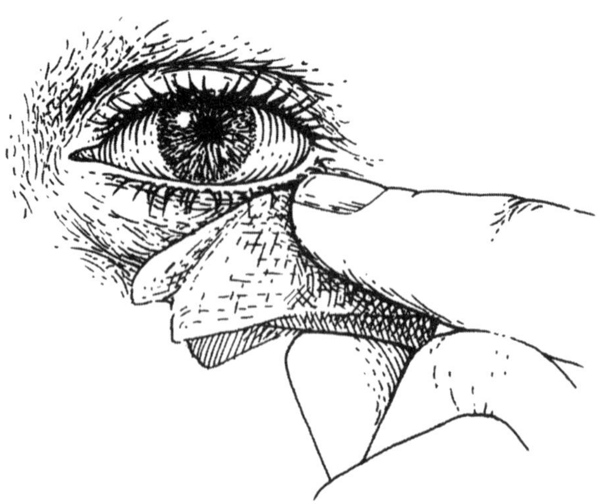

Devices

Contact Lenses: Soft contact lenses can absorb water-soluble drugs and release them to the eye over prolonged periods of time. This has the clinical advantage of promoting sustained-release of solutions or suspensions that would otherwise be removed quickly from the external ocular tissues. Soft contact lenses as drug delivery devices are used occasionally in the management of dry eye disorders.

Corneal Shields: Noncross-linked, homogenized, porcine, or bovine scleral collagen shields are available. These devices are placed as a bandage on the cornea following surgery or injury, protecting and lubricating the cornea. Topical antibiotics have been used in conjunction with the shield to promote healing of corneal ulcers.

Cotton Pledgets: Small pieces of cotton can be saturated with ophthalmic solutions and placed in the conjunctival sac. These devices allow a prolonged ocular contact time with solutions that are normally administered topically into the eye. The clinical use of pledgets usually is reserved for the administration of mydriatic solutions such as cocaine or phenylephrine. This drug delivery method promotes maximum mydriasis in an attempt to break posterior synechiae or to dilate sluggish pupils.

Filter Paper Strips: Sodium fluorescein, lissamine green, and rose bengal dyes are commercially available as drug-impregnated filter paper strips. The strips help ensure sterility of sodium fluorescein which, when prepared in solution, can be easily contaminated with *Pseudomonas aeruginosa*. These dyes are used diagnostically to disclose corneal injuries, infections such as herpes simplex, and dry eye disorders.

Artificial Tear Inserts: A rod-shaped pellet of hydroxypropyl cellulose without preservative (*Lacrisert*) is inserted into the inferior conjunctival sac with a specially designed applicator. Following placement, the device absorbs fluid, swells, and then releases the nonmedicated polymer to the eye for up to 24 hours. The device is designed as a sustained-release artificial tear for the treatment of dry eye disorders.

GENERAL CONSIDERATIONS IN TOPICAL OPHTHALMIC DRUG THERAPY
Proper administration is essential to optimal therapeutic response. In many instances, health professionals may be too casual when instructing patients on proper use of ophthalmics. The administration technique used often determines drug safety and efficacy.
♦ The normal eye retains ≈ 10 mcL of fluid (adjusted for blinking). The average dropper delivers 25 to 50 mcL/drop. There is no value in instilling > 1 properly placed drop.
♦ Minimize systemic absorption of ophthalmic drops by compressing the canaliculus and lacrimal sacs for 3 to 5 minutes after instillation. This retards passage of drops via the nasolacrimal duct into areas of potential absorption, such as nasal and pharyngeal mucosa.
♦ Because of rapid lacrimal drainage and limited eye capacity, if multiple-drop therapy is indicated, the best interval between drops is 5 minutes. This ensures that the first drop is not flushed away by the second or that the second is not diluted by the first.
♦ Factors that may increase absorption from ophthalmic dose forms include lax eyelids of some patients, usually the elderly, which creates a greater reservoir for retention of drops, and hyperemic or diseased eyes.
♦ Eyecup use is discouraged because of risk of contamination and spreading disease.
♦ Ophthalmic suspensions mix with tears less rapidly and remain in the cul-de-sac longer than solutions.
♦ Ophthalmic ointments maintain contact between the drug and ocular tissues by slowing the clearance rate to as little as 0.5% per minute. Ophthalmic ointments provide maximum contact between drug and external ocular tissues.
♦ Ophthalmic ointments may impede delivery of other ophthalmic drugs to the affected site by serving as a barrier to contact.
♦ Ointments may blur vision during the waking hours. Use with caution in conditions where visual clarity is critical (eg, operating motor equipment, reading) or use at bedtime.
♦ Monitor expiration dates closely. Do not use outdated medication.
♦ Solutions and ointments are frequently misused. Do not assume that patients know how to maximize safe and effective use of these agents. Combine appropriate patient education and counseling with prescribing and dispensing of ophthalmics.

ORAL ADMINISTRATION

Although most ocular diseases respond to topical therapy, some disorders require systemic drug administration to achieve adequate therapeutic levels of drug in ocular tissue. Oral administration of certain drugs may be the most effective route of drug delivery. Examples of commonly used oral medications include the following: Carbonic anhydrase inhibitors for the treatment of glaucoma, corticosteroids for Graves ophthalmopathy, analgesics for the management of pain associated with refractive surgery or ocular injury, antibiotic therapy of preseptal cellulitis, and antihistamine therapy for acute allergic angioneurotic edema of the eyelids.

PARENTERAL ADMINISTRATION

Intramuscular (IM) and intravenous (IV) injections are occasionally used for the treatment of ocular disorders. Hydroxocobalamin (vitamin B_{12} [eg, *Hydro Cobex*]) and some antibiotics (eg, penicillin) may be administered through the IM route. The continuous IV infusion of various antibiotics may be required for the treatment of endophthalmitis and other severe ocular infections.

PERIOCULAR/PERIBULBAR ADMINISTRATION

Drugs can be injected locally into the periocular tissues when higher concentrations of drugs are required than can be delivered to the eye by topical, oral, or parenteral administration. Periocular drug administration includes injections under the bulbar conjunctiva (subconjunctival), under Tenon's capsule (sub-Tenon's), and behind the globe itself (retrobulbar). Drugs most often delivered in this manner include corticosteroids and antibiotics. Local anesthetics are commonly administered via retrobulbar or peribulbar injection prior to cataract extraction and other intraocular surgical procedures.

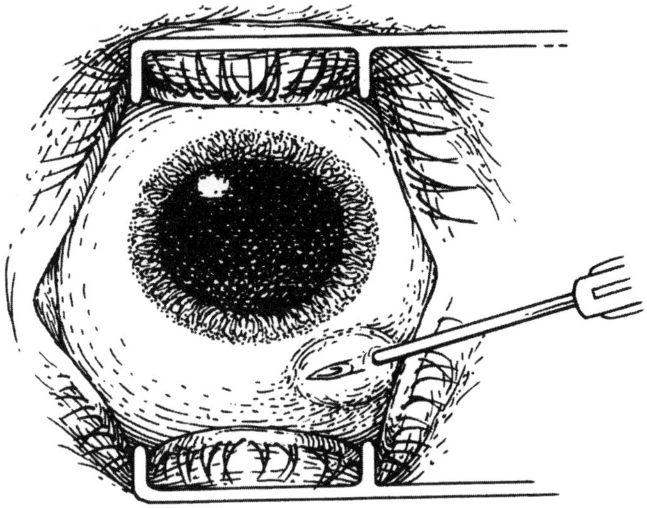

INTRACAMERAL ADMINISTRATION

Although the term "intracameral" technically denotes injection of drug into the globe, contemporary usage of the term implies administering the drug directly into the anterior chamber of the eye. This is most commonly associated with cataract extraction, during which a viscoelastic substance is injected into the anterior chamber to protect the corneal endothelium.

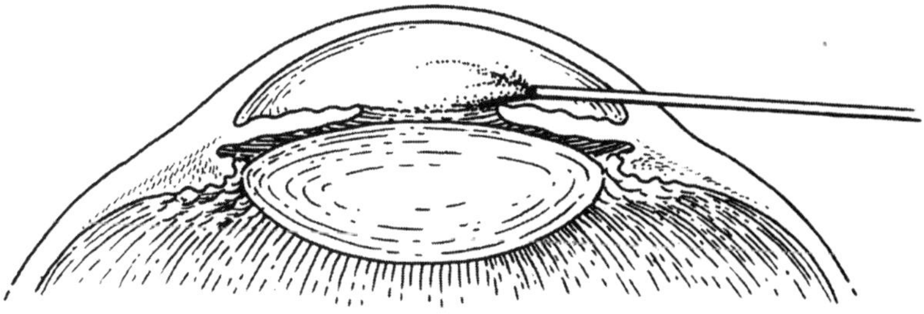

INTRAVITREAL ADMINISTRATION

The intravitreal injection of drugs is primarily reserved as a heroic effort to rescue eyes with severe acute or chronic intraocular inflammation or eyes that have failed to respond to more conservative therapy. Intravitreal antibiotics may be the treatment of choice for endophthalmitis. Intravitreal liquid silicone is used for the treatment of complicated retinal detachment. Intravitreal ganciclovir has been used with some success in treating cytomegalovirus retinitis in patients with acquired immunodeficiency syndrome (AIDS). A ganciclovir implant (*Vitrasert*) is available that delivers the antiviral agent continuously to the vitreous and retina for periods of 4 to 6 months. Intravitreal fluocinolone is available as an implant (*Retisert*) to deliver steroid at a constant rate to the posterior segment of the eye for 2 to 3 years. Pegaptanib (*Macugen*) and other anti-VEGF agents are injected intravitreally to limit progression of choroidal neovascularization associated with neovascular age-related macular degeneration.

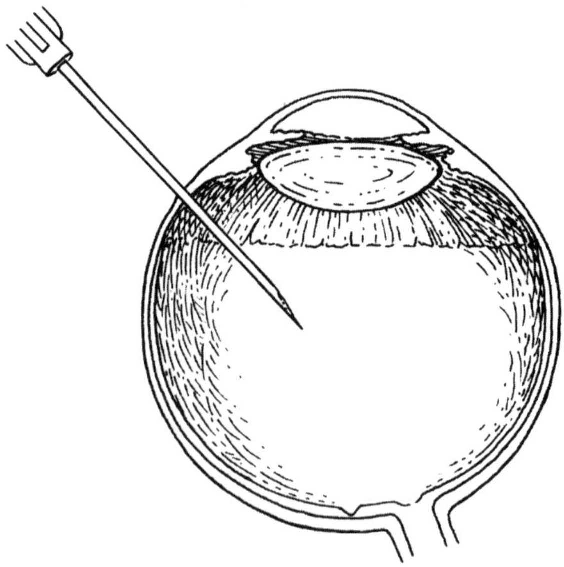

For More Information

Bartlett JD, Jaanus SD, eds. *Clinical Ocular Pharmacology*, ed. 5. St. Louis, MO: Elsevier; 2008.

Bartlett JD, Wesson MD, Swiatocha J, Woolley T. Efficacy of a pediatric cycloplegic administered as a spray. *J Am Optom Assoc.* 1993;64:617-621.

Bourlais CL, Acar L, Zia H, et al. Ophthalmic drug delivery systems-recent advances. *Prog Retin Eye Res.* 1998;17:33-58.

Chang M, Dunn JP. Ganciclovir implant in the treatment of cytomegalovirus retinitis. *Expert Rev Med Devices.* 2005;2:421-427.

Fraunfelder FT. Drug-packaging standards for eye drop medications. *Arch Ophthalmol.* 1988;106:1029.

Fraunfelder FT. Extraocular fluid dynamics: How best to apply topical ocular medication. *Trans Am Ophthalmol Soc.* 1976;74:457.

Gragoudas ES, Adamis AP, Cunningham ET Jr, et al. Pegaptanib for neovascular age-related macular degeneration. *N Engl J Med.* 2004;351:2805-2816.

Holekamp NM, Thomas MA, Pearson A. The safety profile of long-term, high-dose intraocular corticosteroid delivery. *Am J Ophthalmol.* 2005;139:533-535.

Jaffe GJ, McCallum RM, Branchaud B, et al. Long-term followup results of a pilot trial of a fluocinolone acetonide implant to treat posterior uveitis. *Ophthalmology.* 2005;112:1192-1198.

Jain MR. Drug delivery through soft contact lenses. *Br J Ophthalmol.* 1988;72:150.

Martin DF, Dunn JP, Davis JL, et al. Use of the ganciclovir implant for the treatment of cytomegalovirus retinitis in the era of potent antiretroviral therapy: recommendations of the international AIDS society–USA panel. *Am J Ophthalmol.* 1999;127:329-339.

Martin DF, Parks DJ, Mellow SD, et al. Treatment of cytomegalovirus retinitis with intraocular sustained-release ganciclovir implant. A randomized controlled clinical trial. *Arch Opthalmol.* 1994;112:1531.

Silbiger J, Stern GA. Evaluation of corneal collagen shields as a drug delivery device for the treatment of experimental *Pseudomonas* keratitis. *Ophthalmology.* 1992;99:889.

Van Santvliet L, Ludwig A. Determinants of eye drop size. *Surv Ophthalmol.* 2004;49:197-213.

Wesson MD, Bartlett JD, Swiatocha J, et al. Efficacy of a cycloplegic administered as a spray. *J Am Optom Assoc.* 1993;64:637.

Zimmerman TJ, Kooner KS, Kandarakis AS, Ziegler LP. Improving the therapeutic index of topically applied ocular drugs. *Arch Ophthalmol.* 1984;102:551-553.

Ophthalmic Dyes

Dyes are used for a variety of diagnostic ocular procedures. Ophthalmic dyes in current use include sodium fluorescein, fluorexon, rose bengal, lissamine green, and indocyanine green. Topical sodium fluorescein and rose bengal have proven valuable for assessment of ocular surface integrity, while IV fluorescein has proven useful for evaluating retinal vascular function. Iodocyanine green is useful for staining internal limiting membranes in macular surgery and anterior capsule during cataract surgery.

FLUORESCEIN SODIUM

Fluorescein sodium is a yellow water-soluble dibasic acid dye of the xanthine series that produces an intense green fluorescent color in alkaline (pH greater than 5) solution. Fluorescein is used to demonstrate defects of corneal epithelium. It does not actually stain tissues, but is useful as an indicator dye. The normal precorneal tear film appears yellow or orange with fluorescein. The intact corneal epithelium resists penetration of water-soluble fluorescein and is not colored by it. Any break in the epithelial barrier permits rapid fluorescein penetration. Whether resulting from trauma, infection, or other causes, epithelial defects of the cornea appear bright green and are easily visualized. If epithelial loss is extensive, topical fluorescein will penetrate into the aqueous and is readily visible biomicroscopically as a green flare.

Fluorescein sodium exhibits a high degree of ionization at physiologic pH. Therefore, it does not penetrate the intact corneal epithelium or form a firm bond with vital tissue. When exposed to light, fluorescein absorbs certain wavelengths and emits fluorescent light of longer wavelength. Factors that can affect its fluorescence include its concentration, the pH of the solution, the presence of other substances, and the intensity and wavelength of the absorbed light. At pH 8, fluorescein reaches its maximum intensity.

Ophthalmic uses of fluorescein include applanation tonometry, detection of foreign bodies, fitting of rigid contact lenses, determination of tear breakup time, Seidel's test, fluorescein angiography, and fluorophotometry.

For topical ocular use, fluorescein may be administered as a solution or by fluorescein-impregnated filter paper strips (eg, *Fluorets*). Because fluorescein in solution is susceptible to bacterial contamination, multidose formulations are dispensed with a preservative such as chlorobutanol. For diagnostic purposes such as applanation tonometry, a local anesthetic is included in the formulation.

Fluorescein-impregnated filter paper strips are useful for routine office procedures such as contact lens fitting and lacrimal system evaluation. Bacterial contamination is minimized when the strips are stored in a dry state. When wetted with saline or an irrigating solution, the dye is released from the strip and can be applied to the eye by gently touching the conjunctiva.

IV fluorescein (fluorescein angiography) is used for detection of vascular abnormalities of the fundus. Following injection into the antecubital vein, the dye appears in the central retinal artery. Integrity of the retina and choroid may be determined.

Oral fluorescein can be administered by mixing fluorescein powder or several vials of 10% injectable fluorescein in a citrus drink over ice. Time of onset of maximal fluorescence is 45 to 60 minutes compared with seconds via the injectable route. Fasting enhances the serum concentration of the dye. Oral fluorescein can be used to study disorders characterized by late leakage of dye, such as cystoid macular edema, to study retinal vascular abnormalities in young diabetic patients, and to document retinal pigment epithelial detachment, central serous choroidopathy, and optic disc edema.

Topical application of fluorescein has been associated with minimum adverse effects. The most common side effect of IV use is nausea. The oral route appears to have the clinical advantage of less frequent side effects.

FLUOREXON

With a molecular size nearly twice that of fluorescein, fluorexon penetrates hydrophilic contact lenses at a much slower rate. Upon ocular instillation, it yields a pale, yellow-brown color. These properties make it useful as an adjunct in the fitting of soft contact lenses, including hybrid designs with a rigid gas-permeable center with a hydrogel surround. However, the dye can stain hydrophilic lenses if significant amounts become trapped between the lens and cornea or if the dye remains in contact with the soft lens for at least 10 minutes. Fluorexon is not recommended for use with high-water content soft lenses since the possibility of discoloration is much greater and more difficult to reverse than with lower-water content lenses.

Fluorexon has a lower fluorescent intensity than fluorescein. For optimum fluorescence, a special yellow filter is recommended. The dye generally causes little or no discomfort when instilled on the eye. Because of its larger molecular size, it is a less effective stain for epithelial defects, erosions, and contact lens-induced effects than fluorescein. Like rose bengal, it will stain degenerated cells and mucus threads.

INDOCYANINE GREEN

Indocyanine green is a tricarbocyanine dye, available commercially under the trade name of *IC-Green*. Its primary use is as a fluorescent dye for retinal and choroidal angiography, and it has proven useful for visualization of choroidal vessels with infrared absorption angiography. Toxic effects have not been associated with IV use of the dye when manufacturer's recommended dosage regimens have been followed.

LISSAMINE GREEN

Lissamine green stains the same structures of the eye as rose bengal, specifically degenerate cells, dead cells, and precipitated mucus a bluish-green color. The dye is useful for assessing dry eye conditions and can be helpful in detecting recurrent corneal erosions and herpetic ulcers. The staining effect is easier to see than rose bengal in red, inflamed, or hemorrhagic eyes, and the effect of the dye appears to last longer.

Instillation of lissamine green into the conjunctival sac is nonirritating to most patients, and no adverse effects or contraindications for its topical ocular use have been observed. Lissamine green is also available as sterile strips.

ROSE BENGAL

An iodine derivative of fluorescein, rose bengal stains cells of the cornea and conjunctiva (including the nuclei and cell walls) a red color. More recent evidence indicates that this dye stains both normal and degenerated or dead cells. Staining will occur whenever there is poor protection of the surface epithelium by the preocular tear film. It appears that rose bengal is not a vital dye and that stained cells actually lose vitality upon exposure to the dye and undergo morphologic changes. It also will stain the mucus of the precorneal tear film. The most common use of rose Bengal is on the differential diagnosis of dry eye syndromes. When applied from a moistened filter paper strip, this dye can aid in the evaluation of keratoconjunctivitis sicca, and other types of lesions such as herpetic keratitis, corneal abrasions, and detection of foreign bodies.

Rose bengal can cause pronounced irritation and discomfort following instillation, particularly in more severely diseased eyes and with use of higher concentrations of dye. Rose bengal can stain eyelids, cheeks, fingers, and clothing in a concentration-dependent manner. Keeping the amount of dye at a minimum and irrigating the eye can help circumvent this problem.

For More Information

Bartlett JD, Jaanus SD, eds. *Clinical Ocular Pharmacology.* 5th ed. St. Louis, MO: Elsevier; 2008.

Berkow JW, Flower RW, Orth D, et al. *Fluorescein and Indocyanine Green Angiography Technique and Interpretation.* 2nd ed. San Francisco, CA: American Academy of Optometry; 1997.

Bron AJ, Evans VE, Smith JA. Grading of corneal and conjunctival staining in the context of other dry eye tests. *Cornea.* 2003;22:640-650.

Feenstra RP, Tseng SC. Comparison of fluorescein and rose bengal staining. *Arch Ophthalmol.* 1992;99:605.

Johnson M, Murphy PJ. The effect of instilled fluorescein solution volume on the values and repeatability of TBUT measurements. *Cornea.* 2005;24:811-817.

Kim J. The use of vital dyes in corneal disease. *Curr Opin Ophthalmol.* 2000;11:241-247.

Kwok AK, Lai TY, Yew DT, et al. Internal limiting membrane staining with various concentrations of indocyanine dye under air in macular surgeries. *Am J Ophthalmol.* 2003;136:223-230.

Lissamine green colored ophthalmic demulcent [package insert]. Dakryon Pharmaceuticals; 1997.

Marques DM, Marques FF, Osher RH. Three-step technique for staining the anterior lens capsule with indocyanine green or trypan blue. *J Cataract Refract Surg.* 2004;30:13-16.

Morris PF. Fluorescein sodium and indocyanine green: Uses and side effects. In: Saine PJ, Tyler ME, eds. *Ophthalmic Photography.* 2nd ed. Boston, MA: Butterworth-Heinemann; 2002.

FLUORESCEIN SODIUM

Actions:

Pharmacology: Sodium fluorescein, a yellow water-soluble dibasic acid xanthine dye, produces an intense green fluorescent color in alkaline (pH greater than 5) solution. Fluorescein demonstrates defects of corneal epithelium. It does not stain tissues, but is a useful indicator dye. Normal precorneal tear film will appear yellow or orange. The intact corneal epithelium resists fluorescein penetration and is not colored. Any break in the epithelial barrier permits rapid penetration. Whether resulting from trauma, infection, or other causes, epithelial corneal defects appear bright green and are easily seen. If epithelial loss is extensive, topical fluorescein penetrates into the aqueous humor and is readily visible biomicroscopically as a green flare.

Indications:

Topical: In fitting contact lenses; in applanation tonometry; diagnosis and detection of corneal stippling, abrasions, ulcerations, herpetic lesions, foreign bodies (not epithelialized), contact lens pressure points; lacrimal drainage tests; wound leakage tests (Seidel's Test).

Injection: Diagnostic aid in ophthalmic angiography, including examination of the fundus; evaluation of the iris vasculature; distinction between viable and nonviable tissue; observation of the aqueous flow; differential diagnosis of malignant and nonmalignant tumors; determination of circulation time and adequacy.

Off-label use(s): Oral fluorography for diagnosis of retinal vascular diseases.

Contraindications:

Hypersensitivity to fluorescein or any other component of the product; do not use with soft contact lenses (lenses may become discolored).

Topical: Not for injection. Do not use in intraocular surgery.

Warnings:

Topical (drops): Discontinue if sensitivity develops. May stain soft contact lenses. Do not touch dropper tip to any surface, as this may contaminate the solution.

Extravasation: Avoid extravasation during injection. The high pH can result in severe local tissue damage. Complications have occurred from extravasation: sloughing of skin, superficial phlebitis, subcutaneous granuloma, and toxic neuritis along the median curve in the antecubital area. Extravasation can cause severe pain in the arm for several hours. When significant extravasation occurs, discontinue injection and use conservative measures to treat damaged tissue and relieve pain (see Warnings).

Hypersensitivity: Exercise caution when administering to patients with a history of hypersensitivity, allergies, or asthma. If signs of sensitivity develop, discontinue use.

Pregnancy: Category C. Avoid parenteral fluorescein angiography during pregnancy, especially in the first trimester. There are no reports of fetal complications during pregnancy.

Lactation: Fluorescein is excreted in breast milk. Use caution when administering to a nursing woman.

Children: Safety and efficacy for use in children have not been established.

Adverse Reactions:

Miscellaneous:

Injection – Nausea; headache; GI distress; vomiting; syncope; hypotension and other symptoms and signs of hypersensitivity; cardiac arrest; basilar artery ischemia; thrombophlebitis at injection site; severe shock; convulsions; death (rare); temporary yellowish skin discoloration. Hives, itching, bronchospasm, anaphylaxis, pyrexia, transient dyspnea, angioneurotic edema, and slight dizziness may occur. A strong taste may develop with use. Urine becomes bright yellow. Skin discoloration fades in 6 to 12 hours, urine fluorescence in 24 to 36 hours. Extravasation at injection site causes intense pain at the site and dull aching pain in the injected arm (see Warnings).

Patient Information:

May cause strong taste with use.

May cause temporary yellowish discoloration of the skin. Urine will turn bright yellow. Discoloration of skin fades in 6 to 12 hours; urine fluorescence fades in 24 to 36 hours.

Soft contact lenses may become stained. Do not wear lenses while fluorescein is being used. Whenever fluorescein is used, flush the eyes with sterile normal saline solution and wait at least 1 hour before replacing the lenses.

Administration and Dosage:

Topical: To detect foreign bodies and corneal abrasions, instill 1 or 2 drops of 2% solution; allow a few seconds for staining. Wash out the excess with sterile irrigating solution.

Strips: Moisten the strip with sterile water, normal saline, or ocular irrigating solution. Gently touch the superior or inferior bulbar conjunctiva or lower cul-de-sac. The patient should blink several times after application.

Applanation tonometry – Anesthetize the eyes. Retract the upper lid and touch the tip of the strip moistened with saline or ocular irrigating solution (eg, *Blinx*) to the bulbar conjunctiva on the temporal side until an adequate amount of stain is available for a clearly defined endpoint reading.

Injection: Inject the contents of the ampule or prefilled syringe rapidly into the antecubital vein after taking precautions to avoid extravasation. A syringe filled with fluorescein is attached to transparent tubing and a 25-gauge scalp vein needle for injection. Insert the needle and draw blood to the hub of the syringe so that a small air bubble separates the blood in the tubing from the fluorescein. With the room lights on, slowly inject the blood back into the vein while watching the skin over the needle tip. If the needle has extravasated, the patient's blood will bulge the skin, and the injection should be stopped before any fluorescein is injected. When assured that extravasation has not occurred, the room light may be turned off and the fluorescein injection completed. Luminescence appears in the retina and choroidal vessels in 9 to 15 seconds and can be observed by standard viewing equipment.

If potential allergy is suspected, an intradermal skin test may be performed prior to IV administration (eg, 0.05 mL injected intradermally to be evaluated 30 to 60 minutes following injection).

In patients with inaccessible veins where early phases of an angiogram are not necessary, such as cystoid macular edema, 1 g fluorescein has been given orally. Ten to 15 minutes are usually required before evidence of dye appears in the fundus.

Adults – 500 to 750 mg injected rapidly into the antecubital vein.

Children – 7.5 mg/kg (3.5 mg/lb) injected rapidly into the antecubital vein.

Have 0.1% epinephrine IM or IV, an antihistamine, soluble steroid, aminophylline IV, and oxygen available.

Storage/Stability: Store at 8° to 30°C (46° to 86°F). Do not use if the solution contains a precipitate. Discard any unused solution. Keep out of the reach of children.

Rx	**AK-Fluor** (Akorn)	**Injection**: 10%	In 5 mL amps and vials.
Rx	**Angiofluor** (OcuSoft)		In 5 mL single-dose vials and boxes of 12 vials.
Rx	**Angiofluor Lite** (OcuSoft)		In 5 mL single-dose vials and boxes of 12 vials.
Rx	**Fluorescite** (Alcon)		In 5 mL amps with syringes.
Rx	**AK-Fluor** (Akorn)	**Injection**: 25%	In 2 mL amps and vials.
Rx	**Angiofluor** (OcuSoft)		In 2 mL single-dose vials and boxes of 12 vials.
Rx	**Angiofluor Lite** (Alliance Pharm)		In 2 mL single-dose vials and boxes of 12 vials.
Rx	**Ful-Glo** (Akorn)	**Strips**: 0.6 mg	In 300s.

FLUOREXON

Actions:

Pharmacology: Fluorexon is a large-molecular weight fluorescent solution for use as a diagnostic and fitting aid for patients with hydrogel (soft) contact lenses. Used with or without lens in place when fluorescein is contraindicated to avoid staining lenses. It may be used with both soft and hard lenses.

Indications:

Contact lens fitting aid: Assessment of proper fitting characteristics of hydrogel lenses. For quickly and accurately locating the optic zone in aphakic or low-plus lenses.

Evaluation of corneal integrity of patients wearing hydrogel contact lenses. In many instances, arcuate staining will show definite correlation with the edge of the optic zone, indicating improper bearing surfaces.

For use in place of sodium fluorescein when conducting the tear breakup time (BUT) test.

For conducting applanation tonometry without removing the lens.

For locating the lathe-cut index markings (toric lenses). Use as directed for fitting contact lenses.

Contraindications:

Hypersensitivity to fluorescein sodium.

Warnings:

Contact lenses: When used with lenses with greater than 55% hydration, some color may remain on lens. Remove by washing repeatedly with soaking solution approved for the lens. Rinse with saline or water. Any residual coloring will wash out with the tear flow when the lens is reinserted in the eye. With highly hydrated lenses, the amount of coloring picked up will vary with exposure. Avoid unnecessary delays in the examination procedure.

Precautions:

Hydrogen peroxide: Do not use hydrogen peroxide solutions to clean or sterilize lenses until all traces of fluorexon are removed because fluorexon molecules may bind to the lens.

Administration and Dosage:

Place 1 drop on the concave surface of the lens and place the lens immediately on the eye. Alternatively, place 1 or 2 drops in the lower cul-de-sac and have the patient blink several times.

As the dye passes under the lens, observe a central dark zone of 6 to 9 mm in diameter (ie, a limbal fluorescent ring about 2 mm wide), which forms after each blink. If such staining pattern cannot be observed immediately, slide the lens upward by gently pushing it with a finger, causing the dye to penetrate under the lens as it slides back into normal position. Additional drops may be used if the fluorescence starts to dissipate after prolonged examination. When the examination is completed, rinse the eye and lens with saline. The lens may be reinserted immediately, as opposed to the long waiting period required after the use of fluorescein.

Begin the examination immediately after instillation of fluorexon drops. The solution tends to dissipate readily with the tear flow, leading to a progressive reduction in fluorescence. Prolonged examination may require sequential application of drops.

Applanation tonometry (without removing lens): After seating the patient at the slit lamp and instilling a drop of fluorexon with a drop of proparacaine or similar topical anesthetic, the contact lens is displaced to one side onto the sclera with the finger and the procedure begun.

otc	**Fluoresoft** (Various, eg, Holles)	**Solution:** 0.35%	In 0.3 mL ampoules (20s).

INDOCYANINE GREEN

Actions:

Pharmacology: Sterile, water-soluble, tricarbocyanine dye with a peak spectral absorption at 800 to 810 nm in blood or blood plasma. Indocyanine green contains up to 5% sodium iodide.

Indocyanine green permits recording of indicator-dilution curves for both diagnostic and research purposes independent of fluctuations in oxygen saturation. In the performance of dye dilution curves, a known amount of dye is usually injected as a single bolus as rapidly as possible via a cardiac catheter into selected sites in the vascular system. A recording instrument (oximeter or densitometer) is attached to a needle or catheter for sampling of the blood-dye mixture from a systemic arterial sampling site.

The peak absorption and emission of indocyanine green lie in a region (800 to 850 nm) where transmission of energy by the pigment epithelium is more efficient than in the region of visible light energy. Because indocyanine green is also nearly 98% bound to blood protein, excessive dye extravasation does not take place in the highly fenestrated choroidal vasculature. Therefore, it is useful in both absorption and fluorescence infrared angiography of the choroidal vasculature when using appropriate filters and film in a fundus camera.

Pharmacokinetics: Following IV injection, indocyanine green is rapidly bound to plasma protein, of which albumin is the principal carrier (95%). Indocyanine green undergoes no significant extrahepatic or enterohepatic circulation; simultaneous arterial and venous blood estimations have shown negligible renal, peripheral, lung, or cerebrospinal uptake of the dye. Indocyanine green is taken up from the plasma almost exclusively by the hepatic parenchymal cells and is secreted entirely into the bile. After biliary obstruction, the dye appears in the hepatic lymph, independent of the bile, suggesting that the biliary mucosa is sufficiently intact to prevent diffusion of the dye, though allowing diffusion of bilirubin. These characteristics make indocyanine green a helpful index of hepatic function.

Indications:

Angiography: For ophthalmic angiography.

Cataract surgery: As an aid to visualization of the anterior lens capsule.

Warnings:

Pregnancy: Category C. It is not known whether indocyanine green can cause fetal harm when administered to a pregnant woman or can affect reproduction capacity. Give to a pregnant woman only if clearly indicated.

Lactation: It is not known whether this drug is excreted in breast milk. Exercise caution when indocyanine green is administered to a nursing woman.

Precautions:

Plasma fractional disappearance: Plasma fractional disappearance rate at the recommended 0.5 mg/kg dose has been reported to be significantly greater in women than in men; however, there was no significant difference in the calculated value for clearance.

Radioactive iodine uptake studies: Do not perform for at least a week following the use of indocyanine green.

Iodide allergy: Contains sodium iodide. Use with caution in individuals who have a history of allergy to iodides.

Drug Interactions:

Drug/Lab test interactions: Heparin preparations containing sodium bisulfite reduce the absorption peak of indocyanine green in blood. Do not use heparin as an anticoagulant for the collection of samples for analysis.

Adverse Reactions:

Anaphylactic or urticarial reactions have also occurred in patients without history of allergy to iodides. If such reactions occur, treat with appropriate agents (eg, epinephrine, antihistamines, corticosteroids).

Administration and Dosage:

Use 40 mg dye in 2 mL of aqueous solvent. In some patients, half the volume has been found to produce angiograms of comparable resolution. Immediately follow the injected dye bolus with a 5 mL bolus of normal saline. This injection regimen is designed to provide delivery of a spatially limited dye bolus of optimal concentration to the choroidal vasculature following IV injection.

Compatibility: Use only the Aqueous Solvent (pH 5.5 to 6.5) provided, which is specially prepared Sterile Water for Injection, to dissolve indocyanine green because there have been reports of incompatibility with some commercially available Water for Injection products.

Storage/Stability: Indocyanine green is unstable in aqueous solution and must be used within 10 hours. However, the dye is stable in plasma and whole blood so that samples obtained in discontinuous sampling techniques may be read hours later. Use sterile techniques in handling the dye solution and in the performance of the dilution curves.

Indocyanine green powder may cling to the vial or lump together because it is freeze-dried in the vials. This is not due to the presence of water.

Rx	**IC-Green** (Akorn)	**Powder for Injection:** 25 mg	In 10 mL amps of aqueous solvent (6s).

LISSAMINE GREEN

Actions:

Pharmacology: Stains dead or degenerated corneal and conjunctival cells and precipitated mucus.

Indications:

For use as a diagnostic agent when superficial corneal or conjunctival tissue change is suspect.

Off-label use(s): Diagnostic aid for dry eye conditions and squamous cell metaplasia.

Contraindications:

Hypersensitivity to lissamine green or any component of the formulation.

Warnings:

Not to be used with soft contact lenses. For external use only. Keep out of reach of children.

Administration and Dosage:

Moisten the lissamine green impregnated tip before application. One or 2 drops of sterile irrigating or saline solution should be used for this purpose. Touch conjunctiva or fornix as required with moistened tip. It is recommended that the patient blink several times after application.

otc	**Lissamine Green** (Cyanacon/ Ocusoft)	**Strips:** 1.5 mg	100 sterile strips per carton.

ROSE BENGAL

Actions:

Pharmacology: Stains dead or degenerated epithelial cells (corneal and conjunctival) and mucus.

Indications:

Suspected corneal/conjunctival damage: A diagnostic agent when superficial corneal or conjunctival tissue damage is suspected. Effective aid for diagnosis of keratitis, squamous cell carcinomas, keratoconjunctivitis sicca, corneal erosions or abrasions, and for the detection of foreign bodies.

Contraindications:

Hypersensitivity to rose bengal or any component of the formulation.

Precautions:

Irritation: The solution may be irritating.

Contact lenses: Whenever rose bengal is used in patients who wear soft contact lenses, flush the eyes thoroughly with sterile normal saline or irrigating solution and wait at least 1 hour before replacing the lens.

Administration and Dosage:

Strips: Thoroughly saturate tip of strip with sterile irrigating solution. Touch bulbar conjunctiva or lower fornix with moistened strip. The patient should blink several times after application.

otc	**Rose Bengal** (Akorn)	**Strips:** 1.3 mg/strip	In 100s.

Local Anesthetics

Although the exact mechanism of action is unknown, local anesthetics prevent the generation and conduction of nerve impulses by reducing sodium permeability, increasing the electrical excitation threshold, slowing the nerve impulse propagation, and reducing the rate of rise of the action potential. Their action is reversible; complete recovery of nerve function occurs with no evidence of structural damage to nerve tissue.

With the exception of cocaine, local anesthetics are synthetic, aromatic, or heterocyclic compounds. Nearly all local anesthetics in current use are weakly basic tertiary amines. The structural components consist of an aromatic lipophilic portion, an intermediate alkyl chain, and a hydrophilic hydrocarbon chain containing nitrogen. The intermediate chain is linked to the aromatic group by either an ester or an amide, which determines certain pharmacologic properties of the molecule.

CLASSIFICATION

Local anesthetics are divided into 2 groups: *esters*, which are derivatives of para-aminobenzoic acid, and *amides*, which are derivatives of aniline. The "ester" local anesthetics are metabolized by hydrolysis of the ester linkage by plasma esterase, probably plasma cholinesterase. The "amide" local anesthetics are metabolized in the liver, then excreted primarily in the urine as metabolites with a small fraction of unchanged drug. Biliary excretion may contribute to the disposition of lidocaine (eg, *Xylocaine*) and mepivacaine (eg, *Carbocaine*). Allergic reactions to local anesthetics occur almost exclusively to anesthetics with ester linkage (see Precautions). All commonly used topical anesthetics are of the ester type (see Table 1: Classification of Local Anesthetics). Cross-sensitivity reactions are rare between proparacaine and the other ester anesthetics.

Table 1: CLASSIFICATION OF LOCAL ANESTHETICS

Ester Linkage	**Amide Linkage** (Amides of benzoic acid)
A. Esters of benzoic acid: Cocaine	A. Lidocaine
B. Esters of meta-aminobenzoic acid: Proparacaine	B. Mepivacaine
C. Esters of para-aminobenzoic acid:	C. Bupivacaine
1. Procaine	
2. Chloroprocaine	
3. Tetracaine	
4. Benoxinate	

In the amine form, local anesthetics tend to be only slightly soluble in water and, therefore, are usually formulated in the form of their hydrochloride salt, which is water soluble. Because local anesthetics are weak bases with a pK_a between 8 and 9, they ionize in solution, enhancing stability and shelf-life. Upon contact with more neutral or alkaline environments (eg, tears), the nonionized form is liberated. The nonionized drug can penetrate tissues, including the cornea.

PHARMACOKINETICS

Various pharmacokinetic parameters of the local anesthetics can be significantly altered by the presence of hepatic or renal disease, addition of epinephrine, factors affecting urinary pH, renal blood flow, route of administration, and patient age. Onset of local anesthesia is dependent on the dissociation constant (pK_a), lipid solubility, pH of the solution, protein binding, and molecular size. In general, local anesthetics with high lipid solubility or low pK_a have a faster onset. The duration of action of local anesthetics is proportional to the drug's contact time with nerve tissue. To prolong contact time of injectable local anesthetics, vasoconstrictors may be added, but such adjuncts are of no benefit when used with topical anesthetics. The use of vasoconstrictors (eg, epinephrine) in conjunction with local anesthetics promotes local hemostasis, decreases systemic absorption, and prolongs the duration of action.

Systemic absorption of local anesthetics affects the cardiovascular system and central nervous system. At blood concentrations achieved with normal therapeutic doses of injectable anesthetics, changes in cardiac conduction, excitability, refractoriness, contractility, and peripheral vascular resistance are minimal. However, toxic blood concentrations depress cardiac conduction and excitability, which may lead to atrioventricular block and, ultimately, to cardiac arrest. In addition, with toxic blood concentrations, myocardial contractility may be depressed and peripheral vasodilation may occur, leading to decreased cardiac output and arterial blood pressure.

Following systemic absorption, toxic blood concentrations of local anesthetics can produce CNS stimulation, depression, or both. Apparent central stimulation may be manifested as restlessness, tremors, and shivering, that may progress to convulsions. Depression and coma may occur, possibly progressing to respiratory arrest. Local anesthetics have a primary depressant effect on the medulla and on higher centers. The depressed stage may occur without a prior stage of CNS stimulation.

Rate of systemic absorption depends on total dose and concentration of drug, vascularity of administration site, and presence of vasoconstrictors. Depending on route of administration, local anesthetics are distributed to some extent to all body tissues. High concentrations are found in highly perfused organs (eg, liver, lungs, heart, brain). The rate and extent of placental diffusion is determined by plasma protein binding, ionization, and lipid solubility. It is the nonionized form of the drug that crosses cellular membranes to the site of action. Fetal:maternal ratios are inversely related to degree of protein binding. Only the free, unbound drug is available for placental transfer. Drugs with the highest protein binding capacity may have the lowest fetal:maternal ratios. Lipid-soluble, nonionized drugs readily enter the fetal blood from the maternal circulation.

OPHTHALMIC USES

Anesthetics in current clinical use have relatively low systemic and ocular toxicity. They have a sufficiently long duration of action, are stable in solution, and usually lack interference with the actions of other drugs. These advantages make local anesthetics useful for such ocular procedures as tonometry, foreign body and suture removal, gonioscopy, nasolacrimal irrigation and probing, and surgical procedures (see Table 2: Ophthalmic Uses of Local Anesthetics).

Table 2: OPHTHALMIC USES OF LOCAL ANESTHETICS	
Injectable	1. Facial nerve block 2. Retrobulbar or peribulbar anesthesia 3. Eyelid infiltration
Topical	1. Gonioscopy 2. Tonometry 3. Fundus contact lens biomicroscopy 4. Evaluation of corneal abrasions 5. Forced duction testing 6. Schirmer tear testing 7. Electroretinography 8. Lacrimal dilation and irrigation 9. Contact lens fitting 10. Superficial foreign body removal 11. Minor surgery of conjunctiva 12. Suture removal 13. Corneal epithelial debridement

For More Information

Bartlett JD, Jaanus SD, eds. *Clinical Ocular Pharmacology.* 5th ed. St. Louis, MO: Elsevier; 2008.

Bellucci R. Anesthesia for cataract surgery. *Curr Opin Ophthalmol.* 1999;10:36-41.

Canavan KS, Dark A, Garrioch MA. Sub-Tenon's administration of local anaesthetic: a review of the technique. *Br J Anaesth.* 2003;90:787-793.

Chandler MJ, Grammer LC, Patterson R. Provocative challenge with local anesthetics in patients with a prior history of reaction. *J Allergy Clin Immunol.* 1987;79:883.

Crandall AS, Zabriskie NA, Patel BC, et al. A comparison of patient comfort during cataract surgery with topical anesthesia versus topical anesthesia and intracameral lidocaine. *Ophthalmology.* 1999;106:60-66.

Cyriac IC, Pineda R. Postoperative complications of periocular anesthesia. *Int Ophthalmol Clin.* 2000;40:85-91.

Dannaker CJ, Maibach HI, Austin E. Allergic contact dermatitis to proparacaine with subsequent cross-sensitization to tetracaine from ophthalmic preparations. *Am J Contact Dermat.* 2001;12:177-179.

Gail H, Kaufman R, Kalveram CM. Adverse reactions to local anesthetics; analysis of 197 cases. *J Allergy Clin Immunol.* 1996;97:933-937.

Ghosh YK, Goodall KL. Postoperative pain relief in vitreoretinal surgery with sub-Tenon bupivacaine 0.75%. *Acta Ophthalmol Scand.* 2005;83:119-120.

Johnston RL, Whitfield LA, Giralt J, et al. Topical versus peribulbar anesthesia, without sedation, for clear corneal phacoemulsification. *J Cataract Refract Surg.* 1998;24:407-410.

Lai MM, Lai JC, Lee WH, et al. Comparison of retrobulbar and sub-Tenon's capsule injection of local anesthetic in vitreoretinal surgery. *Ophthalmology.* 2005;112:574-579.

Rizzo L, Marini M, Rosati C, et al. Peribulbar anesthesia: a percutaneous single injection technique with a small volume of anesthetic. *Anesth Analg.* 2005;100:94-96.

Rosenwasser GO. Complications of topical ocular anesthetics. *Int Ophthalmol Clin.* 1989;29:153.

Ruschen H, Celaschi D, Bunce C, et al. Randomised controlled trial of sub-Tenon's block versus topical anaesthesia for cataract surgery: a comparison of patient satisfaction. *Br J Ophthalmol.* 2005;89:291-293.

Sobol WM, McCrary JA. Ocular anesthetic properties and adverse reactions. *Int Ophthalmol Clin.* 1989;29:195.

Stoelting RK, Hillier SC. *Pharmacology and Physiology in Anesthetic Practice.* 4th ed. Philadelphia, PA: Lippincott Williams & Wilkins; 2005.

LOCAL ANESTHETICS, INJECTABLE

Actions:

Pharmacology: These agents prevent generation and conduction of nerve impulses by inhibiting ionic fluxes, increasing electrical excitation threshold, slowing nerve impulse propagation, and reducing rate of rise of action potential. Progression of anesthesia is related to the diameter, myelination, and conduction velocity of affected nerve fibers.

The use of vasoconstrictors (eg, epinephrine) with local anesthetics promotes local hemostasis, decreases systemic absorption, and prolongs duration of action.

Pharmacokinetics: Various pharmacokinetic parameters can be significantly altered by presence of hepatic or renal disease, addition of epinephrine, factors affecting urinary pH, renal blood flow, administration route, and age of the patient.

Injectable Local Anesthetics Pharmacokinetics

Anesthetic	Onset (minutes)	Duration (hours)	Equivalent anesthetic concentration (%)	pK_a	Partition coefficient[1]	Systemic protein binding (%)
ESTERS						
Procaine[2]	2-5	0.25-1	2	9.1	0.02	5.8[3]
(w/epinephrine)	nd	0.5-1.5				
Chloroprocaine[2]	6-12	0.5	2	9	0.14	nd
(w/epinephrine)	nd	0.5-1.5				
AMIDES						
Lidocaine[2]	< 2	0.5-1	1	7.9	2.9	64.3
(w/epinephrine)	< 2	2-6				
Mepivacaine[2]	3-5	0.75-1.5	1	7.8	0.8	77.5[4]
(w/epinephrine)	nd	2-6				
Bupivacaine[2]	5	2-4	0.25	8.2	27.5	95.6[4]
(w/epinephrine)	nd	3-7				

[1] n-Heptane/Buffer, pH 7.4. nd - No data.
[2] Values in this line are for infiltrative anesthesia.
[3] Nerve homogenate binding.
[4] Plasma protein binding.

Local anesthetics are divided into 2 groups: *esters,* which are derivatives of para-aminobenzoic acid, and *amides,* which are derivatives of aniline. The "ester" local anesthetics are metabolized by hydrolysis of the ester linkage by plasma esterase, probably plasma cholinesterase. The "amide" local anesthetics are metabolized primarily in the liver, then excreted primarily in the urine as metabolites with a small fraction of unchanged drug. Hypersensitivity reactions may occur with local anesthetics of the ester type (see Warnings).

Indications:

Refer to individual product listings.

Ophthalmic Uses of Local Anesthetics

Route	Use
Injectable	Facial nerve block
	Retrobulbar or peribulbar anesthesia
	Eyelid infiltration

Contraindications:

Hypersensitivity to local anesthetics, para-aminobenzoic acid (esters only), or parabens.

Warnings:

Head and neck area: Small doses of local anesthetics injected into the head and neck area, including retrobulbar, dental, and stellate ganglion blocks, may produce adverse reactions similar to systemic toxicity seen with unintentional intravascular injections of larger doses. The injection procedures require the utmost care. Confusion, convulsions, respiratory depression or arrest, and cardiovascular stimulation or depression have occurred. These reactions may be caused by intra-arterial injection of the local anesthetic with retrograde flow to cerebral circulation. They also may be caused by puncture of the dural sheath of the optic nerve during retrobulbar block with diffusion of any local anesthetic along the subdural space to the midbrain. Observe patient carefully. Monitor respiration and circulation. Do not exceed dosage recommendations.

Ophthalmic – When local anesthetic solutions are used for retrobulbar block, complete corneal anesthesia usually precedes onset of clinically acceptable external ocular muscle akinesia. Therefore, presence of akinesia rather than anesthesia alone should determine readiness of the patient for surgery.

Cardiovascular reactions – Cardiovascular reactions are depressants. They may be the result of direct drug effect, the result of vasovagal reaction, particularly if the patient is in the sitting position. Failure to recognize premonitory signs such as sweating, feeling of faintness, and changes in pulse or sensorium may result in progressive cerebral hypoxia and seizure or serious cardiovascular catastrophe. Place patient in recumbent position and administer oxygen. Vasoactive drugs may be administered IV.

Hypersensitivity: Hypersensitivity reactions, including anaphylaxis, may occur in a small segment of the population allergic to para-aminobenzoic acid derivatives (eg, procaine, tetracaine, benzocaine). The amide-type local anesthetics have not shown cross-sensitivity with the esters. Hypersensitivity reactions and anaphylaxis have occurred rarely with lidocaine. Administer ester-type local anesthetics cautiously to patients with abnormal or reduced levels of plasma esterases.

Renal function impairment: Use mepivacaine with caution in patients with renal disease.

Hepatic function impairment: Because amide-type local anesthetics are metabolized primarily in the liver, patients with hepatic disease, especially severe hepatic disease, may be more susceptible to potential toxicity. Use cautiously in such patients.

Elderly: Repeated doses may cause accumulation of the drug or its metabolites or slow metabolic degradation. Give reduced doses.

Pregnancy: Category B (lidocaine). *Category C* (bupivacaine, chloroprocaine, mepivacaine). Safety for use in pregnant women, other than those in labor, has not been established.

Lactation: Safety for use in the nursing mother has not been established. It is not known whether local anesthetic drugs are excreted in breast milk.

Children: Because of lack of clinical experience, administering bupivacaine to children less than 12 years of age is not recommended. Reduce dosages in children to be commensurate with age, body weight, and physical condition.

Precautions:

Dosage: Use the lowest dosage that results in effective anesthesia to avoid high plasma levels and serious adverse effects. Inject slowly with frequent aspirations before and during the injection to avoid intravascular injection. Perform syringe aspirations before and during each supplemental injection using continuous (intermittent) catheter techniques.

Inflammation or sepsis: Use local anesthetic procedures with caution when there is inflammation or sepsis in the region of proposed injection.

CNS toxicity: Monitor cardiovascular and respiratory vital signs and state of consciousness after each injection. Restlessness, anxiety, incoherent speech, lightheadedness, numbness and tingling of the mouth and lips, metallic taste, tinnitus, dizziness, blurred vision, tremors, twitching, depression, or drowsiness may be early signs of CNS toxicity.

Malignant hyperthermia: Many drugs used during anesthesia are considered potential triggering agents for familial malignant hyperthermia. It is not known whether amide-type local anesthetics trigger this reaction and the need for supplemental general anesthesia cannot be predicted in advance; therefore, have a standard protocol for management available.

Vasoconstrictors: Use solutions containing a vasoconstrictor with caution in areas of the body supplied by end arteries or having otherwise compromised blood supply. Use with extreme caution in patients whose medical history and physical evaluation suggest the existence of hypertension, peripheral vascular disease, arteriosclerotic heart disease, cerebral vascular insufficiency, or heart block; these individuals may exhibit exaggerated vasoconstrictor response.

Debilitated patients, acutely ill patients, children, obstetric delivery patients, and patients with increased intra-abdominal pressure: repeated doses may cause accumulation of the drug or its metabolites or slow metabolic degradation. Give reduced doses. Use anesthetics with caution in patients with severe disturbances of cardiac rhythm, hypotension, shock, or heart block. Local anesthetics should also be used with caution in patients with impaired cardiovascular function because they may be less able to compensate for functional changes associated with the prolongation of A-V conduction produced by these drugs.

Sulfite sensitivity: Some of these products contain sulfites. Sulfites may cause allergic-type reactions (eg, hives, itching, wheezing, anaphylaxis) in certain susceptible people. Although the overall prevalence of sulfite sensitivity in the general population is probably low, it is seen more frequently in asthmatics or in atopic nonasthmatic people.

Drug Interactions:

Intercurrent use: Mixtures of local anesthetics are sometimes employed to compensate for the slower onset of one drug and the shorter duration of action of the second drug. Toxicity is probably additive with mixtures of local anesthetics, but some experiments suggest synergisms. Exercise caution regarding toxic equivalence when mixtures of local anesthetics are employed.

Prior use of chloroprocaine may interfere with subsequent use of bupivacaine. For this reason and because safety of intercurrent use of bupivacaine and chloroprocaine has not been established, such use is not recommended.

Some preparations contain vasoconstrictors. Keep this in mind when using concurrently with other drugs that may interact with vasoconstrictors.

Injectable Local Anesthetic Drug Interactions			
Precipitant drug	Object drug*		Description
Local anesthetics	Sulfonamides	⬇	The para-aminobenzoic acid metabolite of procaine, chloroprocaine, and tetracaine inhibits the action of sulfonamides. Therefore, do not use procaine, chloroprocaine, or tetracaine in any condition in which a sulfonamide drug is employed.

* ⬇ = Object drug decreased.

Adverse Reactions:

The most common acute adverse reactions are related to the CNS and cardiovascular systems. These are generally dose-related and may result from rapid absorption from the injection site, diminished tolerance, or unintentional intravascular injection.

Cardiovascular: Myocardial depression, hypotension (with spinal anesthesia because of vasomotor paralysis and pooling of blood in the venous bed), decreased cardiac output, heart block, syncope, bradycardia, ventricular arrhythmias (including tachycardia and fibrillation), cardiac arrest, and fetal bradycardia (see Warnings).

CNS: Restlessness, anxiety, dizziness, tinnitus, blurred vision, nausea, vomiting, chills, pupil constriction, or tremors may occur, possibly proceeding to convulsions (approximately 0.1% of local anesthetic epidural administrations). Excitement may be transient or absent, with depression being the first manifestation. This may quickly be followed by drowsiness merging into unconsciousness and respiratory arrest.

Postspinal headache; meningismus; arachnoiditis; palsies; apprehension; double vision; euphoria; sensation of heat, cold, or numbness; and spinal nerve paralysis (spinal anesthesia) also have occurred.

Dermatologic: Cutaneous lesions, urticaria, pruritus, erythema, angioneurotic edema (including laryngeal edema). Skin testing is of limited value.

Overdosage:

Acute emergencies from local anesthetics are generally related to high plasma levels encountered during therapeutic use or because of unintended subarachnoid injection.

Management: The first consideration is prevention.

Convulsions – Convulsions, as well as underventilation or apnea, are caused by unintentional subarachnoid injection; maintain patent airway and assist or control ventilation with oxygen and a delivery system capable of permitting immediate positive airway pressure by mask. Evaluate circulation. If convulsions persist despite respiratory support and the status of the circulation permits, give small increments of an ultra short-acting barbiturate (eg, thiopental) or a benzodiazepine (eg, diazepam) IV. Circulatory depression may require administration of IV fluids and a vasopressor. If not treated immediately, convulsions and cardiovascular depression can result in hypoxia, acidosis, bradycardia, arrhythmias, and cardiac arrest. Underventilation or apnea may produce these same signs and also lead to cardiac arrest if ventilatory support is not instituted. If cardiac arrest occurs, institute standard cardiopulmonary resuscitative measures.

Endotracheal intubation may be indicated.

Administration and Dosage:

The administered dose of local anesthetic varies with the procedure, vascularity of the tissues, depth of anesthesia, degree of required muscle relaxation, duration of anesthesia desired, and the physical condition of the patient. Reduce dosages for children, elderly and debilitated patients, and patients with cardiac or liver disease.

Infiltration or regional block anesthesia: Always inject slowly, with frequent aspirations, to prevent intravascular injection.

For detailed administration and dosage, refer to specific manufacturers' labeling.

Individual drug monographs are on the following pages.

BUPIVACAINE HYDROCHLORIDE and BUPIVACAINE COMBINATIONS

For complete prescribing information, refer to the Injectable Local Anesthetics group monograph.

Indications:

Retrobulbar block: 0.75% solution.

Rx	**Bupivacaine Hydrochloride** (Abbott)	**Injection:** 0.75%	In 20 mL amps.
Rx	**Sensorcaine MPF** (Astra Zeneca)		In 30 mL amps and 10 and 30 mL vials.
Rx	**Sensorcaine MPF** (Astra Zeneca)	**Injection:** 0.75% with 1:200,000 epinephrine	In 30 mL vials.[1]

[1] With sodium metabisulfite.

LIDOCAINE HYDROCHLORIDE and LIDOCAINE COMBINATIONS

For complete prescribing information, refer to the Injectable Local Anesthetics group monograph.

Indications:

Retrobulbar or transtracheal injection: 4% solution.

Rx	**Xylocaine MPF** (Astra Zeneca)	**Injection:** 4%	In 5 mL ampules and 5 mL disp. syringe with laryngotracheal cannula.
Rx	**Xylocaine** (Astra Zeneca)	**Injection:** 0.5% with 1:200,000 epinephrine	In 50 mL multiple-dose vials.[1]
Rx	**Xylocaine** (Astra Zeneca)	**Injection:** 1% with 1:100,000 epinephrine	In 10, 20, and 50 mL multiple-dose vials.[1]
Rx	**Xylocaine MPF** (Astra Zeneca)	**Injection:** 1% with 1:200,000 epinephrine	In 30 mL ampules, and 10 and 30 mL single-dose vials.[2]
Rx	**Xylocaine MPF** (Astra Zeneca)	**Injection:** 1.5% with 1:200,000 epinephrine	In 5 and 30 mL ampules, and 10 and 30 mL single-dose vials.[2]
Rx	**Xylocaine** (Astra Zeneca)	**Injection:** 2% with 1:100,000 epinephrine	In 20 and 50 mL multiple-dose vials.[1]
Rx	**Xylocaine MPF** (Astra Zeneca)	**Injection:** 2% with 1:200,000 epinephrine	In 20 mL ampules, and 10 and 20 mL single-dose vials.[2]

[1] With methylparaben.
[2] With sodium metabisulfite.

MEPIVACAINE HYDROCHLORIDE

For complete prescribing information, refer to the Injectable Local Anesthetics group monograph.

Indications:

Peripheral nerve block: 1% or 2% solution.

Infiltration: 0.5% (via dilution) or 1% solution.

Rx	**Polocaine** (Astra Zeneca)	**Injection:** 1%	In 50 mL vials.
Rx	**Polocaine MPF** (Astra Zeneca)		In 30 mL vials.
Rx	**Polocaine MPF** (Astra Zeneca)	**Injection:** 1.5%	In 30 mL vials.
Rx	**Polocaine** (Astra Zeneca)	**Injection:** 2%	In 50 mL vials.
Rx	**Polocaine MPF** (Astra Zeneca)		In 20 mL vials.

LOCAL ANESTHETICS, TOPICAL

Actions:

Pharmacology: Local anesthetics stabilize the neuronal membrane so the neuron is less permeable to ions. This prevents the initiation and transmission of nerve impulses, thereby producing the local anesthetic action.

Studies indicate that local anesthetics influence permeability of the nerve cell membrane by limiting sodium ion permeability by closing the pores through which the ions migrate in the lipid layer of the nerve cell membrane. This limitation prevents the fundamental change necessary for generation of the action potential.

Pharmacokinetics: Tetracaine and proparacaine are approximately equally potent. They have a rapid onset of anesthesia beginning within 13 to 30 seconds following instillation; the duration of action is 15 to 20 minutes.

Indications:

Corneal anesthesia of short duration (eg, tonometry, gonioscopy, removal of corneal foreign bodies and sutures); short corneal and conjunctival procedures; cataract surgery; conjunctival and corneal scraping for diagnostic purposes; paracentesis of the anterior chamber.

Ophthalmic Uses of Local Anesthetics

Route	Use
Topical	Gonioscopy
	Tonometry
	Fundus contact lens biomicroscopy
	Evaluation of corneal abrasions
	Forced duction testing
	Schirmer tear testing
	Electroretinography
	Lacrimal dilation and irrigation
	Contact lens fitting
	Superficial foreign body removal
	Minor surgery of conjunctiva
	Suture removal
	Corneal epithelial debridement

Contraindications:

Hypersensitivity to similar drugs (ester-type local anesthetics), para-aminobenzoic acid or its derivatives, or to any other ingredient in these preparations; prolonged use, especially for self-medication (not recommended).

Warnings:

For topical ophthalmic use only: Prolonged use may diminish duration of anesthesia, retard wound healing, and cause corneal epithelial erosions (see Adverse Reactions).

Systemic toxicity: Systemic toxicity is rare with topical ophthalmic application of local anesthetics. It usually occurs as CNS stimulation followed by CNS and cardiovascular depression.

Protection of the eye: Protection of the eye from irritating chemicals, foreign bodies, and rubbing during the period of anesthesia is very important. Advise the patient to avoid touching the eye until anesthesia has worn off.

Pregnancy: Category C. Safety for use during pregnancy has not been established. Use only when clearly needed and when potential benefits outweigh potential hazards to the fetus.

Lactation: Safety for use during lactation has not been established. Use only when clearly needed and when potential benefits outweigh potential hazards to the infant.

Children: Safety and efficacy for use in children have been well established through clinical experience, although no studies exist.

Precautions:

Reduced plasma esterase: Use caution in patients with abnormal or reduced levels of plasma esterases.

Use cautiously and sparingly in patients with known allergies, cardiac disease, or hyperthyroidism.

Adverse Reactions:

Prolonged ophthalmic use of topical anesthetics has been associated with corneal epithelial erosions, retardation or prevention of healing of corneal erosions, and reports of severe keratitis and permanent corneal opacification with accompanying visual loss and scarring or corneal perforation. Inadvertent damage may be done to the anesthetized cornea and conjunctiva by rubbing an eye to which topical anesthetics have been applied.

Tetracaine:

Miscellaneous – Transient stinging, burning, and conjunctival redness may occur. A rare, severe, immediate-type allergic corneal reaction has been reported. It is characterized by acute diffuse epithelial keratitis with filament formation and sloughing of large areas of necrotic epithelium, diffuse stromal edema, descemetitis, and iritis.

Rarely, local reactions including lacrimation, photophobia, and chemosis have occurred.

Proparacaine:

Miscellaneous – Local or systemic sensitivity occurs occasionally. At recommended concentration and dosage, proparacaine usually produces little or no initial irritation, stinging, burning, conjunctival redness, or lacrimation. However, some local irritation and stinging may occur several hours after instillation.

Rarely, a severe, immediate-type, hyperallergic corneal reaction may occur, which includes acute, intense, and diffuse epithelial keratitis, a gray, ground-glass appearance, sloughing of large areas of necrotic epithelium, corneal filaments, and, sometimes, iritis with descemetitis.

Allergic contact dermatitis with drying and fissuring of the fingertips, softening and erosion of the corneal epithelium, and conjunctival congestion and hemorrhage have been reported.

Patient Information:

Avoid continuous or prolonged use.

Avoid touching or rubbing the eye until the anesthesia has worn off because inadvertent damage may be done to the anesthetized cornea and conjunctiva.

To avoid contamination, do not touch dropper tip to any surface. Replace cap after using.

Do not use if discolored, cloudy, or if it contains a precipitate. Protect from light.

Individual drug monographs are on the following pages.

PROPARACAINE HYDROCHLORIDE

For complete prescribing information, refer to the Topical Local Anesthetics group monograph.

Administration and Dosage:

Deep anesthesia as in cataract extraction: 1 drop every 5 to 10 minutes for 5 to 7 doses.

Removal of sutures: Instill 1 or 2 drops 2 or 3 minutes before removal of sutures.

Removal of foreign bodies: Instill 1 or 2 drops prior to operating.

Tonometry: Instill 1 or 2 drops immediately before measurement.

Storage/Stability: Store at 8° to 24°C (46° to 75°F). Protect from light.

Rx	**Proparacaine Hydrochloride** (Various, eg, Bausch & Lomb, Falcon)	**Solution:** 0.5%	In 15 mL.
Rx	**AK-TAINE** (Akorn)		In 15 mL.[1,2]
Rx	**Alcaine** (Various, eg, Alcon)		In 15 mL *Drop-Tainers.*[3,4]
Rx	**Ophthetic** (Various, eg, Allergan)		In 15 mL.[1,2]
Rx	**Paracaine** (OCuSOFT)		In 15 mL.[1,3]

[1] Refrigerate.
[2] With 0.01% benzalkonium Cl, glycerin, and sodium chloride.
[3] With glycerin and 0.01% benzalkonium Cl.
[4] Refrigerate after opening.

TETRACAINE HYDROCHLORIDE

For complete prescribing information, refer to the Topical Local Anesthetics group monograph.

Administration and Dosage:

Solution: Instill 1 or 2 drops. Not for prolonged use.

Storage/Stability: Store at 8° to 27°C (46° to 80°F). Protect from light.

Rx	**Tetracaine Hydrochloride** (Various, eg, Bausch & Lomb)	**Solution:** 0.5%	In 2 and 15 mL.
Rx	**Tetcaine** (OCuSOFT)		In 15 mL.

MISCELLANEOUS LOCAL ANESTHETIC COMBINATIONS

For complete prescribing information, refer to the Topical Local Anesthetics group monograph.

Indications:

For procedures in which a topical ophthalmic anesthetic agent in conjunction with a disclosing agent is indicated: corneal anesthesia of short duration (eg, tonometry, gonioscopy, removal of corneal foreign bodies); short corneal and conjunctival procedures.

Administration and Dosage:

Removal of foreign bodies or sutures; tonometry: 1 to 2 drops (in single instillations) in each eye before the procedure.

Deep ophthalmic anesthesia:

Proparacaine/Fluorescein – Instill 1 drop in each eye every 5 to 10 minutes for 5 to 7 doses. Use of an eye patch is recommended.

Benoxinate/Fluorescein – Instill 2 drops into each eye at 90-second intervals for 3 instillations.

Storage/Stability: Protect from light.

Rx	**Flucaine** (OCuSOFT)	**Solution:** 0.5% proparacaine hydrochloride and 0.25% fluorescein sodium	In 5 mL.[1,2]
Rx	**Altafluor** (Altaire)	**Solution:** 0.4% benoxinate hydrochloride and 0.25% fluorescein sodium	In 5 mL with dropper.[1,3]
Rx	**Fluress** (Various, eg, Akorn)		In 5 mL with dropper.[3]
Rx	**Flurox** (OCuSOFT)		In 5 mL with dropper.[1,3]
Rx	**FluraSafe** (Altaire)	**Solution:** 0.4% benoxinate hydrochloride and 0.35% fluorexon disodium	In 6 mL with dropper.[1,4]

[1] Refrigerate.
[2] With glycerin, povidone, polysorbate 80, 0.01% thimerosal.
[3] With povidone, boric acid, 1% chlorobutanol.
[4] With povidone, boric acid, 0.5% chlorobutanol.

Mydriatics and Cycloplegics

Mydriatics are drugs that dilate the pupil. Adrenergic agonists are used for routine dilation of the pupil. Phenylephrine (eg, *Neo-Synephrine*) and epinephrine (eg, *Epifrin*) are the only direct-acting adrenergic agents available that produce mydriasis without cycloplegia. However, epinephrine is not used clinically for its mydriatic effects.

Anticholinergic agents administered topically to the eye for purposes of inhibiting accommodation are termed *cycloplegics*. Their primary use is for cycloplegic refraction and in the treatment of uveitis. Because these agents also inhibit action of the iris sphincter muscle, they are effective mydriatics. Of the cholinergic blocking agents, only tropicamide (eg, *Mydriacyl*) is used routinely for mydriasis. For most dilation procedures, the adrenergic or anticholinergic agents can be used alone or in combination for maximum mydriasis.

MYDRIATICS

Phenylephrine Hydrochloride

Phenylephrine is a synthetic alpha-receptor agonist that is structurally similar to epinephrine. Following topical application on the eye, it contracts the iris dilator muscle and smooth muscle of the conjunctival arterioles, causing pupillary dilation and "blanching" of the conjunctiva. Mueller's muscle of the upper eyelid may be stimulated, widening the palpebral fissure.

For pupillary dilation, concentrations of 2.5% and 10% are commercially available. Maximum dilation occurs within 45 to 60 minutes, depending on the concentration used or number of drops instilled. The pupil size usually returns to predrug levels within 4 to 6 hours. Because phenylephrine has little or no effect on the ciliary muscle, mydriasis occurs without cycloplegia.

Phenylephrine 1% solution can be used in diagnosis of Horner syndrome. Significant mydriasis can occur in the eye with a postganglionic lesion as compared with one with a normal innervation.

The mydriatic response to phenylephrine may be affected in situations that alter corneal epithelial integrity. Corneal abrasions or trauma from such procedures as tonometry or gonioscopy, as well as prior instillation of a topical anesthetic, can enhance its pharmacologic effect. Concentrations as small as 0.125%, as present in OTC decongestants, can cause mydriasis if the corneal epithelium is damaged.

Because the topical instillation of phenylephrine can be accompanied by clinically significant ocular and systemic side effects, cardiovascular effects in particular, avoid use of the 10% concentration if possible. The 2.5% concentration is generally recommended for routine dilation, especially in infants and the elderly. Use the drug with caution in patients with cardiac disease, hypertension, arteriosclerosis, and diabetes. It is contraindicated in patients taking tricyclic antidepressants (eg, amitriptyline [eg, *Elavil*]), MAO inhibitors (eg, phenelzine [*Nardil*]), reserpine, guanethidine (*Ismelin*), and methyldopa (eg, *Aldomet*).

Hydroxyamphetamine 1% has been combined with tropicamide 0.25% (*Paremyd*) as a combination formulation for mydriasis. *Paremyd* produces a mydriatic effect equivalent to phenylephrine 2.5% followed by tropicamide 0.5% for the first 45 to 60 minutes. Pupil size is sufficient for binocular indirect ophthalmoscopy. The effect is independent of age, skin, or iris color.

CYCLOPLEGIC MYDRIATICS

Commonly used cycloplegic mydriatics include the following: atropine (eg, *Isopto Atropine*), homatropine (eg, *Isopto Homatropine*), scopolamine (eg, *Isopto Hyoscine*), cyclopentolate (eg, *Cyclogyl*), and tropicamide (eg, *Tropicacyl*).

Objective and subjective refractive procedures are employed to determine the nature of the refractive error. Under normal circumstances, this is best accomplished without interference from topically applied drugs that might adversely affect examination results. However, under some circumstances, the instillation of cycloplegics may enable a more accurate refractive examination.

Use in Esotropia

Children with strabismus, especially esotropia, should receive a cycloplegic examination. It is important to uncover the full amount of hyperopia in young patients with suspected accommodative esotropia so that plus lenses can relieve the effort placed on the accommodative-convergence system. Some clinicians use cycloplegics in children who exhibit myopia for the first time to rule out accommodative spasm (pseudomyopia) as the underlying etiology. Patients who are unresponsive or inconsistent in their responses to subjective refraction will often benefit from cycloplegia. Cycloplegic refraction also is indicated to confirm the refractive amount in patients who exhibit symptoms of malingering or conversion reaction. Refraction of young children and infants is usually more accurate and easier with cycloplegics because these patients may fixate any distance during the examination. Patients with suspected latent hyperopia will also benefit from cycloplegic refraction.

Contraindications: Cycloplegics cause pupillary dilation; therefore, they are contraindicated in patients with extremely narrow anterior chamber angles or a history of angle-closure glaucoma. Use atropine with caution in patients with Down syndrome and in patients receiving systemic anticholinergic drugs. Patients allergic to atropine can usually be given scopolamine, which will enable similar examination results.

Drug selection: Atropine provides the most effective cycloplegia of any currently available anticholinergic drug and is indicated for the cycloplegic retinoscopy of infants and children up to 4 years of age with suspected accommodative esotropia. The use of atropine allows determination of the maximum amount of hyperopia.

Cyclopentolate has become the drug of choice for the cycloplegic refraction of strabismic patients over 4 years of age and nonstrabismic patients of any age. Although atropine is still preferred for patients less than 4 years of age with suspected accommodative esotropia, there is a trend toward the use of cyclopentolate in these patients.

Clinical procedures: The use of atropine for the refractive examination of patients with suspected accommodative esotropia requires that the medication be instilled at home 1 to 3 days prior to the office visit. This allows time for maximum cycloplegia to occur.

Cyclopentolate is used in the practitioner's office and is instilled 30 to 60 minutes prior to refractive examination. Once maximum cycloplegia has occurred, retinoscopy or subjective refraction is performed. Considerable skill and judgment are required to interpret the findings and prescribe a useful refractive correction.

Use in Uveitis

Uveitis is an inflammation of the iris, ciliary body, or choroid of the eye. The inflammation can be limited to the anterior structures or the posterior structures of the eye, or both; the clinical features depend on the site of involvement. Uveitis can be classified based on the anatomic site of inflammation. For example, uveitis involving the iris only is termed iritis. Another method to classify the uveal inflammation is based on whether it affects the anterior or posterior structures of the eye. Uveitis can also be classified as either granulomatous or nongranulomatous. Any clinical classification system has considerable overlap, but these classifications provide the opportunity to differentiate various clinical presentations and predict the natural course of the uveal inflammation.

Etiology: Uveitis is thought to be an immune-complex disease with T-cell antigen dysfunction playing a major role. Idiopathic anterior uveitis is the most common clinical presentation. Human leukocyte antigen (HLA) studies are being undertaken to identify individuals who might be predisposed to recurrent episodes of uveitis or whose uveitis might be associated with other conditions. Systemic disorders are often associated with uveitis and include collagen diseases such as rheumatoid arthritis, ankylosing spondylitis, and systemic lupus erythematosus. Other systemic causes include metabolic diseases, granulomatous diseases, and infectious diseases such as herpes zoster and herpes simplex.

Diagnosis: The signs and symptoms of uveitis depend largely on the anatomic site of inflammation. Anterior uveitis is characterized by conjunctival hyperemia, the distribution of which often follows a circumcorneal pattern. The pupil is frequently miotic, and there is almost always an anterior chamber reaction manifested by cells and flare. The intraocular pressure may be reduced, and there are often keratic precipitates on the corneal endothelium as seen with the slit lamp. Symptoms include ocular pain, photophobia, and blurred vision. Consider cases of anterior uveitis that are bilateral, recurrent, or resistant to treatment for more extensive diagnostic evaluation for the presence of underlying systemic disease.

Posterior uveitis is characterized by little or no pain, and although there can be some anterior chamber reaction, inflammation of the vitreous (vitritis) is most prominent. If the macula is involved or if the vitreous is sufficiently hazy to diminish vision, visual acuity will be affected.

Drug selection: Cycloplegics are useful in the treatment of anterior uveitis because they often prevent posterior synechiae. Cycloplegia places the ciliary body and iris at rest, reducing many of the associated symptoms, and cycloplegics also reduce the anterior chamber reaction. Cyclopentolate, homatropine, and atropine are the most commonly used cycloplegic agents for the treatment of uveitis.

Topical corticosteroids are usually administered in conjunction with cycloplegic therapy. In severe cases, periocular or oral steroids may also be considered; immunosuppressive agents can be used in cases where corticosteroids may not be effective. If uveitic glaucoma ensues, antiglaucoma therapy is usually initiated.

For More Information

Bartlett JD, Jaanus SD, eds. *Clinical Ocular Pharmacology.* 5th ed. St. Louis, MO: Elsevier; 2008.

Cooper J, Feldman JM, Jaanus SD, et al. Pupillary dilation and fundoscopy with 1% hydroxyamphetamine plus 0.25% tropicamide (*Paremyd*) versus tropicamide 0.5% or 1% as a function of iris and skin pigmentation and age. *J Am Optom Assoc.* 1996;67:669-675.

Egashira SM, Kish LL, Twelker JD, et al. Comparison of cyclopentolate versus tropicamide cycloplegia in children. *Optom Vis Sci.* 1993;70:1019-1026.

Manny RE, Fern KD, Zervas HJ, et al. 1% cyclopentolate hydrochloride: another look at the time course of cycloplegia using an objective measure of the accommodative response. *Optom Vis Sci.* 1993;70:651-665.

Manny RE, Hussein M, Scheiman M, et al. Tropicamide 1%: an effective cycloplegic agent for myopic children. *Invest Ophthalmol Vis Sci.* 2001;42:1728-1735.

Mirshahi A, Kohnen T. Acute psychotic reaction caused by topical cyclopentolate use for cycloplegic refraction before refractive surgery: case report and review of the literature. *J Cataract Refract Surg.* 2003;29:1026-1030.

PHENYLEPHRINE HYDROCHLORIDE

Actions:

Pharmacology: Phenylephrine ophthalmic solution possesses predominantly α-adrenergic effects. In the eye, phenylephrine acts locally as a potent vasoconstrictor and mydriatic by constricting ophthalmic blood vessels and the radial muscle of the iris. The ophthalmic usefulness of phenylephrine is because of its rapid effect and moderately prolonged action.

Actions of different concentrations of phenylephrine are shown in the following table:

Phenylephrine Hydrochloride			
	Mydriasis/Vasoconstriction		
Strength of solution (%)	Maximal (min)	Recovery time (hr)	Paralysis of accommodation
0.12	30 to 90	-	-
2.5	15 to 60	3	trace
10	10 to 60	6	slight

Although rare, systemic absorption of sufficient quantities of phenylephrine may lead to systemic alpha-adrenergic effects, such as rise in blood pressure that may be accompanied by a reflex atropine-sensitive bradycardia.

Indications:

2.5% and 10%: Decongestant and vasoconstrictor and for pupil dilation in uveitis (posterior synechiae), open-angle glaucoma, refraction without cycloplegia, prior to surgery, ophthalmoscopic examination (funduscopy).

Contraindications:

Hypersensitivity to any component of the formulation; narrow-angle glaucoma or individuals with a narrow (occludable) angle who do not have glaucoma; in low birth weight infants and in some elderly adults with severe arteriosclerotic cardiovascular or cerebrovascular disease; during intraocular operative procedures when the corneal epithelial barrier has been disturbed.

Phenylephrine 10%: In infants, small children with low body weights, debilitated or elderly patients, and patients with aneurysms. The administration of phenylephrine is contraindicated in patients with long-standing, insulin-dependent diabetes, hypertensive patients receiving reserpine or guanethidine, advanced arteriosclerotic changes, idiopathic orthostatic hypotension, and in patients with a known history of organic cardiac disease.

In individuals with an intraocular lens implant, the administration of 10% phenylephrine is contraindicated because of the possibility of dislodging the lens.

Warnings:

Phenylephrine 10%: There have been rare reports of the development of serious cardiovascular reactions, including ventricular arrhythmias and myocardial infarctions. These episodes, some fatal, have usually occurred in elderly patients with preexisting cardiovascular diseases.

Elderly: Use with caution. Because of the strong action of phenylephrine 2.5% to 10% on the dilator muscle, older individuals also may develop transient pigment floaters in the aqueous humor 30 to 45 minutes following administration. The appearance may be similar to anterior uveitis or microscopic hyphema.

Rebound miosis occurs in some elderly patients. Subsequent instillation of phenylephrine may produce less mydriasis than the initial instillation. This may be of clinical importance when dilating pupils prior to retinal detachment or cataract surgery. Exercise caution not to overdose these patients.

Pregnancy: Category C. Safety for use has not been established. Use only if clearly needed and potential benefits to the mother outweigh potential hazards to the fetus.

Lactation: It is not known whether this drug is excreted in breast milk. Use caution when phenylephrine hydrochloride is administered to a nursing woman.

Children: Safety and efficacy for use in children have not been established. Phenylephrine 2.5% has been used for a "1 application method" in combination with a preferred rapid-acting cycloplegic (see Administration and Dosage). Phenylephrine 10% is contraindicated in infants.

Precautions:

Systemic absorption: Exceeding recommended dosages or applying phenylephrine 2.5% to 10% to an instrumented, traumatized, diseased, or postsurgical eye or adnexa, or to patients with suppressed lacrimation, as during anesthesia, may result in the absorption of sufficient quantities to produce a systemic vasopressor response.

A significant elevation in blood pressure is rare but has been reported following conjunctival instillation of recommended doses of phenylephrine 10%. Use with caution in children of low body weight, the elderly, and patients with insulin-dependent diabetes, hypertension, hyperthyroidism, generalized arteriosclerosis, or cardiovascular disease. Carefully monitor the posttreatment blood pressure of these patients and any patients who develop symptoms (see Contraindications).

The hypertensive effects of phenylephrine may be treated with an alpha-adrenergic blocking agent, such as phentolamine mesylate, 5 to 10 mg IV, repeated as necessary.

Narrow-angle glaucoma: Ordinarily, mydriatics are contraindicated in glaucoma patients. However, when temporary pupil dilation may free adhesions, or when intrinsic vessel vasoconstriction may lower IOP, this may temporarily outweigh danger from coincident dilation.

Corneal effects: If the corneal epithelium has been denuded or damaged, corneal clouding may occur if phenylephrine 10% is instilled. This may be especially serious following corneal epithelium removal during retinal detachment surgery or vitrectomy. The corneas of diabetic patients may manifest epithelial ulcerations as well as a slow rate of re-epithelialization. Use of phenylephrine in such corneas may be especially hazardous.

Rebound congestion: Rebound congestion may occur with extended use of ophthalmic vasoconstrictors.

Sulfite sensitivity: Some of these products contain sulfites. Sulfites may cause allergic-type reactions (eg, hives, itching, wheezing, anaphylaxis) in certain susceptible people. Although the overall prevalence of sulfite sensitivity in the general population is low, it is seen more frequently in asthmatics or in atopic nonasthmatic people. Specific products containing sulfites are identified in the product listings.

Drug Interactions:

Anesthetics: Use anesthetics that sensitize the myocardium to sympathomimetics (eg, cyclopropane or halothane) cautiously. Local anesthetics can increase ocular absorption of topical drugs. Exercise caution when applying prior to use of phenylephrine.

Beta-adrenergic blocking agents: Systemic side effects may occur more readily in patients taking these drugs. A severe hypertensive episode and fatal intracranial hemorrhage possibly associated with ophthalmic use of phenylephrine was reported in 1 patient taking propranolol for hypertension.

MAOIs: When given with, or up to 21 days after MAOIs, exaggerated adrenergic effects may result. Supervise and adjust dosage carefully. The pressor response of adrenergic agents may also be potentiated by tricyclic antidepressants, propranolol, reserpine, guanethidine, methyldopa, and anticholinergics (see Adverse Reactions).

Adverse Reactions:

Cardiovascular: Palpitations; tachycardia; cardiac arrhythmia; hypertension; collapse; extrasystoles; ventricular arrhythmias (ie, premature ventricular contractions); reflex bradycardia; coronary occlusion; subarachnoid hemorrhage; myocardial infarction; stroke; death associated with cardiac reactions. Headache or browache may occur.

> *Phenylephrine 10%* – Significant elevation of blood pressure is rare but can occur after conjunctival instillation. Exercise caution with elderly patients and children of low body weight. Carefully monitor the blood pressure of these patients (see Warnings and Contraindications). There have been rare reports of the development of serious cardiovascular reactions, including ventricular arrhythmias and myocardial infarctions. These episodes, some fatal, have usually occurred in elderly patients with preexisting cardiovascular diseases.

Ophthalmic: Transitory stinging on initial instillation; blurring of vision; mydriasis; increased redness; irritation; discomfort; punctate keratitis; lacrimation; increased IOP. May cause rebound miosis and decreased mydriatic response to therapy in the elderly.

Miscellaneous: Headache; blanching; sweating; dizziness; nausea; nervousness; drowsiness; weakness; hyperglycemia.

Patient Information:

Potentially hazardous tasks: May cause temporary blurred vision. Observe caution while driving or performing other hazardous tasks.

If severe eye pain, headache, vision changes, acute eye redness, or pain with light exposure occur, discontinue use and consult a physician.

To avoid contamination, do not touch dropper tip to any surface. Replace cap after using.

Do not use if solution changes color or becomes cloudy.

Administration and Dosage:

Vasoconstrictors and pupil dilation: Instill a drop of topical anesthetic. Follow in a few minutes with 1 drop of the 2.5% or 10% phenylephrine. The anesthetic prevents stinging and consequent dilution of solution by lacrimation. It may be necessary to repeat the instillation after 1 hour, again preceded by a topical anesthetic.

Uveitis: The formation of synechiae may be prevented by using the 2.5% or 10% solution and atropine to produce wide dilation of the pupil. However, the vasoconstrictor effect of phenylephrine may be antagonistic to the increase of local blood flow in uveal infection.

To free recently formed posterior synechiae, instill 1 drop of the 2.5% or 10% solution to the upper surface of the cornea. Continue treatment the following day, if necessary. In the interim, apply hot compresses for 5 or 10 minutes, 3 times daily using 1 drop of 1% or 2% solution of atropine sulfate before and after each series of compresses.

Glaucoma: Instill 1 drop of 10% solution on the upper surface of the cornea as often as necessary. The 2.5% and 10% solutions have been used in conjunction with miotics in patients with open-angle glaucoma. Phenylephrine reduces the difficulties experienced by the patient because of the small field produced by miosis. Hence, there may be marked improvement in visual acuity after using phenylephrine with miotic drugs.

Surgery: When a short-acting mydriatic is needed for wide dilation of the pupil before intraocular surgery, the 2.5% or 10% solution may be instilled from 30 to 60 minutes before the operation.

Refraction: Prior to determination of refractive errors, the 2.5% solution may be used effectively with homatropine HBr, atropine sulfate, cyclopentolate, tropicamide hydrochloride, or a combination of homatropine and cocaine hydrochloride.

> *Adults* – Instill 1 drop of the preferred cycloplegic in each eye; follow in 5 minutes with 1 drop phenylephrine 2.5% solution and in 10 minutes with another drop of the cycloplegic. In 50 to 60 minutes, the eyes are ready for refraction.
>
> Because adequate cycloplegia is achieved at different time intervals after the necessary number of drops, different cycloplegics will require different waiting periods.
>
> *Children* – Instill 1 drop of atropine sulfate 1% in each eye; follow in 10 to 15 minutes with 1 drop of phenylephrine 2.5% solution and in 5 to 10 minutes with a second drop of atropine sulfate 1%. In 1 to 2 hours, the eyes are ready for refraction.
>
> For a "1 application method," combine 2.5% phenylephrine solution with a cycloplegic, such as cyclopentolate, to elicit synergistic action. The additive effect varies depending on the patient. Therefore, when using a "1 application method," it may be desirable to increase the concentration of the cycloplegic.

Ophthalmoscopic examination: Phenylephrine is rarely used alone for mydriasis. Maximum dilation is achieved in 45 to 60 minutes.

Diagnostic procedures: Heavily pigmented irides may require larger doses in all the following procedures:

Retinoscopy – When dilation of the pupil without cycloplegic action is desired, the 2.5% solution may be used alone.

Blanching test – Instill 1 to 2 drops of the 2.5% solution in the injected eye. After 5 minutes, examine for perilimbal blanching. If blanching occurs, the congestion is superficial and probably does not indicate iritis.

Storage/Stability: Prolonged exposure to air or strong light may cause oxidation and discoloration. Do not use if solution changes color, becomes cloudy, or contains a precipitate.

Rx	**Phenylephrine Hydrochloride** (Various, eg, Bausch & Lomb, Falcon)	**Solution**: 2.5%	In 2, 5, and 15 mL.
Rx	**AK-Dilate** (Akorn)		In 2 and 15 mL.[1]
Rx	**Mydfrin 2.5%** (Alcon)		In 3 and 5 mL *Drop-Tainers*.[2]
Rx	**Neofrin 2.5%** (OCuSOFT)		In 2, 5, and 15 mL.[2]
Rx	**Phenylephrine Hydrochloride** (Various, eg, Novartis Ophthalmic)	**Solution**: 10%	In 1, 2, and 5 mL.
Rx	**AK-Dilate** (Akorn)		In 2 and 5 mL.[1]
Rx	**Neofrin 10%** (OCuSOFT)		In 5 and 15 mL.[1]

[1] With benzalkonium chloride.
[2] With 0.01% benzalkonium chloride, EDTA, sodium bisulfite.

CYCLOPLEGIC MYDRIATICS

Actions:

Pharmacology: Anticholinergic agents (cholinergic antagonists) block the responses of the sphincter muscle of the iris and the muscle of the ciliary body to cholinergic stimulation, producing pupillary dilation (mydriasis), and paralysis of accommodation (cycloplegia).

Cycloplegic Mydriatics					
	Mydriasis		Cycloplegia		
Drug	Peak (minutes)	Recovery (days)	Peak (minutes)	Recovery (days)	Solution available
Atropine	30-40	7-10	60-180	6-12	0.5%-2%
Cyclopentolate	30-60	1	25-75	0.25-1	0.5%-2%
Homatropine	40-60	1-3	30-60	1-3	2%-5%
Scopolamine	20-30	3-7	30-60	3-7	0.25%
Tropicamide	20-40	0.25	20-35	0.25	0.25%-1%

Indications:

Mydriasis/Cycloplegia: For cycloplegic refraction and for dilating the pupil in inflammatory conditions of the iris and uveal tract. See individual monographs for specific indications.

Contraindications:

Primary glaucoma or a tendency toward glaucoma (eg, narrow anterior chamber angle); hypersensitivity to belladonna alkaloids or any component of the products; adhesions (synechiae) between the iris and the lens; children who have previously had a severe systemic reaction to atropine.

Warnings:

For topical ophthalmic use only: Not for injection.

Glaucoma: Determine the intraocular tension and the depth of the angle of the anterior chamber before and during use to avoid glaucoma attacks.

Elderly: Use these products with caution in the elderly and others where increased IOP may be encountered.

Pregnancy: Category C (atropine, cyclopentolate, homatropine). Safety for use during pregnancy has not been established. Give to a pregnant woman only if clearly needed.

Lactation: Atropine and homatropine may be detectable, in very small amounts, in breast milk. Although this is controversial, according to the American Academy of Pediatrics, these agents are compatible with breastfeeding. It is not known if cyclopentolate is excreted in breast milk. Exercise caution when administering to a nursing woman.

Children: Excessive use in children and in certain susceptible individuals may produce systemic toxic symptoms. Use with extreme caution in infants and small children.

> *Tropicamide and cyclopentolate* – May cause CNS disturbances that may be dangerous in infants and children. Keep in mind the possibility of psychotic reaction and behavioral disturbance caused by hypersensitivity to anticholinergic drugs. Use with extreme caution. Increased susceptibility to cyclopentolate has been reported in infants, young children, and in children with spastic paralysis or brain damage. Feeding intolerance may follow ophthalmic use of this product in neonates. It is recommended that feeding be withheld for 4 hours after examination. Do not use in concentrations greater than 0.5% in small infants.

Precautions:

Systemic effects: Avoid excessive systemic absorption by compressing the lacrimal sac by digital pressure during and for 2 to 3 minutes after instillation.

Down syndrome/Children with brain damage: Use cycloplegics with caution. These patients may demonstrate a hyperreactive response to topical atropine.

Hazardous tasks: May produce drowsiness, blurred vision, or sensitivity to light (caused by dilated pupils); observe caution while driving or performing other tasks requiring alertness, coordination, or physical dexterity.

Sulfite sensitivity: Some of these products contain sulfites that may cause allergic-type reactions (eg, hives, itching, wheezing, anaphylaxis) in certain susceptible people. Although the overall prevalence of sulfite sensitivity in the general population is probably low, it is seen more frequently in asthmatics or in atopic nonasthmatic people. Specific products containing sulfites are identified in the product listings.

Adverse Reactions:

Local: Increased intraocular pressure; transient stinging/burning; irritation with prolonged use (eg, allergic lid reactions, hyperemia, follicular conjunctivitis, blepharoconjunctivitis, vascular congestion, edema, exudate, eczematoid dermatitis).

Systemic: Dryness of the mouth and skin; blurred vision; photophobia with or without corneal staining; tachycardia; headache; parasympathetic stimulation; somnolence; visual hallucinations.

Other toxic manifestations of anticholinergic drugs include the following: skin rash; abdominal distention in infants; unusual drowsiness; hyperpyrexia; vasodilation; urinary retention; diminished GI motility; decreased secretion in salivary and sweat glands, pharynx, bronchi, and nasal passages. Severe manifestations of toxicity include the following: coma; medullary paralysis; death. Severe reactions are manifested by hypotension with progressive respiratory depression.

Cyclopentolate and tropicamide have been associated with psychotic reactions and behavioral disturbances in children. Ataxia, incoherent speech, restlessness, hallucinations, hyperactivity, seizures, disorientation as to time and place, and failure to recognize people have occurred with cyclopentolate. CNS disturbances also have occurred in children with tropicamide.

Overdosage:

Ocular: If ocular overdosage occurs, flush eye(s) with water or normal saline. Use of a topical miotic may be required. If accidentally ingested, induce emesis or gastric lavage.

Systemic: If symptoms develop (see Adverse Reactions), patients usually recover spontaneously when the drug is discontinued. In cases of severe toxicity, give physostigmine salicylate (see individual monograph in the Agents for Glaucoma chapter). Have atropine 1 mg available for immediate injection if physostigmine causes bradycardia, convulsions, or bronchoconstriction.

Cyclopentolate toxicity: Cyclopentolate toxicity may produce exaggerated symptoms (see Adverse Reactions). When administration of the drug product is discontinued, the patient usually recovers spontaneously. In case of severe manifestations of toxicity, the antidote of choice is physostigmine salicylate.

Children – Slowly inject physostigmine salicylate 0.5 mg IV. If toxic symptoms persist and no cholinergic symptoms are produced, repeat at 5-minute intervals to a maximum cumulative dose of 2 mg.

Adults and adolescents – Slowly inject physostigmine salicylate 2 mg IV. A second dose of 1 to 2 mg may be given after 20 minutes if no reversal of toxic manifestations has occurred.

Patient Information:

To avoid contamination, do not touch dropper tip to any surface. Replace cap after using.

May cause blurred vision. Do not drive or engage in any hazardous activities while the pupils are dilated.

May cause sensitivity to light. Protect eyes in bright illumination during dilation.

Keep out of the reach of children. These drugs should not be taken orally. Wash your hands and the child's hands following administration.

If eye pain occurs, discontinue use and consult physician immediately.

Individual drug monographs are on the following pages.

ATROPINE SULFATE

For complete prescribing information, refer to the Cycloplegic Mydriatrics group monograph.

Indications:

Mydriasis/Cycloplegia: For cycloplegic refraction or pupil dilation in acute inflammatory conditions of iris and uveal tract.

Administration and Dosage:

Solution:

Adults - Uveitis – Instill 1 or 2 drops into the eye(s) up to 4 times daily.

Children - Uveitis – Instill 1 or 2 drops of 0.5% solution into the eye(s) up to 3 times daily.

Refraction – Instill 1 or 2 drops of 0.5% solution into the eye(s) twice daily for 1 to 3 days before examination.

Ointment: Apply a small amount in the conjunctival sac up to 3 times daily.

Compress the lacrimal sac by digital pressure during and for 2 to 3 minutes after instillation.

Individuals with heavily pigmented irides may require larger doses.

Storage/Stability: Keep away from heat.

Rx	**Atropine Sulfate Ophthalmic** (Various, eg, Bausch & Lomb)	**Ointment**: 1%	In 3.5.
Rx	**Atropine Sulfate** (Various, eg, Alcon, Bausch & Lomb, Fougera)	**Solution**: 1%	In 2, 5, and 15 mL.

CYCLOPENTOLATE HYDROCHLORIDE

For complete prescribing information, refer to the Cycloplegic Mydriatics group monograph.

Indications:

Mydriasis/Cycloplegia: For mydriasis and cycloplegia in diagnostic procedures and acute inflammatory condition of the iris and uveal tract.

Administration and Dosage:

Adults: Instill 1 or 2 drops of 0.5%, 1%, or 2% solution into eye(s). Repeat in 5 to 10 minutes, if necessary. Complete recovery usually occurs in 24 hours.

Children: Instill 1 or 2 drops of 0.5%, 1%, or 2% solution into each eye. Follow in 5 to 10 minutes with a second application of 0.5% or 1% solution, if necessary.

Small infants: Instill 1 drop of 0.5% solution into each eye. Observe patient closely for at least 30 minutes following instillation.

Compress the lacrimal sac by digital pressure during and for 2 to 3 minutes after instillation.

Individuals with heavily pigmented irides may require higher strengths.

Storage/Stability: Store at 8° to 27°C (46° to 80°F).

Rx	**Cyclogyl** (Alcon)	**Solution:** 0.5%	In 15 mL *Drop-Tainers*.[1]
Rx	**Cyclopentolate Hydrochloride** (Various, eg, Bausch & Lomb)	**Solution:** 1%	In 2 and 15 mL.
Rx	**AK-Pentolate** (Akorn)		In 2, 5, and 15 mL.[1]
Rx	**Cylate** (OCuSOFT)		In 2 and 15 mL.[1]
Rx	**Cyclogyl** (Alcon)		In 2, 5, and 15 mL.[1]
Rx	**Cyclogyl** (Alcon)	**Solution:** 2%	In 2, 5, and 15 mL *Drop-Tainers*.[1]

[1] With 0.01% benzalkonium chloride, EDTA, boric acid.

HOMATROPINE HYDROBROMIDE

For complete prescribing information, refer to the Cycloplegic Mydriatics group monograph.

Indications:

Mydriasis/Cycloplegia: A moderately long-acting mydriatic and cycloplegic for refraction, and in the treatment of inflammatory conditions of the uveal tract. For preoperative and postoperative states when mydriasis is required.

Lens opacity: As an optical aid in some cases of axial lens opacities.

Administration and Dosage:

Uveitis: Instill 1 or 2 drops into the eye(s) up to every 3 to 4 hours.

Refraction: Instill 1 or 2 drops into the eye(s); repeat in 5 to 10 minutes if necessary.

Individuals with heavily pigmented irides may require larger doses.

Children: Use only the 2% strength.

Compress the lacrimal sac by digital pressure during and for 2 to 3 minutes after instillation.

Storage/Stability: Store at 8° to 24°C (46° to 75°F).

Rx	**Isopto Homatropine** (Alcon)	**Solution:** 2%	In 5 mL *Drop-Tainers.*[1]
Rx	**Homatropine HBr** (Various, eg, OCuSOFT)	**Solution:** 5%	In 2 and 5 mL.
Rx	**Isopto Homatropine** (Alcon)		In 5 and 15 mL *Drop-Tainers.*[2]

[1] With 0.01% benzalkonium chloride, 0.5% hydroxypropyl methylcellulose, polysorbate 80.
[2] With 0.005% benzethonium chloride, 0.5% hydroxypropyl methylcellulose.

SCOPOLAMINE HYDROBROMIDE (Hyoscine Hydrobromide)

For complete prescribing information, refer to the Cycloplegic Mydriatics group monograph.

Indications:

Mydriasis/Cycloplegia: For cycloplegia and mydriasis in diagnostic procedures.

Iridocyclitis: For preoperative and postoperative states in the treatment of iridocyclitis.

Administration and Dosage:

Uveitis: Instill 1 or 2 drops into the eye(s) up to 4 times daily.

Refraction: Instill 1 or 2 drops into the eye(s) 1 hour before refracting.

Compress the lacrimal sac by digital pressure during and for 2 to 3 minutes after instillation.

Storage/Stability: Protect from light. Store at 8° to 27°C (46° to 80°F).

Rx	**Isopto Hyoscine** (Alcon)	**Solution:** 0.25%	In 5 and 15 mL *Drop-Tainers.*[1]

[1] With 0.01% benzalkonium chloride, 0.5% hydroxypropyl methylcellulose.

TROPICAMIDE

For complete prescribing information, refer to the Cycloplegic Mydriatics group monograph.

Indications:

Mydriasis/Cycloplegia: For mydriasis and cycloplegia in diagnostic purposes.

Administration and Dosage:

Refraction: Instill 1 or 2 drops of 1% solution into the eye(s); repeat in 5 minutes. If patient is not seen within 20 to 30 minutes, instill an additional drop to prolong mydriatic effect.

Examination of fundus: Instill 1 or 2 drops of 0.5% solution 15 to 20 minutes prior to examination. Compress the lacrimal sac by digital pressure during and for 2 to 3 minutes after instillation to avoid excessive absorption.

Individuals with heavily pigmented irides may require larger doses.

Storage/Stability: Store away from heat. Do not refrigerate.

Rx	**Tropicamide** (Various, eg, Bausch & Lomb, Falcon)	**Solution:** 0.5%	In 15 mL.
Rx	**Mydral** (OCuSOFT)		In 15 mL.[1]
Rx	**Tropicacyl** (Akorn)		In 2 and 15 mL.
Rx	**Tropicamide** (Various, eg, Falcon)	**Solution:** 1%	In 3 and 15 mL.
Rx	**Mydriacyl** (Alcon)		In 3 and 15 mL *Drop-Tainers.*[1]
Rx	**Mydral** (OCuSOFT)		In 2 and 15 mL.[1]
Rx	**Tropicacyl** (Akorn)		In 2 and 15 mL.[2]

[1] With 0.01% benzalkonium chloride, EDTA.
[2] With 0.1% benzalkonium chloride, EDTA.

MYDRIATIC COMBINATIONS

These combinations induce mydriasis that is greater than that of either drug used alone at the concentrations present in these combination formulations. See individual monographs for complete prescribing information.

Indications:

Cyclomydril: Production of mydriasis.

Murocoll-2: For mydriasis, cycloplegia, and to break posterior synechiae in iritis.

Paremyd: Production of mydriasis.

Administration and Dosage:

Cyclomydril: Instill 1 drop into each eye every 5 to 10 minutes, not to exceed 3 times.

Murocoll-2:

> *Mydriasis* – Instill 1 or 2 drops into eye(s); repeat in 5 minutes, if necessary.
>
> *Postoperatively* – Instill 1 or 2 drops into the eye(s) 3 or 4 times daily.

Paremyd: Instill 1 drop into each eye, repeat as necessary.

Rx	**Cyclomydril** (Alcon)	**Solution**: 0.2% cyclopentolate hydrochloride and 1% phenylephrine hydrochloride.	In 2 and 5 mL *Drop-Tainers.*[1]
Rx	**Paremyd** (Akorn)	**Solution**: 0.25% tropicamide and 1% hydroxyamphetamine HBr	In 15 mL.[2]
Rx	**Murocoll-2** (Bausch & Lomb)	**Drops**: 0.3% scopolamine HBr and 10% phenylephrine hydrochloride.	In 5 mL.[3]

[1] With 0.01% benzalkonium chloride, EDTA, boric acid.
[2] With 0.005% benzalkonium chloride, 0.015% EDTA, NaCl.
[3] With 0.01% benzalkonium chloride, sodium metabisulfite, EDTA.

Antiallergy and Decongestant Agents

Release of histamine, prostaglandins, leukotrienes, various cytokines, and other less well-defined mediators from the mast cell during an allergic reaction can cause a variety of uncomfortable symptoms and sometimes life-threatening complications. Drug therapy is often successful in satisfactorily relieving associated signs and symptoms, especially when ocular tissues are affected.

Type I hypersensitivity reactions, also known as anaphylactic, immediate, or IgE-mediated reactions, occur when an antigen such as a drug or pollen is reintroduced into an individual who has been previously exposed to the antigen. Upon initial exposure to the antigen, IgE antibodies are produced that attach to mast cells and make the cells susceptible to rupture when the patient is again exposed to the same antigen. Disruption (degranulation) of mast cells causes a release of large quantities of inflammatory mediators, including histamine, prostaglandins, leukotrienes, and eosinophil chemotactic factor. Histamine activates H_1 receptors on blood vessels, causing vasodilation. These dilated blood vessels leak fluid, causing tissues to swell. Common symptoms and signs of local Type I reactions include redness, swelling, and itching. Such reactions occur in hay fever, allergic conjunctivitis, asthma, bee stings, and other chemical and toxin sensitivities (eg, penicillin). The following ocular diseases are characterized by Type I hypersensitivity reactions and may be treated with antihistamines or mast cell stabilizers.

ALLERGIC CONDITIONS

Seasonal Allergic Conjunctivitis

Allergic conjunctivitis can result from a variety of exogenous antigens and is often a component of more widespread allergic states. Airborne pollens, dust, and other environmental contaminants constitute the largest single group of agents responsible for the disorder. Ophthalmic drugs and their preservatives/excipients that may cause allergic conjunctivitis include neomycin, sulfonamides, atropine, and thimerosal. A careful patient history along with the typical appearance of conjunctival chemosis and hyperemia, together with itching and tearing, are necessary for the proper etiologic diagnosis.

Vernal Conjunctivitis

Affecting primarily adolescent males, vernal conjunctivitis is a bilateral inflammation involving the upper tarsal conjunctiva and sometimes the limbal conjunctiva. The disease is seasonal and has peak activity during the warm months of the year. It is characterized by the formation of large papillae having the appearance of cobblestones on the upper tarsal conjunctiva. Papillary hypertrophy can occur at the limbus and is characterized by a gelatinous thickening of the superior limbus. Tear histamine levels are significantly higher than in normal patients. Symptoms include intense itching during warm months and often a thick, ropy discharge. If the cornea becomes involved, photophobia may be marked. Significant papillary involvement of the upper lids may result in ptosis.

Atopic Keratoconjunctivitis

Atopic keratoconjunctivitis represents a hypersensitivity state caused by predispositional, constitutional, or hereditary factors rather than by acquired hypersensitivity to specific antigens. Patients usually have a personal or family history of allergy, especially asthma or hay fever. Atopic dermatitis is characterized by patches of thickened, excoriated, lichenified skin that is usually dry and itchy. Ocular findings are characterized by conjunctival hyperemia and chemosis. Corneal involvement is not uncommon and may be evident as a classic shield ulcer or pannus.

Giant Papillary Conjunctivitis

Giant papillary conjunctivitis (GPC) is a specific conjunctival inflammatory reaction to materials on contact lenses (eg, protein), but has also been reported in patients wearing methylmethacrylate ocular prostheses. The condition is characterized by papillary hypertrophy and primarily affects the upper tarsal conjunctiva. Although the condition is similar in appearance to that of vernal conjunctivitis, it probably represents a chronic conjunctival inflammatory reaction to denatured proteins that are adherent to the anterior lens surface. Lens bulk (thickness and diameter) may also play a part. Once the conjunctival changes reach a certain point, itching, lens instability, mucoid discharge, and contact lens intolerance occur.

DECONGESTANTS

The vasoconstrictor effect of the adrenergic agonists (ie, phenylephrine, imidazole derivatives) makes them useful as topical ocular decongestants. Following instillation, conjunctival vessels constrict within minutes, causing the eye to whiten. Minor ocular irritation can be temporarily relieved.

Because of the relatively low concentrations required for ocular decongestion, phenylephrine and the imidazole derivatives generally do not cause systemic adverse reactions. These products are designed for short-term use because they may mask symptoms of more serious ocular problems such as bacterial or other infections. If the condition does not respond to use of these products within 48 hours, a more serious condition should be suspected.

Phenylephrine

Phenylephrine (eg, *Neo-Synephrine*), a synthetic amine structurally similar to epinephrine, has been used in OTC products at concentrations of 0.12% or 0.125%, which cause vasoconstriction with little or no pupillary dilation in eyes with intact corneal epithelium. Because a potential for mydriasis does exist at low concentrations, phenylephrine is contraindicated in eyes predisposed to angle-closure glaucoma. Prolonged or excessive use can result in rebound conjunctival hyperemia. The eye may become more congested and red as the effect of the drug begins to subside.

Phenylephrine can exhibit variable efficacy because it is subject to oxidation on exposure to air, light, or heat. The solution may show no evidence of discoloration. To prolong shelf-life, antioxidants such as sodium bisulfite may be added to the formulation.

Imidazole Derivatives

The imidazole derivatives, naphazoline (eg, *Naphcon*), tetrahydrozoline (eg, *Visine*), and oxymetazoline (eg, *Visine L.R.*), differ structurally from phenylephrine by replacement of the benzene ring with an unsaturated ring. Concentrations used for ocular vasoconstriction do not alter pupil size or raise intraocular pressure in the normal eye.

The imidazole derivatives do not differ significantly in their ability to relieve conjunctival congestion. After instillation, the blanching effect occurs within minutes and may last up to several hours. These agents are generally more stable in solution than phenylephrine, and have a longer shelf-life and duration of action. Imidazole derivatives are buffered to a pH of 6.2 and may sting upon initial instillation.

ANTIHISTAMINES, MAST CELL STABILIZERS, AND NSAIDS

Because many of the signs and symptoms associated with Type I hypersensitivity reactions are caused by the release of histamine from mast cells, antihistamines can be effective in relieving at least some signs and symptoms and provide patient comfort. Several H_1-receptor antagonists have been formulated for topical ocular use.

More recently developed ophthalmic antihistamines have a dual mechanism of action. They block the action of histamine on H_1 receptors and also prevent the release of other mediators from cells involved in allergic reactions. Currently available ophthalmic formulations include olopatadine (*Pataday, Patanol*), ketotifen (*Zaditor*), and azelastine (*Optivar*). Relief of symptoms usually occurs within minutes.

The newest member of the dual mechanism of action topical antihistamines is epinastine (*Elestat*). The clinical indication is itching associated with allergic conjunctivitis. It does not penetrate the blood brain barrier; therefore, central nervous system adverse reactions should not occur with prolonged administration. During clinical trials, the most frequently reported ocular effects were burning sensation, hyperemia, folliculosis, and pruritus. Systemic adverse reactions included upper respiratory infections and headache.

Mast cell stabilizers also can be useful for certain ocular allergic signs and symptoms. Cromolyn sodium (*Crolom*) and lodoxamide tromethamine (*Alomide*) are currently FDA-approved for the management of vernal keratoconjunctivitis. Nedocromil (*Alocril*) and pemirolast (*Alamast*) are approved for seasonal allergic conjunctivitis. Nedocromil has a relatively faster onset of action than the other mast cell stabilizers. Some relief of symptoms can be achieved approximately 15 minutes following instillation. Pemirolast can provide symptomatic relief within days but may require several weeks.

Ketorolac tromethamine (*Acular*) is the first NSAID approved for topical ocular use in seasonal allergic conjunctivitis (see the Anti-inflammatory Agents chapter). It can alleviate the ocular itching as well as other signs and symptoms that accompany the condition.

COMBINATION PRODUCTS

In addition to vasoconstrictors, ocular decongestants may also contain preservatives, antihistamines, viscosity-increasing agents, buffers, and astringents. Because preservatives may induce allergic reactions in some patients, unit-dose preservative-free products are being formulated.

PHARMACOLOGIC MANAGEMENT

Antihistamines can be given with or without decongestants and are administered topically or orally, depending on the degree of involvement. Mast cell stabilizers, such as nedocromil (*Alocril*) and pemirolast (*Alamast*), can provide relief of itching and provide protection throughout the allergy season. Cromolyn sodium (*Crolom*) is also effective and can even be used prophylactically. For severe reactions or when rapid relief of symptoms is warranted, topical, such as loteprednol (*Alrex*), or oral corticosteroids may be justified.

For More Information

Bartlett JD, Jaanus SD, eds. *Clinical Ocular Pharmacology*. 5th ed. St. Louis, MO: Elsevier; 2008.

Bielory L. Role of antihistamines in ocular allergy. *Am J Med*. 2002;113(suppl 9A):34S-37S.

Bielory L. Allergic diseases of the eye. *Med Clin North Am*. 2006;90:129-148.

Cook EG, Stahl JL, Barney NP, et al. Mechanisms of antihistamines and mast cell stabilizers in ocular allergic inflammation. *Curr Drug Targets Inflamm Allergy*. 2002;1:167-180.

Fiscella RG, Jensen MK. Ophthalmic disorders. In: Berardi RR, ed. *Handbook of Non-Prescription Drugs—An Interactive Approach or Self-Care*. 14th ed. Washington, DC: American Pharmacists Association; 2004:659-689.

Leonardi A. Emerging drugs for ocular allergy. *Expert Opin Emerg Drugs*. 2005;10:505-520.

McGill JL. A review of the use of olopatadine in allergic conjunctivitis. *Int Ophthalmol*. 2004;25:171-179.

Ono SJ, Abelson MB. Allergic conjunctivitis; update on pathophysiology and prospects for future treatment. *J Allergy Clin Immunol*. 2005;115:118-122.

Shulman DG, Lothringer LL, Rubin JM, et al. A randomized, double-masked, placebo-controlled, parallel study of loteprednol etabonate 0.2% in patients with seasonal allergic conjunctivitis. *Ophthalmology*. 1999;106:362-369.

DECONGESTANTS

Actions:

Pharmacology: The effects of sympathomimetic agents on the eye are concentration-dependent and include: pupil dilation and vasoconstriction (alpha-adrenergic effects).

Higher concentrations of drug (ie, phenylephrine 2.5% and 10%) cause vasoconstriction and pupillary dilation for diagnostic eye exams, during surgery, and to prevent synechiae formation in uveitis. Weak concentrations of phenylephrine (0.12%) and other alpha-adrenergic agonists (naphazoline; tetrahydrozoline) are used as ophthalmic decongestants (vasoconstriction of conjunctival blood vessels) and for symptomatic relief of minor eye irritations.

Ophthalmic Vasoconstrictors

Vasoconstrictor	Duration of action (hr)	Available concentration	Prescription status
Naphazoline	3 to 4	0.012%	otc
		0.02%	otc
		0.03%	otc
		0.1%	Rx
Oxymetazoline	4 to 6	0.025%	otc
Phenylephrine	0.5 to 1.5	0.12%	otc
	—	2.5%	Rx
	—	10%	Rx
Tetrahydrozoline	1 to 4	0.05%	otc

Indications:

Refer to individual product listings for specific indications.

Contraindications:

Hypersensitivity to any of these agents; narrow-angle glaucoma or anatomically narrow (occludable) angle with no glaucoma; prior to peripheral iridectomy in eyes capable of angle closure because mydriatic action may precipitate angle closure.

Phenylephrine 10%: Infants and patients with aneurysms.

Warnings:

Anesthetics: Discontinue prior to use of anesthetics that sensitize the myocardium to sympathomimetics (eg, cyclopropane, halothane).

Local anesthetics can increase absorption of topically applied drugs; exercise caution when applying prior to use of phenylephrine. However, use of a local anesthetic prior to phenylephrine 2.5% or 10% may prevent stinging and enhance ocular drug penetration.

Overuse: Overuse may produce rebound vasodilation and increased redness of the eye.

Phenylephrine 10%: There have been rare reports of the development of serious cardiovascular reactions, including ventricular arrhythmias and myocardial infarctions. These episodes, some fatal, usually have occurred in elderly patients with preexisting cardiovascular diseases.

Pregnancy: Category C. Safety for use in pregnancy is not established. Use only if clearly needed and if the potential benefits outweigh the potential hazards to the fetus.

Lactation: Safety for use during breastfeeding has not been established. Use caution when administering to a nursing woman.

Children: Safety and efficacy have not been established. Phenylephrine 10% is contraindicated in infants.

Precautions:

Narrow-angle glaucoma: Ordinarily, any mydriatic is contraindicated in patients with angle-closure glaucoma. However, when temporary pupil dilation may free adhesions, these advantages may temporarily outweigh danger from coincident pupil dilation.

Rebound congestion: Rebound congestion may occur with frequent or extended use of ophthalmic vasoconstrictors. Rebound miosis has occurred in older people 1 day after receiving phenylephrine; reinstallation produced a reduction in mydriasis.

Systemic absorption: Exceeding recommended dosages of these agents or applying phenylephrine 2.5% to 10% solutions to the traumatized, diseased, or postsurgical eye or adnexa, or to patients with suppressed lacrimation, as during anesthesia, may result in the absorption of sufficient quantities to produce a systemic vasopressor response.

Pigment floaters: Older individuals may develop transient pigment floaters in the aqueous humor 30 to 45 minutes after instillation of phenylephrine. The appearance may be similar to anterior uveitis or to a microscopic hyphema.

Use with caution in children of low body weight, in elderly elderly patients, and in the presence of hypertension, diabetes, hyperthyroidism, cardiovascular abnormalities, or arteriosclerosis.

Hazardous tasks: Phenylephrine may cause temporary blurred or unstable vision; observe caution while driving or performing other hazardous tasks.

Sulfite sensitivity: Some of these products contain sulfites that may cause allergic-type reactions (eg, hives, itching, wheezing, anaphylaxis) in certain susceptible people. Although the overall prevalence of sulfite sensitivity in the general population is low, it is seen more frequently in asthmatics or in atopic nonasthmatic people.

Drug Interactions:

Ophthalmic Sympathomimetic Drug Interactions			
Precipitant drug	Object drug*		Description
Anesthetics	Ophthalmic sympathomimetics	↑	Use with caution anesthetics that sensitize the myocardium to sympathomimetics (eg, cyclopropane, halothane). Local anesthetics can increase absorption of topical drugs; exercise caution when applying prior to use of phenylephrine.

Ophthalmic Sympathomimetic Drug Interactions			
Precipitant drug	Object drug*		Description
Beta-blockers	Ophthalmic sympatho-mimetics	↑	Systemic adverse reactions may occur more readily in patients taking these drugs.
MAOIs	Ophthalmic sympatho-mimetics	↑	When given with, or up to 21 days after MAOIs, exaggerated adrenergic effects may result. Supervise and adjust dosage carefully.

* ↑ = Object drug increased.

Also consider drug interactions that may occur with systemic use of the sympathomimetics.

Adverse Reactions:

Ophthalmic: Transitory stinging on initial instillation; blurring of vision; mydriasis; increased redness; irritation; discomfort; punctate keratitis; lacrimation; increased IOP.

Phenylephrine may cause rebound miosis and decreased mydriatic response to therapy in older people.

Cardiovascular: Palpitation; tachycardia; cardiac arrhythmia; hypertension; collapse; extrasystoles; ventricular arrhythmias (ie, premature ventricular contractions); reflex bradycardia; coronary occlusion; subarachnoid hemorrhage; myocardial infarction; stroke; death associated with cardiac reactions. Headache or browache may occur.

> *Phenylephrine 10%* – Significant elevation of blood pressure is rare but can occur after conjunctival instillation. Exercise caution with elderly patients and children of low body weight. Carefully monitor the blood pressure of these patients (see Warnings and Precautions). There have been rare reports of the development of serious cardiovascular reactions, including ventricular arrhythmias and myocardial infarctions. These episodes, some fatal, have usually occurred in elderly patients with preexisting cardiovascular diseases.

Miscellaneous: Blanching; sweating; dizziness; nausea; nervousness; drowsiness; weakness; hyperglycemia.

Patient Information:

Do not use for more than 48 to 72 hours without consulting a physician.

If irritation, blurring, or redness persists, or if severe eye pain, headache, vision changes, floating spots, dizziness, decrease in body temperature, drowsiness, acute eye redness, or pain with light exposure occur, discontinue use and consult a physician.

Do not use if you have glaucoma except under the advice of a physician.

Refer to the Dosage Forms and Administration chapter for more complete information.

Hazardous tasks: Phenylephrine may cause temporary blurred or unstable vision; observe caution while driving or performing other hazardous tasks.

Individual drug monographs are on the following pages.

NAPHAZOLINE HYDROCHLORIDE

For complete prescribing information, refer to the Decongestants group monograph.

Indications:

Redness: To soothe, refresh, and remove redness caused by minor eye irritation such as smoke, smog, sun glare, allergies, or swimming.

Administration and Dosage:

Instill 1 or 2 drops into the conjunctival sac of affected eye(s) every 3 to 4 hours, up to 4 times daily.

Storage/Stability: Do not use if solution changes color or becomes cloudy.

otc	**20/20 Eye Drops** (S.S.S.)	**Solution**: 0.012%	In 15 mL.[1]
otc	**Clear Eyes** (Allscripts)		In 15 mL.[2]
otc	**Naphcon** (Alcon)		In 15 mL.[3]
Rx	**Naphazoline Hydrochloride** (Various, eg, S.S.S.)	**Solution**: 0.1%	In 15 mL.
Rx	**AK-Con** (Various, eg, Akorn)		In 15 mL.[3]
Rx	**Albalon** (Allergan)		In 15 mL.[4]
Rx	**Vasocon Regular** (Novartis Ophthalmics)		In 15 mL.[5]

[1] With benzalkonium chloride 0.01%, glycerin 0.4%, zinc sulfate 0.25%, EDTA.
[2] With benzalkonium chloride, EDTA, glycerin 0.2%, boric acid.
[3] With benzalkonium chloride 0.01%, EDTA.
[4] With benzalkonium chloride 0.004%, EDTA, polyvinyl alcohol 1.4%.
[5] With benzalkonium chloride, polyvinyl alcohol, EDTA, PEG-8000.

OXYMETAZOLINE HYDROCHLORIDE

For complete prescribing information, refer to the Decongestants group monograph.

Indications:

Redness: For the relief of redness of the eye caused by minor eye irritations.

Administration and Dosage:

Adults and children at least 6 years of age: Instill 1 or 2 drops in the affected eye(s) every 6 hours.

Storage/Stability: Do not use if solution changes color or becomes cloudy.

otc	**Visine L.R.** (Pfizer)	**Solution**: 0.025%	In 15 and 30 mL.[1]

[1] With benzalkonium chloride 0.01%, EDTA 0.1%.

PHENYLEPHRINE HYDROCHLORIDE

For complete prescribing information, refer to the Decongestants group monograph.

Indications:

0.12%: A decongestant to provide relief of minor eye irritations.

Administration and Dosage:

Minor eye irritations: Instill 1 or 2 drops of the 0.12% solution in eye(s) up to 4 times daily as needed.

Storage/Stability: Prolonged exposure to air or strong light may cause oxidation and discoloration. Do not use if solution changes color, becomes cloudy, or contains a precipitate.

otc	**Relief** (Allergan)	**Solution:** 0.12%	Preservative free. In 15 mL.[1]

[1] With polyvinyl alcohol 1.4%, EDTA.

TETRAHYDROZOLINE HYDROCHLORIDE

For complete prescribing information, refer to the Decongestants group monograph.

Indications:

Redness: For relief of redness of the eye caused by minor irritations.

Burning/Irritation: For temporary relief of burning and irritation caused by dryness of the eye or discomfort caused by minor irritations or to exposure to wind or sun.

Administration and Dosage:

Instill 1 or 2 drops into eye(s) up to 4 times a day.

Storage/Stability: Do not use if solution changes color or becomes cloudy.

otc	**Tetrahydrozoline Hydrochloride** (Rugby)	**Solution:** 0.05%	In 15 and 30 mL.
otc	**Collyrium Fresh** (Wyeth-Ayerst)		In 15 mL.[1]
otc	**Altazine Irritation Relief** (Altaire)		In 15 mL.[2]
otc	**Altazine Moisturizing Relief** (Altaire)		In 15 mL.[3]
otc	**Eyesine** (Akorn)		In 15 mL.[4]
otc	**Geneyes** (Ivax)		In 15 and 22.5 mL.[5]
otc	**Murine Tears Plus** (Prestige/ Medtech)		In 15 and 30 mL.[6]
otc	**Optigene 3** (Pfeiffer)		In 15 mL.[5]
otc	**Visine** (Various, eg, Pfizer)		In 15and 30 mL.[5]
otc	**Visine A.C.** (Pfizer)		In 15 mL.[7]
otc	**Visine Advanced Relief** (Pfizer)		In 15 and 30 mL.[8]

[1] With benzalkonium chloride 0.01%, EDTA 0.1%, glycerin 1%.
[2] With benzalkonium chloride, zinc sulfate 0.25%.
[3] With benzalkonium chloride, 1% dextran 70, 1% polyethylene glycol 400, povidone 1%.
[4] With benzalkonium chloride 0.01%, EDTA.
[5] With benzalkonium chloride 0.01%, EDTA 0.1%.
[6] With benzalkonium chloride, EDTA, polyvinyl alcohol 1.4%, povidone 0.6%.
[7] With benzalkonium chloride 0.01%, EDTA 0.1%, zinc sulfate 0.25%.
[8] With benzalkonium chloride, 1% polyethylene glycol 400, povidone 1%, dextran 70 1%, EDTA.

ANTIHISTAMINES

Actions:

Pharmacology: Antihistamines can be used alone or in combination with decongestants to provide relief of ocular irritation or congestion for the treatment of allergic or inflammatory ocular conditions. Antihistamines counteract the effects of histamine, a chemical released in the body in response to an antigen-antibody reaction that causes redness, itching, and irritation of tissues, and can cause watery eyes, runny nose, and sneezing.

Indications:

To provide relief of symptoms of allergic conjunctivitis (eg, watering, itching eyes).

Contraindications:

Hypersensitivity to any component of the formulation; with monoamine oxidase inhibitor use.

Warnings:

Elderly: Elderly patients may require lower doses of oral antihistamines. Antihistamines are more likely to cause dizziness, sedation, confusion, and decreased blood pressure in elderly patients.

Pregnancy: Category C. Safety for use has not been established. Use only if clearly needed and if the potential benefits to the mother outweigh the potential hazards to the fetus.

Lactation: Antihistamines appear in breast milk. Breast-feeding should be discouraged while using these medications.

Children: Antihistamine overdosage in children may cause hallucinations, convulsions, and death. Antihistamines may decrease mental alertness. They produce hyperactivity in children. Use caution in children younger than 12 years of age.

Precautions:

Use with caution in the presence of asthma, coronary artery disease, digestive tract obstruction, enlarged prostate, glaucoma (narrow-angle), heart disease, hypertension, hyperthyroidism, irregular heartbeat, liver disease, peptic ulcer, pregnancy, urinary bladder obstruction.

Glaucoma: Because they can produce angle closure, use with caution in people with narrow angle or a history of glaucoma.

Topical antihistamines: Topical antihistamines are potential sensitizers and may produce a local sensitivity reaction.

Drug Interactions:

Alcohol, sedatives (sleeping pills), tranquilizers, antianxiety medications, and narcotic pain relievers all are known to react with oral antihistamines. The following drugs and drug classes also interact with antihistamines: anticoagulants, epinephrine, fluconazole, isocarboxazid, itraconazole, ketoconazole, macrolides, metronidazole, miconazole, phenelzine, procarbazine, selegiline, tranylcypromine.

Adverse Reactions:

Ophthalmic: Blurred and double vision; eye pain; dryness; sensitivity to light.

Systemic: Stomach ache; constipation; appetite changes; nausea; vomiting; diarrhea; drowsiness; dizziness; mental confusion; decreased coordination; fatigue; headache; sleeplessness; sleepiness; sore throat; pharyngitis; cough; dry nose, throat, and mouth; thickening of mucus in respiratory tract; wheezing; stuffiness.

Cardiovascular: Irregular heartbeat; palpitations; hypotension.

Miscellaneous: Difficult urination; urine retention; ringing in the ears; rash; hives; excessive perspiration; chills.

Patient Information:

May cause drowsiness or dizziness. Use caution while driving or performing tasks requiring mental alertness. Avoid alcohol and other sedatives, hypnotics, tranquilizers, etc.

Elderly patients are more likely to experience dizziness, sedation, decreased coordination, mental confusion, and fainting when they take antihistamines.

May produce unexpected excitation, restlessness, irritability, and insomnia in rare instances. This is most likely in children and elderly patients.

Do not use for several days before allergy skin testing.

To avoid contamination, do not touch tip of the container to any surface. Replace cap after using.

Individual drug monographs are on the following pages.

AZELASTINE HYDROCHLORIDE

Actions:

Pharmacology: Azelastine hydrochloride is a relatively selective histamine H_1 antagonist and an inhibitor of the release of histamine and other mediators from cells (eg, mast cells) involved in the allergic response. Based on in vitro studies using human cell lines, inhibition of other mediators involved in allergic reactions (eg, leukotrienes and PAF) has been demonstrated with azelastine hydrochloride. Decreased chemotaxis and activation of eosinophils has also been demonstrated.

Pharmacokinetics: Systemic absorption of azelastine following ocular administration is relatively low. A study in symptomatic patients receiving one drop of azelastine 0.06 to 0.12 mg in each eye 2 to 4 times daily demonstrated plasma concentrations of azelastine generally to be between 0.02 and 0.25 ng/mL after 56 days of treatment. Three of 19 patients had quantifiable amounts of N-desmethylazelastine that ranged from 0.25 to 0.87 ng/mL at day 56.

Based on IV and oral administration, the elimination half-life, steady-state volume of distribution, and plasma clearance were 22 hours, 14.5 L/kg and 0.5 L/hr/kg, respectively. Approximately 75% of an oral dose of radiolabeled azelastine was excreted in feces with less than 10% as unchanged azelastine. Azelastine is oxidatively metabolized to the principal metabolite, N-desmethylazelastine, by the CYP–450 enzyme system. In vitro studies in human plasma indicate that the plasma protein binding of azelastine and N-desmethylazelastine are approximately 88% and 97%, respectively. It has a pH of approximately 5 to 6.5 and an osmolality of approximately 271 to 312 mOsmol/L.

Clinical Trials: In a conjunctival antigen challenge study, azelastine was more effective than its vehicle in preventing itching associated with allergic conjunctivitis. Azelastine had a rapid (within 3 minutes) onset of effect and a duration of action of approximately 8 hours for the prevention of itching.

In environmental studies, adult and pediatric patients with seasonal allergic conjunctivitis were treated with azelastine for 2 to 8 weeks. In these studies, azelastine was more effective than its vehicle in relieving itching associated with allergic conjunctivitis.

Indications:

Allergic conjunctivitis: Treatment of itching of the eye associated with allergic conjunctivitis.

Contraindications:

Known or suspected hypersensitivity to any of its components.

Warnings:

For ocular use only. Not for injection or oral use.

Carcinogenesis: Azelastine administered orally for 24 months was not carcinogenic in rats and mice at doses up to 30 mg/kg/day and 25 mg/kg/day, respectively. Based on a 30 mcL drop size, these doses were approximately 25,000 and 21,000 times higher than the maximum recommended ocular human use level of 0.001 mg/kg/day for a 50 kg adult.

Mutagenesis: Azelastine showed no genotoxic effects in the Ames test, DNA repair test, mouse lymphoma forward mutation assay, mouse micronucleus test, or chromosomal aberration test in rat bone marrow.

Fertility impairment: Reproduction and fertility studies in rats showed no effect on male or female fertility at oral doses up to 25,000 times the maximum recommended ocular human use level. At 68.6 mg/kg/day (57,000 times the maximum recommended ocular human use level), the duration of the estrous cycle was prolonged and copulatory activity and the number of pregnancies were decreased. The numbers of corpora lutea and implantations were decreased; however, the implantation ratio was not affected.

Elderly: No overall differences in safety or efficacy have been observed between elderly and younger adult patients.

Pregnancy: Category C. Azelastine has been shown to be embryotoxic, fetotoxic, and teratogenic (external and skeletal abnormalities) in mice at an oral dose of 68.6 mg/kg/day (57,000 times the recommended ocular human use level). At an oral dose of 30 mg/kg/day (25,000 times the recommended ocular human use level), delayed ossification (undeveloped metacarpus) and the incidence of the 14th rib were increased in rats. At 68.6 mg/kg/day (57,000 times the recommended ocular human use level), azelastine caused resorption and fetotoxic effects in rats. The relevance to humans of these skeletal findings noted at only high drug exposure levels is unknown.

There are no adequate and well-controlled studies in pregnant women. Azelastine should be used during pregnancy only if the potential benefit to the mother justifies the potential risk to the fetus.

Lactation: It is not known whether azelastine is excreted in human breast milk. Because many drugs are excreted in human milk, exercise caution when administering to a breast-feeding woman.

Children: Safety and efficacy have not been established in children younger than 3 years of age.

Adverse Reactions:

In controlled multiple-dose studies where patients were treated for up to 56 days, the most frequently reported adverse reactions were transient eye burning/stinging (approximately 30%), headaches (approximately 15%), and bitter taste (approximately 10%). The occurrence of these events was generally mild.

The following reactions were reported in 1% to 10% of patients: asthma, conjunctivitis, dyspnea, eye pain, fatigue, influenza-like symptoms, pharyngitis, pruritus, rhinitis, and temporary blurring. Some of these reactions were similar to the underlying disease being studied.

Patient Information:

Do not touch the dropper tip to any surface, the eyelids, or surrounding areas to prevent contaminating the dropper tip and the solution. Keep bottle tightly closed when not in use. This product is sterile when packaged.

Do not wear contact lens if the eye is red. Azelastine should not be used to treat contact lens-related irritation. The preservative in azelastine, benzalkonium chloride, may be absorbed by soft contact lenses. Patients who wear soft contact lenses and whose eyes are not red should wait at least 10 minutes after instilling azelastine before they insert their contact lenses.

Administration and Dosage:

The recommended dose is 1 drop instilled into each affected eye twice a day.

Storage/Stability: Store upright between 2° and 25°C (36° and 77°F).

Rx	**Optivar** (MedPointe)	**Solution:** 0.05%	In 6 mL.[1]

[1] With benzalkonium chloride 0.125 mg, disodium edetate dihydrate, hydroxypropylmethylcellulose, sorbitol solution, sodium hydroxide.

CROMOLYN SODIUM

Actions:

Pharmacology: In vitro and in vivo animal studies have shown that cromolyn inhibits the degranulation of sensitized mast cells that occurs after exposure to specific antigens. Cromolyn acts by inhibiting the release of histamine and other mediators from the mast cell.

Another activity demonstrated in vitro is the capacity of cromolyn to inhibit the degranulation of nonsensitized rat mast cells by phospholipase A and the subsequent release of chemical mediators. In another study, cromolyn did not inhibit the enzymatic activity of released phospholipase A on its specific substrate.

Cromolyn has no intrinsic vasoconstrictor, antihistaminic, or anti-inflammatory activity.

Pharmacokinetics: Cromolyn is poorly absorbed. When multiple doses of cromolyn ophthalmic solution are instilled into normal rabbit eyes, less than 0.07% of the dose is absorbed into the systemic circulation (presumably by way of the eye, nasal passages, buccal cavity, and GI tract). Trace amounts (less than 0.01%) of the dose penetrate into the aqueous humor, and clearance from this chamber is virtually complete within 24 hours after treatment is stopped.

In healthy volunteers, analysis of drug excretion indicates that approximately 0.03% of cromolyn is absorbed following administration to the eye.

Indications:

Conjunctivitis: Treatment of vernal keratoconjunctivitis, vernal conjunctivitis, and vernal keratitis.

Contraindications:

Hypersensitivity to cromolyn or to any of the other ingredients.

Warnings:

Stinging/Burning: Patients may experience a transient stinging or burning sensation following instillation of cromolyn.

Duration/Frequency of therapy: The recommended frequency of administration should not be exceeded. Symptomatic response to therapy (decreased itching, tearing, redness, and discharge) is usually evident within a few days, but longer treatment for up to 6 weeks is sometimes required. Once symptomatic improvement has been established, continue therapy for as long as needed to sustain improvement.

Contact lens use: As with all ophthalmic preparations containing benzalkonium chloride, users of soft (hydrophilic) contact lenses should refrain from wearing lenses while under treatment with cromolyn ophthalmic solution. Wear can be resumed within a few hours after discontinuation of the drug.

Concomitant therapy: If required, corticosteroids may be used concomitantly with cromolyn ophthalmic solution.

Pregnancy: Category B. In animals receiving parenteral cromolyn, adverse fetal effects (increased resorption and decreased fetal weight) were noted only at the very high parenteral doses that produced maternal toxicity. There are no adequate and well-controlled studies in pregnant women. Use during pregnancy only if clearly needed.

Lactation: It is not known whether this drug is excreted in breast milk. Exercise caution when cromolyn is administered to a breast-feeding woman.

Children: Safety and efficacy in children younger than 4 years of age have not been established.

Adverse Reactions:

The most frequently reported adverse reaction is transient ocular stinging or burning upon instillation. Other adverse reactions (infrequent) include conjunctival infection; wateriness; itchiness; dryness around the eye; puffiness; irritation; styes.

Patient Information:

Advise patients that the effect of cromolyn therapy is dependent on its administration at regular intervals, as directed.

Do not wear soft contact lenses while using cromolyn.

Administration and Dosage:

Instill 1 or 2 drops in each eye 4 to 6 times a day at regular intervals. One drop contains approximately 1.6 mg of cromolyn sodium.

Rx	**Cromolyn Sodium** (Various, eg, Akorn, Falcon, Teva)	**Solution:** 4%	In 10 and 15 mL.
Rx	**Crolom** (Bausch & Lomb)		In 10 mL bottle with controlled drop tip.[1]
Rx	**Opticrom** (Allergan)		In 10 mL opaque polyethylene eye drop bottles.[2]

[1] With benzalkonium chloride 0.01%, EDTA 0.1%, hydrochloric acid and/or sodium hydroxide.
[2] With benzalkonium chloride 0.01%, EDTA 0.1%.

EMEDASTINE DIFUMARATE

Actions:

Pharmacology: Emedastine is a relatively selective histamine H_1-antagonist. In vivo studies have shown concentration-dependent inhibition of histamine-induced increase in conjunctival vascular permeability in the conjunctiva following topical ocular administration.

Pharmacokinetics: Following topical administration, emedastine has low systemic exposure.

Clinical Trials: Patients with allergic conjunctivitis treated with emedastine for 6 weeks gained relief of redness, itching, and other symptoms as compared with placebo therapy.

Indications:

Allergic conjunctivitis: Temporary relief of the signs and symptoms of allergic conjunctivitis.

Contraindications:

Hypersensitivity to emedastine difumarate or any of its component products.

Warnings:

Topical (ophthalmic) use only: Not for injection or oral use.

Pregnancy: Category B. At 70,000 times the maximum recommended ocular human use level, emedastine difumarate increased the incidence of external, visceral, and skeletal anomalies in rats. There are no adequate and well-controlled studies in pregnant women. Use this drug during pregnancy only if clearly needed.

Lactation: Oral emedastine has been identified in rat milk. It is not known whether topical ocular administration could result in sufficient systemic absorption to produce detectable quantities in breast milk. Exercise caution when administering to a breast-feeding woman.

Children: Safety and efficacy in children younger than 3 years old have not been established.

Adverse Reactions:

Headache (11%); abnormal dreams, asthenia, bad taste, blurred vision, burning or stinging, corneal infiltrates, corneal staining, dermatitis, discomfort, dry eyes, foreign body sensations, hyperemia, keratitis, pruritus, rhinitis, sinusitis, tearing (less than 5%).

Patient Information:

To prevent contaminating the dropper tip, take care not to touch the eyelids or surrounding areas with the dropper tip of the bottle.

Keep the bottle tightly closed when not in use. Do not use if the solution has become discolored.

Do not wear contact lenses if eyes become red. Do not use emedastine to treat contact-lens related irritation. The preservative in emedastine, benzalkonium chloride, may be absorbed by soft contact lenses. Patients who wear soft contact lenses and whose eyes are not red should wait at least 10 minutes after instilling emedastine before inserting contacts.

Administration and Dosage:

One drop in the affected eye(s) up to 4 times a day.

Storage/Stability: Store at 4° to 30°C (39° to 86°F). Keep lid tightly closed.

Rx	**Emadine** (Alcon)	**Ophthalmic suspension:** 0.05%	In 5 mL *Drop-Tainers.*[1]

[1] With benzalkonium 0.01%, tromethamine, sodium chloride, hydroxypropyl methylcellulose, hydrochloric acid/sodium hydroxide.

EPINASTINE HYDROCHLORIDE

Actions:

Pharmacology: Epinastine is a topically active, direct H_1-receptor antagonist and an inhibitor of the release of histamine from the mast cell. Epinastine is selective for the histamine H_1-receptor and has affinity for the histamine H_2-receptor. Epinastine also possesses affinity for the α_1, α_2, and 5-HT_2-receptors. Epinastine does not penetrate the blood/brain barrier and, therefore, is not expected to induce adverse reactions of the central nervous system.

Pharmacokinetics: Fourteen subjects with allergic conjunctivitis received 1 drop of epinastine ophthalmic solution in each eye twice daily for 7 days. On day 7, average maximum epinastine plasma concentrations of approximately 0.04 ng/mL were reached after about 2 hours, indicating low systemic exposure. While these concentrations represented an increase over those seen following a single dose, the day 1 and day 7 area under the concentration-time curve (AUC) values were unchanged, indicating that there is no increase in systemic absorption with multiple dosing. Epinastine is 64% bound to plasma proteins. The total systemic clearance is approximately 56 L/hr, and the terminal plasma elimination half-life is about 12 hours. Epinastine is mainly excreted unchanged. About 55% of an intravenous dose is recovered unchanged in the urine, with about 30% in feces. Less than 10% is metabolized. The renal elimination is mainly via active tubular secretion.

Clinical Trials: Epinastine 0.05% has been shown to be significantly superior to vehicle for improving ocular itching in patients with allergic conjunctivitis in clinical studies using 2 different models: 1) conjunctival antigen challenge (CAC), where patients were dosed and then received antigen instilled into the inferior conjunctival fornix; and 2) environmental field studies, where patients were dosed and evaluated during allergy season in their natural habitat. Results demonstrated a rapid onset of action for epinastine 0.05% within 3 to 5 minutes after conjunctival antigen challenge. Duration of effect was 8 hours, making a twice daily regimen suitable. This dosing regimen was shown to be safe and effective for up to 8 weeks, without evidence of tachyphylaxis.

Indications:

Allergic conjunctivitis: For the prevention of itching associated with allergic conjunctivitis.

Contraindications:

Hypersensitivity to epinastine or to any of the other ingredients.

Warnings:

Topical (ophthalmic) use only: Not for injection or oral use.

Mutagenesis: Positive results were seen with early batches of epinastine in 2 in vitro chromosomal aberration studies conducted in the 1980s with human peripheral lymphocytes and with V79 cells, respectively.

Fertility impairment: Decreased fertility in female rats was observed at an oral dose up to approximately 90,000 times the maximum recommended ocular human dose (MROHD).

Pregnancy: Category C. In an embryofetal developmental study in pregnant rats, maternal toxicity with no embryofetal effects was observed at an oral dose that was approximately 150,000 times the MROHD. Total resorptions and abortion were observed in an embryofetal study in pregnant rabbits at an oral dose that was approximately 55,000 times the MROHD. In both studies, no drug-induced teratogenic effects were noted.

Epinastine reduced pup body weight gain following an oral dose to pregnant rats that was approximately 90,000 times the MROHD.

There are, however, no adequate and well-controlled studies in pregnant women. Because animal reproduction studies are not always predictive of human response, epinastine should be used during pregnancy only if the potential benefit justifies the potential risk to the fetus.

Lactation: A study in lactating rats revealed excretion of epinastine in the breast milk. It is not known whether this drug is excreted in human milk. Because many drugs are excreted in human milk, caution should be exercised when epinastine is administered to a breast-feeding woman.

Children: Safety and efficacy in children younger than 3 years of age have not been established.

Adverse Reactions:

Some of these reactions were similar to the underlying disease being studied.

Ophthalmic: Burning sensation in the eye, folliculosis, hyperemia, pruritus (1% to 10%).

Miscellaneous: Infection (cold symptoms and upper respiratory infections) (10%); headache, rhinitis, sinusitis, increased cough, pharyngitis (1% to 3%).

Patient Information:

To prevent contaminating the solution, take care not to touch the eye or surroundings areas, fingers, or any other surface with the dropper tip of the bottle. Serious damage to the eye and subsequent loss of vision may result from using contaminated solutions.

Do not wear contact lenses if eyes are red. Do not use epinastine to treat contact lens-related irritation. The preservative in epinastine, benzalkonium chloride, may be absorbed by soft contact lenses. Contact lenses should be removed prior to instillation of the solution and may be reinserted after 10 minutes following its administration.

Keep the bottle tightly closed when not in use.

Administration and Dosage:

One drop in each eye twice a day. Treatment should be continued throughout the period of exposure (until the pollen season is over or until exposure to the offending allergen is terminated), even when symptoms are absent.

Storage/Stability: Store at 15° to 25°C (59° to 77°F). Keep bottle tightly closed and out of the reach of children.

Rx	**Elestat** (Allergan)	**Solution:** 0.05%	In 5 mL opaque, white plastic bottles with dropper tips and caps.[1]

[1] With benzalkonium chloride 0.01%, EDTA, sodium chloride, sodium phosphate monobasic, hydrochloric acid/sodium hydroxide.

KETOTIFEN FUMARATE

Actions:

Pharmacology: Ketotifen is a relatively selective, noncompetitive histamine H_1-receptor antagonist and mast cell stabilizer. Ketotifen inhibits the release of mediators from cells involved in hypersensitivity reactions. Decreased chemotaxis and activation of eosinophils has also been demonstrated.

In human conjunctival allergen challenge studies, topical ketotifen was significantly more effective than placebo in preventing ocular itching associated with allergic conjunctivitis. The onset of action occurs rapidly with an effect seen within minutes of administration.

Indications:

Allergic conjunctivitis: Temporary prevention of itching of the eye caused by allergic conjunctivitis.

Contraindications:

Hypersensitivity to any component of this product.

Warnings:

Route of administration: For topical ophthalmic use only. Not for injection or oral use.

Pregnancy: Category C. It is not known whether ketotifen fumarate can cause fetal harm when administered to a pregnant woman or can affect reproductive capacity. There are no adequate and well-controlled studies in pregnant women. Use during pregnancy only if the potential benefits outweigh the potential hazards to the fetus.

Lactation: Ketotifen has been identified in the breast milk of rats following oral administration. It is not known whether topical ocular administration could result in sufficient systemic absorption to produce detectable quantities in breast milk. Caution should be exercised when ketotifen is administered to a breast-feeding woman.

Children: Safety and efficacy in children younger than 3 years of age have not been established.

Adverse Reactions:

In controlled clinical studies, conjunctival injection, headaches, and rhinitis were reported at an incidence of 10% to 25%. The occurrence of these adverse reactions was generally mild. Some of these reactions were similar to the underlying ocular disease being studied.

Ophthalmic: Allergic reaction, burning or stinging, conjunctivitis, discharge, dry eyes, eye pain, eyelid disorder, itching, keratitis, lacrimation disorder, mydriasis, photophobia, and rash (less than 5%).

Miscellaneous: Flu syndrome; pharyngitis (less than 5%).

Patient Information:

To prevent contaminating the dropper tip and solution, do not touch the eyelids or surrounding areas with the dropper tip of the bottle. Keep the bottle tightly closed when not in use.

Do not wear contact lenses if eyes are red. The preservative in ketotifen, benzalkonium chloride, may be absorbed by soft contact lenses. Ketotifen should not be used to treat contact lens-related irritation. Patients who wear contact lenses and whose eyes are not red should wait at least 10 minutes after instilling ketotifen before they insert their contact lenses.

Administration and Dosage:

The recommended dose is 1 drop twice daily in the affected eye(s) every 8 to 12 hours.

Storage/Stability: Store between 4° to 25°C (39° to 77°F).

Rx	**Zaditor** (Novartis)	**Solution:** 0.25 mg/mL (0.345 mg/mL ketotifen fumarate)	In 5 mL.[1]

[1] With benzalkonium chloride 0.01%, glycerol, sodium hydroxide/hydrochloric acid.

LODOXAMIDE TROMETHAMINE

Actions:

Pharmacology: Lodoxamide is a mast cell stabilizer that inhibits, in vivo, the Type I immediate hypersensitivity reaction. Lodoxamide therapy inhibits the increases in cutaneous vascular permeability that are associated with reagin or IgE and antigen-mediated reactions. In vitro, lodoxamide stabilizes rodent mast cells, prevents release of mast cell inflammatory mediators, and inhibits eosinophil chemotaxis. Although lodoxamide's precise mechanism of action is unknown, the drug may prevent calcium influx into mast cells upon antigen stimulation.

Lodoxamide has no intrinsic vasoconstrictor, antihistaminic, cyclooxygenase inhibition, or other anti-inflammatory activity.

Pharmacokinetics: The disposition of lodoxamide was studied in 6 healthy adult volunteers receiving a 3 mg oral dose. Urinary excretion was the major route of elimination. The elimination half-life was 8.5 hours in urine. In a study in 12 healthy adult volunteers, topical administration of 1 drop in each eye 4 times per day for 10 days did not result in any measurable lodoxamide plasma levels at a detection limit of 2.5 ng/mL.

Indications:

Treatment of vernal keratoconjunctivitis, vernal conjunctivitis, and vernal keratitis.

Off-label use(s): Treatment of seasonal allergic conjunctivitis.

Contraindications:

Hypersensitivity to any component of this product.

Warnings:

For ophthalmic use only: Not for injection.

Contact lenses: As with all ophthalmic preparations containing benzalkonium chloride, instruct patients not to wear soft contact lenses during treatment with lodoxamide.

Pregnancy: Category B. There are no adequate and well-controlled studies in pregnant women. Use during pregnancy only if clearly needed.

Lactation: It is not known whether lodoxamide is excreted in breast milk. Exercise caution when administering to a breast-feeding woman.

Children: Safety and efficacy in children younger than 2 years of age have not been established.

Precautions:

Burning/Stinging: Patients may experience a transient burning or stinging upon instillation of lodoxamide. Should these symptoms persist, advise the patient to contact their health care provider.

Adverse Reactions:

Ophthalmic: Transient burning, stinging, or discomfort upon instillation (approximately 15%); ocular itching/pruritus, blurred vision, dry eye, tearing/discharge, hyperemia, crystalline deposits, foreign body sensation (1% to 5%); corneal erosion/ulcer, scales on lid/lash, eye pain, ocular edema/swelling, ocular warming sensation, ocular fatigue, chemosis, corneal abrasion, anterior chamber cells, keratopathy/keratitis, blepharitis, allergy, sticky sensation, epitheliopathy (less than 1%).

Systemic: Headache (1.5%); heat sensation, dizziness, somnolence, nausea, stomach discomfort, sneezing, dry nose, rash (less than 1%).

Overdosage:

Overdose of an oral preparation of 120 to 180 mg resulted in a temporary sensation of warmth, profuse sweating, diarrhea, light-headedness, and a feeling of stomach distension; no permanent adverse reactions were observed. Adverse reactions reported following oral administration of 0.1 to 10 mg included a feeling of warmth or flushing, headache, dizziness, fatigue, sweating, nausea, loose stools, and urinary frequency/urgency. Consider emesis in the event of accidental ingestion.

Administration and Dosage:

Adults and children older than 2 years of age: Instill 1 to 2 drops in each affected eye 4 times daily for up to 3 months.

Rx	**Alomide** (Alcon)	**Solution:** 0.1%	In 10 mL *Drop-Tainers.*

NEDOCROMIL SODIUM

Actions:

Pharmacology: Nedocromil is a mast cell stabilizer that inhibits the release of mediators from cells involved in hypersensitivity reactions. Decreased chemotaxis and decreased activation of eosinophils and other inflammatory cells including neutrophils and basophils have also been demonstrated. In vitro studies with adult human bronchoalveolar cells showed that nedocromil sodium inhibits histamine release from a population of mast cells having been defined as belonging to the mucosal subtype and beta-glucuronidase release from macrophages. Nedocromil has a quick onset of action (within 15 to 30 minutes) which differentiates it from cromolyn.

Pharmacokinetics: Nedocromil exhibits low systemic absorption. When administered as a 2% ophthalmic solution in adult human volunteers, less than 4% of the total dose was systemically absorbed following multiple dosing. Absorption is mainly through the nasolacrimal duct rather than through the conjunctiva. It is not metabolized and is eliminated primarily unchanged in urine (70%) and feces (30%). It has a pH of 4 to 5.5.

Indications:

Treatment of itching associated with allergic conjunctivitis.

Contraindications:

Hypersensitivity to nedocromil or any component of this product.

Warnings:

Contact lenses: Users of contact lenses should refrain from wearing lenses while exhibiting the signs and symptoms of allergic conjunctivitis.

Carcinogenesis: A 2-year inhalation carcinogenicity study of nedocromil sodium at a dose of 24 mg/kg/day (approximately 400 times the maximum recommended human daily ocular dose on a mg/kg basis) in Wistar rats showed no carcinogenic potential.

Mutagenesis: Nedocromil showed no mutagenic potential in the Ames Salmonella/microsome plate assay, mitotic gene conversion in *Saccharomyces cerevisiae*, mouse lymphoma forward mutation, and mouse micronucleus assays.

Fertility impairment: Reproduction and fertility studies in mice and rats showed no effects on male and female fertility at a subcutaneous dose of 100 mg/kg/day (greater than 1,600 times the maximum recommended human daily ocular dose).

Elderly: No overall differences in safety or efficacy have been observed between elderly and younger patients.

Pregnancy: Category B. There are no adequate and well-controlled studies in pregnant women. Use during pregnancy only if clearly needed.

Lactation: After IV administration to lactating rats, nedocromil was excreted in milk. It is not known whether this drug is excreted in human breast milk. Exercise caution when administering to a breast-feeding woman.

Children: Safety and efficacy in children younger than 3 years of age have not been established.

Adverse Reactions:

The most frequently reported adverse reaction was headache (approximately 40%). Other adverse reactions include: ocular burning, irritation and stinging, unpleasant taste, nasal congestion (10% to 30%); asthma, conjunctivitis, eye redness, photophobia, rhinitis (1% to 10%).

Patient Information:

Avoid placing nedocromil solution directly on the cornea (the area just over the pupil), because it is especially sensitive. The administration of eye drops will be more comfortable if placed just inside the lower eyelid.

To avoid contamination of the solution, do not touch the dropper tip to the eye, fingers, or any other surface. Replace cap after use. It is recommended that any remaining contents be discarded after the treatment period prescribed by the physician.

Do not use with any other ocular medication unless directed by a physician. Do not wear contact lenses during treatment with nedocromil.

Administration and Dosage:

The recommended dosage is 1 or 2 drops in each eye twice a day. Nedocromil should be used at regular intervals.

Treatment should be continued throughout the period of exposure (ie, until the pollen season is over or until exposure to the offending allergen is terminated), even when symptoms are absent.

Storage/Stability: Store between 2° to 25°C (36° to 77°F). Store in original carton.

Rx	**Alocril** (Allergan)	**Solution:** 2%	In 5 mL bottle with a controlled dropper tip.[1]

[1] With benzalkonium chloride 0.01%, sodium chloride 0.5%, edetate disodium 0.05%.

OLOPATADINE HYDROCHLORIDE

Actions:

Pharmacology: Olopatadine is a relatively selective H_1-receptor antagonist that inhibits, in vivo and in vitro, the Type I immediate hypersensitivity reaction. It has no effect on alpha-adrenergic, dopamine, muscarinic type 1 and 2, and serotonin receptors.

Pharmacokinetics: Olopatadine was shown to have low systemic exposure in humans following topical ocular administration. Olopatadine was evaluated in 2 studies of healthy volunteers given 0.15% solution once every 12 hours for 2 weeks. The plasma concentrations were generally below 0.5 ng/mL. Higher concentrations were typically found within 2 hours of dosing and ranged from 0.5 to 1.3 ng/mL. Urinary excretion was the primary route of elimination. The half-life was approximately 3 hours.

Approximately 60% to 70% of the parent drug was recovered in the urine, with mono-desmethyl and N-oxide detected at low concentrations.

Olopatadine 0.1% was significantly more effective than its vehicle in preventing ocular itching associated with allergic conjunctivitis when challenged with an antigen initially and up to 8 hours after dosing.

Indications:

Allergic conjunctivitis: For the temporary prevention of itching of the eye.

Contraindications:

Hypersensitivity to any component of this product.

Warnings:

For topical ophthalmic use only. Not for injection.

Pregnancy: Category C. Rats treated at doses 93,750 times and rabbits treated at doses 62,500 times the maximum recommended ocular human use level showed a decrease in the number of live fetuses. There are no adequate and well-controlled studies in pregnant women. Use during pregnancy only if the potential benefits outweigh the potential hazards to the fetus.

Lactation: Olopatadine has been identified in the milk of nursing rats following oral administration. It is not known whether topical ocular administration could result in sufficient systemic absorption to produce detectable quantities in human breast milk. Exercise caution when administering to a breast-feeding woman.

Children: Safety and efficacy in children younger than 3 years of age have not been established.

Adverse Reactions:

Ophthalmic: Burning or stinging; dry eye; foreign body sensation; hyperemia; keratitis; lid edema; pruritus.

Systemic: Headache (7%); asthenia; cold syndrome; pharyngitis; rhinitis; sinusitis; taste perversion.

Patient Information:

To prevent contaminating the dropper tip and solution, take care not to touch the eyelids or surrounding areas with the dropper tip of the bottle.

Administration and Dosage:

The recommended dosage for 0.1% olopatadine is 1 to 2 drops in each affected eye 2 times per day every 6 to 8 hours. The recommended dosage for 0.2% olopatadine is once daily.

Storage/Stability: Keep bottle tightly closed when not in use. Store between 4° to 30°C (39° to 86°F).

Rx	**Patanol** (Alcon)	**Ophthalmic solution:** 0.1%	In 5 mL *Drop-Tainers.*[1]
Rx	**Olopatadine Hydrochloride** (Alcon)	**Ophthalmic solution:** 0.2%	In 2.5 mL fill in 4 mL bottle.[2]
Rx	**Pataday** (Alcon)		In 2.5 mL *Drop-Tainers.*[1]

[1] With benzalkonium chloride 0.01%.
[2] With benzalkonium chloride 0.01%, EDTA, povidone, dibasic sodium phosphate, sodium chloride, hydrochloric acid/sodium hydroxide.

PEMIROLAST POTASSIUM

Actions:

Pharmacology: Pemirolast is a mast cell stabilizer that inhibits the in vivo Type I immediate hypersensitivity reaction. In vitro and in vivo studies have demonstrated that pemirolast inhibits the antigen-induced release of inflammatory mediators (eg, histamine, leukotriene C_4, D_4, E_4) from human mast cells. In addition, pemirolast inhibits the chemotaxis of eosinophils into ocular tissue and blocks the release of mediators from human eosinophils. Although the precise mechanism of action is unknown, the drug has been reported to prevent calcium influx into mast cells upon antigen stimulation.

Pharmacokinetics: Topical ocular administration of 1 to 2 drops of pemirolast in each eye 4 times daily in 16 healthy volunteers for 2 weeks resulted in detectable concentrations in the plasma. The mean peak plasma level of 4.7 $\pm$ 0.8 ng/mL occurred at 0.42 $\pm$ 0.05 hours and the mean half-life was 4.5 $\pm$ 0.2 hours. When a single pemirolast 10 mg dose was taken orally, a peak plasma concentration of 0.723 mcg/mL was reached. Following topical administration, approximately 10% to 15% of the dose was excreted unchanged in the urine.

Clinical Trials: In clinical environmental studies, pemirolast was significantly more effective than placebo after 28 days in preventing ocular itching associated with allergic conjunctivitis.

Indications:

Prevention of itching of the eye caused by allergic conjunctivitis. Symptomatic response to therapy (decreased itching) may be evident within a few days but frequently requires longer treatment (up to 4 weeks).

Contraindications:

Hypersensitivity to any component of this product.

Warnings:

For topical ophthalmic use only. Not for injection or oral use.

Mutagenesis: Pemirolast was not mutagenic or clastogenic when tested in a series of bacterial and mammalian tests for gene mutation and chromosomal injury in vitro, nor was it clastogenic when tested in vivo in rats.

Fertility impairment: Pemirolast had no effect on mating and fertility in rats at oral doses up to 250 mg/kg (approximately 20,000-fold the human dose at 2 drops/eye, 40 mcL/drop, 4 times daily for a 50 kg adult). A reduced fertility and pregnancy index occurred in the F_1 generation when F_0 dams were treated with 400 mg/kg pemirolast during late pregnancy and lactation period (approximately 30,000-fold the human dose).

Pregnancy: Category C. Pemirolast caused an increased incidence of thymic remnant in the neck, interventricular septal defect, fetuses with wavy rib, splitting of thoracic vertebral body, and reduced numbers of ossified sternebrae, sacral and caudal vertebrae, and metatarsi when rats were given oral doses at least 250 mg/kg (approximately 20,000-fold the human dose at 2 drops/eye, 40 mcL/drop, 4 times daily for a 50 kg adult) during organogenesis. Increased incidence of dilation of renal pelvis/ureter in the fetuses and neonates was also noted when rats were given an oral dose of 400 mg/kg pemirolast (approximately 30,000-fold the human dose). There are no adequate and well-controlled studies in pregnant women. Use during pregnancy only if the benefit outweighs the risk.

Lactation: Pemirolast is excreted in the milk of lactating rats at concentrations higher than those in plasma. It is not known whether pemirolast is excreted in breast milk. Exercise caution when administering to a breast-feeding woman.

Children: Safety and efficacy in children younger than 3 years of age have not been established.

Adverse Reactions:

The most common adverse reactions were headache, rhinitis, cold/flu symptoms (10% to 25%). These adverse reactions were generally mild.

Ophthalmic: Burning, dry eye, foreign body sensation, ocular discomfort (less than 5%).

Miscellaneous: Allergy, back pain, bronchitis, cough, dysmenorrhea, fever, sinusitis, sneezing/nasal congestion (less than 5%).

Patient Information:

To prevent contaminating the dropper tip and solution, do not touch the eyelids or surrounding areas with the dropper tip. Keep the bottle tightly closed when not in use.

Do not wear contact lenses if eye is red. Pemirolast should not be used to treat contact lens-related irritation. The preservative in this solution, lauralkonium chloride, may be absorbed by soft contact lenses. Patients who wear soft contact lenses and whose eyes are not red should wait at least 10 minutes after instilling the solution before inserting their contact lenses.

Administration and Dosage:

The recommended dose is 1 to 2 drops in each affected eye 4 times daily.

Storage/Stability: Store at 15° to 25°C (59° to 77°F).

Rx	**Alamast** (Johnson & Johnson Vision Care)	**Solution:** 0.1%	In 10 mL bottles with a controlled dropper tip.[1]

[1] With lauralkonium chloride 0.005%, glycerin, dibasic sodium phosphate, monobasic sodium phosphate, phosphoric acid, or sodium hydroxide.

OPHTHALMIC DECONGESTANT/ANTIHISTAMINE COMBINATIONS

In these combinations:

Naphazoline hydrochloride has decongestant actions. See individual monograph for further information.

Hydroxypropyl methylcellulose and **polyvinyl alcohol** increase the viscosity of the solution, thereby increasing contact time.

Pheniramine maleate and **antazoline** are antihistamines.

Indications:

Itching/Redness: Temporary relief of the minor eye symptoms of itching and redness caused by pollen, animal hair, etc.

Warnings:

Antihistamines: Topical antihistamines are potential sensitizers and may produce a local sensitivity reaction. Because they may produce angle closure, use with caution in people with a narrow angle or a history of glaucoma.

Administration and Dosage:

Recommendations vary. Refer to manufacturer package insert for instructions.

		Decongestant	Antihistamine	
otc	**Naphcon-A Solution** (Alcon)	naphazoline hydrochloride 0.025%	pheniramine maleate 0.3%	In 15 mL *Drop-Tainers.*[1]
otc	**Opcon-A Solution** (Bausch & Lomb)	naphazoline hydrochloride 0.027%	pheniramine maleate 0.315%	In 15 mL.[2]
otc	**Vasocon-A Solution** (Novartis)	naphazoline hydrochloride 0.05%	antazoline phosphate 0.5%	In 15 mL.[3]
otc	**Visine•A** (Visine)	naphazoline hydrochloride 0.025%	pheniramine maleate 0.3%	In 15 mL.[4]

[1] With benzalkonium chloride 0.01%, EDTA 0.01%.
[2] With hydroxypropyl methylcellulose 0.5%, benzalkonium chloride 0.01%, 0.1% EDTA, boric acid.
[3] With benzalkonium chloride 0.01%, PEG-8000, polyvinyl alcohol, EDTA.
[4] With benzalkonium chloride 0.01%, EDTA 0.1%, boric acid, sodium borate.

ANTI-INFLAMMATORY AGENTS

CORTICOSTEROIDS

Since their introduction into ocular therapy, corticosteroids have been useful in the control of inflammatory and immunologic diseases of the eye. The anti-inflammatory effects of corticosteroids are nonspecific, and they inhibit inflammation to a variety of inciting agents of mechanical, chemical, or immunologic nature. Due to their broad spectrum of activity, they are used extensively in pre- and postocular surgery.

In general, corticosteroids appear to be more effective in acute rather than chronic conditions. Degenerative diseases are usually completely refractory to corticosteroid therapy. Corticosteroids are generally not considered appropriate therapy for mild ocular allergies because other modalities can be effective (see the Antiallergy and Decongestant Agents chapter).

The beneficial effects of these agents on inflammation are numerous and include the following:

- Reduction in capillary permeability and cellular exudation;
- Inhibition of degranulation of mast cells, basophils, and neutrophils. Stabilization of intracellular membranes of these cells inhibits release of hydrolytic enzyme and other mediators of inflammation such as histamines, bradykinins, and platelet-activating factor;
- Suppression of lymphocyte proliferation;
- Inhibition of phospholipase A synthesis, resulting in decreased synthesis of prostaglandins and leukotrienes; and
- Inhibition of cell-mediated immune responses.

Clinical use and experimental data indicate that corticosteroids differ in their ability to suppress inflammation. This has been attributed, in part, to differences in their ability to penetrate the corneal epithelium. Acetate and alcohol formulations are sparingly soluble in water and are formulated for topical ocular use as suspensions. Phosphate derivatives are highly soluble in aqueous media and are formulated as solutions. The suspension formulations of acetate and alcohol derivatives exhibit biphasic solubility and can therefore better penetrate the lipid-rich layers of the cornea. It has also been suggested that corticosteroid particles in suspension persist in the cul-de-sac for longer periods of time and thus contact of the drug with the ocular surface is prolonged. For topical ocular use, prednisolone (eg, *AK-Pred*), fluorometholone (eg, *FML Liquifilm*, *Flarex*), and dexamethasone (eg, *Decadron Phosphate*) can be effective in inflammations involving the lids, conjunctiva, cornea, iris, and ciliary body. In severe forms of anterior uveitis, topical therapy may require supplementation with periocular injection or systemic corticosteroids.

Chorioretinitis and optic neuritis are usually treated with systemic or periocular administration, or both. Medrysone (*HMS*), which appears to exhibit limited corneal penetration, is recommended for minor reactions involving the lids and conjunctiva. Its efficacy has not been demonstrated in iritis or uveitis.

More recently, a group of compounds with similar anti-inflammatory activity but less propensity to raise intraocular pressure has been synthesized. The first to become available are loteprednol etabonate and rimexolone (*Vexol*). Rimexolone is presently indicated for treatment of anterior uveitis and for postoperative inflammation following cataract surgery. Loteprednol etabonate is a product of the so-called "soft drug" design developed by Bodor to enhance drug efficacy and minimize adverse effects. Although loteprednol is structurally similar to prednisolone, the ketone group at position 20 is absent. This modification in the molecule allows for the synthetic production of a therapeutically active, but metabolically unstable, compound that is rapidly inactivated following administration.

Loteprednol etabonate has shown clinical efficacy for various inflammatory conditions affecting the eye, including giant papillary conjunctivitis, postoperative inflammation, and seasonal allergic conjunctivitis. The relatively low incidence, transient nature, and reversibility of ocular pressure increase reported thus far with loteprednol and rimexolone indicate that they can provide an additional treatment choice for ocular inflammatory condition. Loteprednol 0.5% (*Lotemax*) has also shown clinical efficacy in various anterior segment inflammations, including giant papillary conjunctivitis. Loteprednol 0.2% (*Alrex*) has been approved for seasonal allergic conjunctivitis.

Corticosteroids also have been formulated with antibiotics. Both prednisolone and dexamethasone have been combined with aminoglycoside antibiotics. A recent addition to these combination formulations is *Zylet* (by Bausch and Lomb) which incorporates the soft steroid loteprednol etabonate 0.5% with tobramycin 0.3%.

The use of corticosteroids in ocular disease remains largely empirical, but some general guidelines include the following:

- Type and location of inflammation determine which route of administration is appropriate;
- Dosage is largely determined by clinical experience and should be reevaluated at frequent intervals during therapy;
- Therapy should be reduced gradually, not discontinued abruptly;
- The minimal effective dose should be used for the shortest time necessary;
- Individualize dosage; and
- Maintain close supervision to assess the effects of therapy on the disease course and possible adverse effects to the patient.

Patient compliance with the drug regimen is important in resolution of the inflammation. Patients should not discontinue use of medication at their own discretion. If suspensions are employed, the patient must shake the bottle sufficiently to maintain the proper concentration of drug.

Adverse effects can occur with all routes of administration and all preparations currently in use. Incidence of adverse effects appears to rise significantly as dosages are increased. Short-term topical ocular therapy usually does not produce significant side effects. Prolonged topical therapy can cause ocular hypertension and glaucoma. Pressure elevation rarely occurs within the first 2 weeks of therapy unless the patient is a "steroid responder." Such patients can experience an increase in IOP within hours after initiation of therapy. Withdrawal of the steroid usually results in baseline IOP readings within 2 to 4 weeks.

NONSTEROIDAL ANTI-INFLAMMATORY AGENTS

Nonsteroidal anti-inflammatory drugs (NSAIDs), also referred to as the "aspirin-like" drugs, include the salicylates, as well as indole, pyrazolone and propionic acid derivatives, and the fenamates. Following oral administration, these agents relieve discomfort associated with rheumatoid arthritis and lupus erythematosus, and reduce fever and alleviate pain that accompanies injury or inflammation.

The mechanism of action of the NSAIDs involves inhibition of cyclo-oxygenase, an enzyme important in synthesis of prostaglandins from their precursor, arachidonic acid. NSAIDs do not inhibit phospholipase A or the lipoxygenase enzyme, which generate the leukotrienes and related compounds that are also involved in the inflammatory response.

Prostaglandins are 20-carbon, unsaturated fatty acid derivatives that are subdivided into groups, designated by letters such as D, E, and F. Evidence indicates that they also act as mediators of inflammation in ocular structures. Prostaglandins can cause vasodilation of ocular blood vessels, disrupt the blood-aqueous barrier, and induce neovascularization and miosis. Some of the prostaglandins such as $PGF_{2\alpha}$ and PGD_2 can lower intraocular pressure whereas others (eg, PGF_2) can raise it.

The topical ocular use of NSAIDs includes maintenance of pupillary dilation during surgery and control of inflammation, photophobia, and pain after cataract extraction and following argon laser trabeculoplasty and photorefractive procedures. Also, reactions associated with nonsurgically induced inflammatory disorders of the eye, such as allergic conjunctivitis and cystoid macular edema, respond to topical ocular application. Currently available nonsteroidal ophthalmic anti-inflammatory drugs include flurbiprofen (eg, *Ocufen*), suprofen (*Profenal*), diclofenac (eg, *Voltaren*), and ketorolac (*Acular*), and the recently approved bromfenac (*Xibrom*), and nepafenac (*Nevanac*). Both are approved for twice daily use.

IMMUNOMODULATORS

Immunosuppressive agents have proven effective in various ocular inflammatory conditions resistant to steroids, or when chronic use of steroids is associated with complications. Currently available agents act as cytotoxic agents to block lymphocyte proliferation or as immunomodulators to block synthesis of lymphokines.

Of the immunomodulators, systemic and various topical formulations of cyclosporine A have been used to treat severe ocular immune-mediated diseases, such as uveitis, chronic vernal keratoconjunctivitis, keratoconjunctivitis sicca, and ocular symptoms of Behcet syndrome. Research studies indicate that topical cyclosporine A reduces cell-mediated inflammatory responses of ocular surface disease by preventing activation of T-lymphocytes.

The availability of cyclosporine A as a topical ophthalmic formulation (*Restasis*) for dry eye associated with keratoconjunctivitis sicca has focused on its role in chronic dry eye disease (CDED). Topical use in patients with moderate to severe dry eye can improve both objective (corneal staining and Schirmer values) and subjective measures (blurred vision, concomitant use of artificial tears, improved patient satisfaction) in both Sjögren and non-Sjögren associated dry eye disease. An increase in goblet cell numbers and a decrease in number of activated lymphocytes within the conjunctiva also have been observed.

The most common ocular side effect during clinical trials with *Restasis* was burning, reported by about 17%. Other less frequently reported events include conjunctival hyperemia, blurring, pruritus, and foreign body sensation.

Restasis is commercially available as a 0.05% ophthalmic emulsion. The recommended dosage is 2 times/day, approximately 12 hours apart. It can be used concomitantly with artificial tears, with a 15 minute interval between instillations.

For More Information

Bartlett JD, Jaanus SD, eds. *Clinical Ocular Pharmacology*. 5th ed. St. Louis, MO: Elsevier; 2008.

Dell SJ, Lowry GM, Northcutt JA, et al. A randomized, double-marked, placebo-controlled parallel study of 0.2% loteprednol etabonate in patients with seasonal allergic conjunctivitis. *J Allergy Clin Immunol*. 1998;102:241-255.

Foster CS, et al. Efficacy and safety of rimexolone 1% ophthalmic suspension vs 1% prednisolone acetate in the treatment of uveitis. *Am J Ophthalmol*. 1996;122:171-182.

Friedlander MH, Howes J. A double-masked, placebo-controlled evaluation of the efficacy and safety of loteprednol etabonate in the treatment of giant papillary conjunctivitis. *Am J Ophthalmol*. 1997;123:455.

Kunert KS, Tisdale AS, Gipson IK. Goblet cell numbers and epithelial proliferation in the conjunctiva of patients with dry eye syndrome treated with cyclosporin. *Arch Opthalmol.* 2002;120:330-337.

The Loteprednol Etabonate Postoperative Study Group 2. A double-masked, placebo-controlled evaluation of 0.5% Loteprednol etabonate in the treatment of postoperative inflammation. *Ophthalmology.* 1998;105:1780-1786.

Schalnus R. Topical nonsteroidal anti-inflammatory therapy in ophthalmology. *Ophthalmologica.* 2003;217:89-98.

Sheppard JD. Dry eye moves beyond palliative therapy. *Manag Care.* 2003;12:6-8.

Tripathi RC, Parapuram SK, Tripathi BJ, et al. Corticosteroids and glaucoma risks. *Drugs Aging.* 1999;15:439-450.

Urban RC, Cotlier E. Corticosteroid-induced cataracts. *Surv Ophthalmol.* 1986;31:102.

TOPICAL CORTICOSTEROIDS

Actions:

Pharmacology: Topical corticosteroids exert an anti-inflammatory action. Aspects of the inflammatory process such as hyperemia, cellular infiltration, vascularization, and fibroblastic proliferation are suppressed. Steroids inhibit inflammatory response to inciting agents of mechanical, chemical, or immunological nature. Topical corticosteroids are effective in acute inflammatory conditions of conjunctiva, sclera, cornea, lids, iris, ciliary body, and anterior segment of the globe; and in ocular allergic conditions. They inhibit edema and capillary dilation. In ocular disease, route depends on site and extent of disorder.

The mechanism of the anti-inflammatory action is thought to be potentiation of epinephrine vasoconstriction, stabilization of lysosomal membranes, retardation of macrophage movement, prevention of kinin release, inhibition of lymphocyte and neutrophil function, inhibition of prostaglandin synthesis, and, in prolonged use, decrease of antibody production.

Inhibiting fibroblastic proliferation may prevent symblepharon formation in chemical and thermal burns. Decreased scarring with clearer corneas after topical corticosteroids is a result of inhibiting fibroblast proliferation and vascularization.

Indications:

Inflammatory conditions: Treatment of steroid-responsive inflammatory conditions of the palpebral and bulbar conjunctiva, lid, cornea, and anterior segment of the globe, such as the following: allergic conjunctivitis; nonspecific superficial keratitis; superficial punctate keratitis; herpes zoster keratitis; iritis; cyclitis; and selected infective conjunctivitis when the inherent hazard of steroid use is accepted to obtain a diminution in edema and inflammation. Rimexolone is also indicated for postoperative inflammation following ocular surgery.

Corneal injury: Also used for corneal injury from chemical, radiation, or thermal burns or penetration of foreign bodies.

Graft rejection: May be used to suppress graft rejection after keratoplasty.

Anterior uveitis.

Contraindications:

Acute superficial herpes simplex keratitis; fungal diseases of ocular structures; vaccinia, varicella, and most other viral diseases of the cornea and conjunctiva; mycobacterial infection of the eye (eg, ocular tuberculosis); diseases caused by microorganisms; hypersensitivity, or following uncomplicated removal of a superficial corneal foreign body.

Medrysone: Not for use in iritis and uveitis; its efficacy has not been demonstrated.

Warnings:

Moderate to severe inflammation: Use higher strengths for moderate to severe inflammations. In difficult cases of anterior segment eye disease, systemic therapy may be required. When deeper ocular structures are involved, use systemic therapy.

Ocular damage: Prolonged use may result in glaucoma, elevated IOP, optic nerve damage, defects in visual acuity and fields of vision, posterior subcapsular cataract formation, or secondary ocular infections from pathogens liberated from ocular tissues. Check IOP and lens frequently. In diseases causing thinning of cornea or sclera, perforation has occurred with topical steroids.

Mustard gas keratitis or Sjögren keratoconjunctivitis: Topical steroids not effective.

Infections: Acute, purulent, untreated eye infection may be masked or activity enhanced by steroids. Fungal infections of the cornea have occurred with long-term local steroid applications. Therefore, suspect fungal invasion in any persistent corneal ulceration where a steroid has been, or is being used.

Stromal herpes simplex keratitis treatment with steroid medication requires great caution; frequent slit-lamp microscopy is mandatory.

Pregnancy: Category C. Use only when clearly needed and when potential benefits to the mother outweigh potential hazards to the fetus.

Lactation: It is not known whether topical steroids are excreted in breast milk. Exercise caution when administering to a nursing mother.

Children: Safety and efficacy have not been established in children.

Precautions:

Sulfite sensitivity: Some of these products contain sulfites that may cause allergic-type reactions (eg, hives, itching, wheezing, anaphylaxis) in certain susceptible people. Although the overall prevalence of sulfite sensitivity in the general population is low, it is seen more frequently in asthmatics or in atopic nonasthmatic people. Specific products containing sulfites are identified in the product listings.

Adverse Reactions:

Glaucoma (elevated IOP) with optic nerve damage, loss of visual acuity, and field defects; posterior subcapsular cataract formation; secondary ocular infection from pathogens, including herpes simplex liberated from ocular tissues; perforation of globe; exacerbation of viral and fungal corneal infections; transient stinging or burning; blurred vision; discharge; discomfort; ocular pain; foreign body sensation; hyperemia; pruritus (rimexolone). Rarely, filtering blebs have occurred with steroid use after cataract surgery.

Other ocular adverse reactions occurring in less than 1% of patients included sticky sensation; increased fibrin; dry eye; conjunctival edema; corneal staining; keratitis; tearing; photophobia; edema; irritation; corneal ulcer; browache; lid margin crusting; corneal edema; infiltrate; corneal erosion.

Miscellaneous: Headache; aggravation or worsening of hypertension; rhinitis; pharyngitis; taste perversion.

Systemic: Systemic side effects may occur with extensive use.

Patient Information:

Medical supervision during therapy is recommended.

To avoid contamination, do not touch applicator tip to any surface. Replace cap after use.

If improvement of the condition being treated does not occur within several days, or if pain, itching, or swelling of the eye occurs, notify the physician. Do not discontinue use without consulting physician. Take care not to discontinue prematurely.

Refer to the Dosage Forms and Routes of Administration chapter for more complete information on administration and use.

Administration and Dosage:

Treatment duration varies with type of lesion and may extend from a few days to several weeks, depending on therapeutic response. Relapse may occur if therapy is reduced too rapidly; taper over several days. Relapses, more common in chronic active lesions than in self-limited conditions, usually respond to retreatment.

Suspensions and solutions: Refer to specific product labeling, because dosage depends on product and indication. Suspension must be vigorously shaken (5X) before instillation or the active ingredient will remain on the bottom of the bottle.

Generally, instill 1 or 2 drops into the conjunctival sac every hour during the day and every 2 hours during the night. When a favorable response is observed, reduce dosage to 1 drop every 4 hours. Later, 1 drop 3 or 4 times daily may suffice to control symptoms. Shake suspension well before use. For postoperative inflammation, instill 1 to 2 drops 4 times daily beginning 24 hours after surgery; continue throughout the first 2 weeks of the postoperative period.

Ointments: Apply a thin coating (approximately 0.5 to 1 inch) in the lower conjunctival sac 3 or 4 times a day. When a favorable response is observed, reduce the number of daily applications to 2, and, later, to 1 as a maintenance dose if sufficient to control symptoms.

Ointments are particularly convenient when an eye pad is used and may be the preparation of choice when prolonged contact of drug with ocular tissues is needed.

For product information on Steroid/Antibiotic Combinations, see the Anti-infective Agents chapter.

Individual drug monographs are on the following pages.

DEXAMETHASONE

Complete prescribing information is found in the Corticosteroids group monograph.

Administration and Dosage:

Storage: Store upright at 8° to 27°C (46° to 80°F).

Rx	**Dexamethasone Sodium Phosphate** (Various, eg, Bausch & Lomb, Falcon, Schein)	**Solution:** dexamethasone phosphate (as sodium phosphate) 0.1%	In 5 mL.
Rx	**AK-Dex** (Various, eg, Akorn)		In 5 mL.[1]
Rx	**Maxidex** (Alcon)	**Suspension:** dexamethasone 0.1%	In 5 and 15 mL *Drop-Tainers.*[2]

[1] With benzalkonium chloride 0.01%, EDTA, hydroxyethylcellulose.
[2] With benzalkonium chloride 0.01%, EDTA, hydroxypropyl methylcellulose 0.5%, polysorbate 80.

FLUOROMETHOLONE

Complete prescribing information is found in the Corticosteroids group monograph.

Administration and Dosage:

Storage: Store at or below 25°C (77°F); protect from freezing.

Rx	**FML** (Allergan)	**Suspension:** fluorometholone alcohol 0.1%	In 1, 5, 10, and 15 mL.[1]
Rx	**Flarex** (Alcon)	**Suspension:** fluorometholone acetate 0.1%	In 5 mL *Drop-Tainers.*[2]
Rx	**eFLone** (Novartis)		In 5 and 10 mL.[2]
Rx	**FML Forte** (Various, eg, Allergan)	**Suspension:** fluorometholone alcohol 0.25%	In 5, 10, and 15 mL.[3]
Rx	**FML S.O.P.** (Various, eg, Allergan)	**Ointment:** 0.1%	In 3.5 g.[4]

[1] With benzalkonium chloride 0.004%, EDTA, polysorbate 80, polyvinyl alcohol 1.4%.
[2] With benzalkonium chloride 0.01%, EDTA, hydroxyethylcellulose, tyloxapol.
[3] With benzalkonium chloride 0.005%, EDTA, polysorbate 80, polyvinyl alcohol 1.4%.
[4] With phenylmercuric acetate 0.0008%, white petrolatum, mineral oil, petrolatum, lanolin alcohol.

LOTEPREDNOL ETABONATE

Complete prescribing information is found in the Corticosteroids group monograph.

Administration and Dosage:

Storage: Store upright at 15° to 25°C (59° to 77°F); do not freeze.

Rx	**Alrex** (Bausch & Lomb)	**Suspension:** loteprednol etabonate 0.2%	In 5 and 10 mL.
Rx	**Lotemax** (Bausch & Lomb)	**Suspension:** loteprednol etabonate 0.5%	In 2.5, 5, 10, and 15 mL.[1]

[1] With EDTA, glycerin, povidone, tyloxapol.

PREDNISOLONE

Complete prescribing information is found in the Corticosteroids group monograph.

Administration and Dosage:

Storage: Protect from freezing.

Rx	**Pred Mild** (Allergan)	**Suspension:** prednisolone acetate 0.12%	In 5 and 10 mL.[1]
Rx	**Econopred Plus** (Alcon)	**Suspension:** prednisolone acetate 1%	In 5 and 10 mL *Drop-Tainers.*[2]
Rx	**Pred Forte** (Allergan)		In 1, 5, 10, and 15 mL.[1]
Rx	**Prednisolone Acetate Ophthalmic** (Falcon)		In 5 and 10 mL.[2]
Rx	**Prednisolone Sodium Phosphate** (Various, eg, Bausch & Lomb)	**Solution:** prednisolone sodium phosphate 1%	In 5, 10, and 15 mL.

[1] With benzalkonium chloride, EDTA, polysorbate 80, hydroxypropyl methylcellulose, sodium bisulfite.
[2] With benzalkonium chloride 0.01%, EDTA, polysorbate 80, hydroxypropyl methylcellulose, glycerin.

RIMEXOLONE

Complete prescribing information is found in the Corticosteroids group monograph.

Administration and Dosage:

Storage: Store upright between 4° and 30°C (40° and 86°F).

Rx	**Vexol** (Alcon)	**Suspension:** 1%	In 5 and 10 mL *Drop-Tainers.*[1]

[1] With benzalkonium chloride 0.01%, polysorbate 80, EDTA in carbopol gel.

NONSTEROIDAL ANTI-INFLAMMATORY AGENTS (NSAIDS)

Actions:

Pharmacology: Bromfenac, diclofenac, flurbiprofen, ketorolac, nepafenac, and suprofen are NSAIDs available as ophthalmic solutions. Flurbiprofen and suprofen are phenylalkanoic acids, diclofenac is a phenylacetic acid, and ketorolac tromethamine is a member of the pyrrolo-pyrolle group; they have analgesic, antipyretic, and anti inflammatory activity. Bromfenac is an NSAID that has anti-inflammatory activity. Nepafenac is a nonsteroidal anti-inflammatory and analgesic prodrug. After topical ocular dosing, nepafenac penetrates the cornea and is converted by ocular tissue hydrolases to amfenac, an NSAID. Their mechanism of action is believed to be through inhibition of the cyclo-oxygenase enzyme that is essential in the biosynthesis of prostaglandins.

In animals, certain prostaglandins are mediators of intraocular inflammation. Prostaglandins produce disruption of the blood-aqueous humor barrier, vasodilation, increased vascular permeability, leukocytosis, and increased intraocular pressure (IOP).

Prostaglandins also appear to play a role in the miotic response produced during ocular surgery by constricting the iris sphincter independently of cholinergic mechanisms. NSAIDs inhibit the miosis induced during the course of cataract surgery.

Nonsteroidal Anti-Inflammatory Ophthalmic Agents

Ophthalmic NSAID	Trade name (manufacturer)	Solution concentration	Ophthalmic indication
Bromfenac	*Xibrom* (Bausch & Lomb)	0.09%	Treatment of postoperative inflammation and the reduction of ocular pain in patients who have undergone cataract extraction.
Diclofenac	*Voltaren* (Ciba Vision)	0.1%	Treatment of postoperative inflammation in patients who have undergone cataract extraction and for the temporary relief of pain and photophobia in patients undergoing corneal refractive surgery.
Flurbiprofen	*Ocufen* (Allergan)	0.03%	Inhibition of intraoperative miosis.
Ketorolac	*Acular LS* (Allergan)	0.4%	Reduction of ocular pain and burning/stinging following corneal refractive surgery.
	Acular (Allergan)	0.5%	Temporary relief of ocular itching caused by seasonal allergic conjunctivitis; treatment of postoperative inflammation in patients who have undergone cataract extraction.
Nepafenac	*Nevanac* (Alcon)	0.1%	Treatment of pain and inflammation associated with cataract surgery.
Suprofen	*Profenal* (Alcon)	1%	Inhibition of intraoperative miosis.

Indications:

Bromfenac: Treatment of postoperative inflammation and the reduction of ocular pain in patients who have undergone cataract extraction.

Diclofenac: Treatment of postoperative inflammation in patients who have undergone cataract extraction and for the temporary relief of pain and photophobia in patients undergoing corneal refractive surgery.

Flurbiprofen, suprofen: Inhibition of intraoperative miosis.

Ketorolac: Temporary relief of ocular itching caused by seasonal allergic conjunctivitis; treatment of postoperative inflammation in patients who have undergone cataract extraction; reduction of ocular pain and burning/stinging following corneal refractive surgery.

Nepafenac: Treatment of pain and inflammation associated with cataract surgery.

Off-label use(s):

Diclofenac – Anti-inflammatory treatment following argon laser trabeculoplasty, treatment of seasonal allergic conjunctivitis, pain associated with radial keratotomy, and photorefractive keratectomy.

Flurbiprofen – Inflammation after cataract or glaucoma laser surgery and uveitis syndromes.

Ketorolac – Treatment of pain associated with corneal trauma; topical treatment of cystoid macular edema.

Suprofen – Topical treatment of contact lens-associated GPC.

Contraindications:

Hypersensitivity to the drugs or any component of the products.

Suprofen: Epithelial herpes simplex keratitis (dendritic keratitis).

Diclofenac, ketorolac: Patients wearing soft contact lenses (see Precautions).

Warnings:

Cross-sensitivity: The potential for cross-sensitivity to acetylsalicylic acid, phenylacetic acid derivatives, and other NSAIDs exists. Therefore, use caution when treating individuals who have previously exhibited sensitivities to these drugs.

Bleeding tendencies: Systemic absorption occurs with drugs applied ocularly. With some NSAIDs, there exists the potential for increased bleeding time due to interference with thrombocyte aggregation. There have been reports that ocularly applied NSAIDs may cause increased bleeding of ocular tissues (including hyphemas) in conjunction with ocular surgery. Use with caution in surgical patients with known bleeding tendencies or in patients taking drugs known to cause bleeding (eg, anticoagulants).

Sulfite sensitivity: Bromfenac contains sodium sulfite, a sulfite that may cause allergic-type reactions, including anaphylactic symptoms and life-threatening or less severe asthmatic episodes, in certain susceptible people. The overall prevalence of sulfite sensitivity in the general population is unknown and probably low. Sulfite sensitivity is seen more frequently in asthmatic than in nonasthmatic people

Pregnancy: Category C (bromfenac, flurbiprofen, ketorolac, nepafenac, suprofen); *Category B* (diclofenac). Flurbiprofen is embryocidal, delays parturition, prolongs gestation, reduces weight, and slightly retards fetal growth in rats at daily oral doses of at least 0.4 mg/kg (approximately 185 times the human daily topical dose).

Oral doses of ketorolac at 1.5 mg/kg (8.8 mg/m^2), which is half of the human oral exposure, administered after gestation day 17 caused dystocia and higher pup mortality in rats. Because of the known effects of prostaglandin-inhibiting drugs on the fetal cardiovascular system, avoid the use of ketorolac during late pregnancy.

Oral doses of suprofen of up to 200 mg/kg/day in animals resulted in an increased incidence of fetal resorption associated with maternal toxicity. There was an increase in stillbirths and a decrease in postnatal survival in pregnant rats treated with at least 2.5 mg/kg/day.

Oral diclofenac in mice and rats crosses the placental barrier. In rats, maternally toxic doses were associated with dystocia, prolonged gestation, and reduced fetal weights, growth, and survival. Because of the known effects of prostaglandin-inhibiting drugs on the fetal cardiovascular system, avoid the use of ophthalmic diclofenac during late pregnancy.

In rats, maternally toxic doses of nepafenac greater than or equal to 10 mg/kg were associated with dystocia, increased postimplantation loss, reduced fetal weights and growth, and reduced fetal survival. Nepafenac has been shown to cross the placental barrier in rats.

Doses of bromfenac 0.9 mg/kg/day in rats caused embryo-fetal lethality, increased neonatal mortality, and reduced postnatal growth. Pregnant rabbits treated with 7.5 mg/kg/day caused increased postimplantation loss.

There are no adequate and well-controlled studies in pregnant women. Use during pregnancy only if the potential benefits to the mother outweigh the potential hazards to the fetus.

Lactation: It is not known whether flurbiprofen or nepafenac is excreted in breast milk. Because of the potential for serious adverse reactions in nursing infants, decide whether to discontinue nursing or to discontinue the drug, taking into account the importance of the drug to the mother.

Suprofen is excreted in breast milk after a single oral dose. Based on measurements of plasma and milk levels in women taking oral suprofen, the milk concentration is approximately 1% of the plasma level. Because systemic absorption may occur from topical ocular administration, consider discontinuing nursing while on suprofen; its safety in human neonates has not been established.

Exercise caution while bromfenac or ketorolac is administered to a nursing woman.

Children: Safety and efficacy for use in children have not been established.

Precautions:

Contact lenses: Patients wearing hydrogel soft contact lenses who have used diclofenac concurrently have experienced ocular irritation manifested by redness and burning.

Ketorolac – Do not administer while patient is wearing contact lenses.

Ocular effects: Use of topical NSAIDs may result in keratitis. In some susceptible patients, continued use of topical NSAIDs may result in epithelial breakdown, corneal thinning, corneal erosion, corneal ulceration, or corneal perforation. These events may be sight threatening. Immediately discontinue use of topical NSAIDs in patients with evidence of corneal epithelial breakdown, and closely monitor them for corneal health.

Renal effects: Use of oral suprofen has been associated with a syndrome of acute flank pain and generally reversible renal insufficiency, which may present as acute uric acid nephropathy. This syndrome occurs in approximately 1 in 3,500 patients and has been reported with as few as 1 to 2 doses of a 200 mg capsule.

Wound healing: Wound healing may be delayed with the use of flurbiprofen and diclofenac.

Drug Interactions:

Acetylcholine chloride and carbachol: Although clinical and animal studies revealed no interference, and there is no known pharmacological basis for an interaction, both of these drugs have reportedly been ineffective when used in patients treated with flurbiprofen or suprofen.

Adverse Reactions:

Sterile infiltrates are increasingly seen when NSAIDS are used in incisional photorefractive surgery without concomitant low dose steroids. The epithelial defect appears to predispose to this adverse effect.

Most frequent: Transient burning and stinging upon instillation (diclofenac 15%, ketorolac approximately 40%); other minor symptoms of ocular irritation.

Diclofenac: Keratitis (28%, although most cases occurred in cataract studies prior to drug therapy); elevated IOP (15%, although most cases occurred postsurgery and prior to drug therapy); dry eye complaints (12% in patients undergoing incisional refractive surgery); discharge; corneal deposits; corneal lesions; itching; irritation; blurred vision; fever; pain; insomnia. The following reactions occurred in 1% or less: Corneal edema; corneal opacity; eyelid disorder; iritis; injection and lacrimation disorder; asthenia; chills; facial edema; vomiting; viral infection; anterior chamber reaction; ocular allergy; nausea.

Ketorolac: Ocular irritation, allergic reactions; superficial keratitis; superficial ocular infections. The following adverse reactions occurred rarely: eye dryness; corneal infiltrates; corneal ulcer; visual disturbance (blurred vision).

Suprofen: Discomfort; itching; redness; allergy, iritis, pain, chemosis, photophobia, irritation, punctate epithelial staining (less than 0.5%).

Overdosage:

Overdosage will not ordinarily cause acute problems. If accidentally ingested, drink fluids to dilute.

Individual drug monographs are on the following pages.

BROMFENAC

Complete prescribing information is found in the NSAIDs group monograph.

Administration and Dosage:

Instill 1 drop to the affected eye(s) 2 times daily beginning 24 hours after cataract surgery and continuing through the first 2 weeks of the postoperative period.

Storage: Store at 15° to 25°C (59° to 77°F).

Rx	**Xibrom** (Bausch & Lomb)	**Solution**: 0.09%	In 5 mL dropper bottles.[1]

[1] With benzalkonium chloride 0.05 mg/mL, EDTA 0.2 mg/mL, povidone 20 mg/mL, and sodium hydroxide.

DICLOFENAC SODIUM

Complete prescribing information is found in the NSAIDs group monograph.

Administration and Dosage:

Cataract surgery: Instill 1 drop in the affected eye 4 times daily, beginning 24 hours after cataract surgery and continuing throughout the first 2 weeks of the postoperative period.

Incisional refractive surgery: Within 1 hour prior to incisional refractive surgery, instill 1 drop to the operative eye(s). Instill a second drop within 15 minutes after surgery. Instill 1 drop to the operative eye(s) 4 times daily beginning 4 to 6 hours after surgery and continuing for up to 3 days as needed.

Storage: Store at 15° to 30°C (59° to 86°F). Protect from light.

Rx	**Voltaren** (Novartis)	**Solution**: 0.1%	In 2.5 and 5 mL dropper bottles.[1]

[1] With EDTA 1 mg/mL, boric acid, polyoxyl 35 castor oil, sorbic acid 2 mg/mL, tromethamine.

FLURBIPROFEN SODIUM

Complete prescribing information is found in the NSAIDs group monograph.

Administration and Dosage:

Instill 1 drop approximately every 30 minutes, beginning 2 hours before surgery (total of 4 drops).

Storage: Store at room temperature.

Rx	**Ocufen** (Allergan)	**Solution**: 0.03%	In 2.5 mL dropper bottles.[1]
Rx	**Flurbiprofen Sodium Ophthalmic** (Various, eg, Bausch & Lomb)		In 2.5 mL.[1]

[1] With polyvinyl alcohol 1.4%, thimerosal 0.005%, EDTA.

KETOROLAC TROMETHAMINE

Complete prescribing information is found in the NSAIDs group monograph.

Administration and Dosage:

Relief of ocular itching: Instill 1 drop (0.25 mg) 4 times a day.

Postoperative inflammation: Instill 1 drop (0.25 mg) in the affected eye(s) 4 times daily beginning 24 hours after cataract surgery and continuing through the first 2 weeks of the postoperative period.

Postcorneal refractive surgery: One drop 4 times/day in the affected eye as needed for pain and burning/stinging for up to 4 days following corneal refractive surgery.

Storage: Store at controlled room temperature 15° to 30°C (59° to 86°F). Protect from light.

Rx	**Acular LS** (Allergan)	**Solution:** 0.4%	In 5 mL bottle w/dropper.[1]
Rx	**Acular** (Allergan)	**Solution:** 0.5%	In 5 mL dropper bottles.[2]
Rx	**Acular PF** (Allergan)		In 12 single-use 0.4 mL vials.[3]

[1] With benzalkonium chloride 0.006%, EDTA 0.015%, octoxynol 40.
[2] With benzalkonium chloride 0.01%, EDTA 0.1%, octoxynol 40.
[3] With ketorolac tromethamine 0.5%.

NEPAFENAC

Complete prescribing information is found in the NSAIDs group monograph.

Administration and Dosage:

Shake well before use. Apply 1 drop to the affected eye(s) 3 times daily beginning 1 day prior to cataract surgery; continue on the day of surgery, and through the first 2 weeks of the postoperative period.

Nepafenac may be administered in conjunction with other topical ophthalmic medications such as beta-blockers, carbonic anhydrase inhibitors, alpha-agonists, cycloplegics, and mydriatics.

Storage: Store at 2° to 25°C (36° to 77°F).

Rx	**Nevanac** (Alcon)	**Solution:** 0.1%	In 3 mL.

SUPROFEN

Complete prescribing information is found in the NSAIDs group monograph.

Administration and Dosage:

On the day of surgery, instill 2 drops into the conjunctival sac at 3 hours, 2 hours and 1 hour prior to surgery. Two drops may be instilled into the conjunctival sac every 4 hours while awake the day preceding surgery.

Storage: Store at room temperature

Rx	**Profenal** (Alcon)	**Solution:** 1%	In In 2.5 mL *Drop-Tainers.*[1]

[1] With 0.005% thimerosal, 2% caffeine and EDTA.

IMMUNOMODULATORS

Actions:

Pharmacology: Cyclosporine is an immunosuppressive agent when administered systemically. In patients whose tear production is presumed to be suppressed because of ocular inflammation associated with keratoconjunctivitis sicca, cyclosporine emulsion is thought to act as a partial immunomodulator. The exact mechanism of action is not known.

Pharmacokinetics: Blood cyclosporin A concentrations were measured using a specific high pressure liquid chromatography-mass spectrometry assay. After topical administration twice daily in humans for up to 12 months, blood concentrations of cyclosporine, in all the samples collected, were below the quantitation limit of 0.1 ng/mL. There was no detectable drug accumulation in blood during 12 months of treatment with the emulsion.

Indications:

Tear production: Indicated to increase tear production in patients whose tear production is presumed to be suppressed because of ocular inflammation associated with keratoconjunctivitis sicca. Increased tear production was not seen in patients currently taking topical anti-inflammatory drugs or using punctal plugs.

Contraindications:

Active ocular infections; known or suspected hypersensitivity to any of the ingredients in the formulation.

Warnings:

Herpes keratitis: Has not been studies in patients with herpes keratitis.

Pregnancy: Category C. There are no adequate and well-controlled studies in pregnant women. Administer to a pregnant woman only if clearly needed.

Lactation: Cyclosporine is known to be excreted in human breast milk following systemic administration, but excretion in human milk after topical treatment has not been investigated. Although blood concentrations are undetectable after topical administration, exercise caution when administering to a nursing woman.

Children: Safety and efficacy have not been established in children below 16 years of age.

Precautions:

For ophthalmic use only.

Adverse Reactions:

The most common adverse event was ocular burning (17%). Other events reported in 1% to 5% of patients included conjunctival hyperemia, discharge, epiphora, eye pain, foreign body sensation, pruritus, stinging, and visual disturbance (most often blurring).

Patient Information:

The emulsion from one individual single-use vial is to be used immediately after opening for administration to one or both eyes, and the remaining contents should be discarded immediately after administration.

Do not allow the tip of the vial to touch the eye or any surface, as this may contaminate the emulsion.

Do not administer while wearing contact lenses. Patients with decreased tear production typically should not wear contact lenses. If contact lenses are worn, they should be removed prior to the administration of the emulsion. Lenses may be reinserted 15 minutes following administration.

Individual drug monographs are on the following pages.

CYCLOSPORINE

Complete prescribing information is found in the Immunomodulators group monograph.

Administration and Dosage:

Invert the unit dose vial a few times to obtain a uniform, white, opaque emulsion before using. Instill 1 drop twice daily in each eye approximately 12 hours apart. Can be used concomitantly with artificial tears, allowing a 15 minute interval between products. Discard vial immediately after use.

Storage: Store at 15° to 25°C (59° to 77°F). Keep out of reach of children.

Rx	**Restasis** (Allergan)	**Emulsion:** 0.05%	In 0.4 mL fill in a 0.9 mL single-use vial. In 32s.[1]

[1] With glycerin and polysorbate 80.

Artificial Tear Solutions and Ocular Lubricants

Availability of synthetic polymers suitable for ocular use has resulted in development of artificial tear solutions, ointments, and other formulations to help alleviate ocular discomfort and maintain integrity of the surface epithelium. Ideally, formulations for dry eyes should be compatible with and substitute for components of the tear film, including lipid, aqueous, and mucin layers. Some products, such as *Soothe*, claim to restore both the lipid and aqueous layer of the tear film.

SOLUTIONS

Lubricant preparations formulated as artificial tear solutions usually contain inorganic electrolytes, preservatives, and water-soluble polymeric systems. Sodium chloride (NaCl), potassium chloride (KCl), various other ions, and boric acid help maintain tonicity and pH of the formulations. Preservatives, including benzalkonium chloride, chlorobutanol, thimerosal, EDTA, methylparaben, and propylparaben, are included in multidose preparations to prevent bacterial contamination. Newer preservative systems, such as stabilized oxychloro complex (*Purite*) and sodium perborate, are effective preservatives that are very well-tolerated, break down to nontoxic components, and cause very little disruption of the ocular surface. Methylcellulose and its derivatives, polyvinyl alcohol (PVA), povidone (PVP), dextran, and propylene glycol can enhance viscosity and promote tear film stability. A more recent advance in artificial tear formulations is the introduction of preservative-free preparations. These formulations can prevent adverse ocular surface effects in patients who use artificial tears frequently or for prolonged periods of time.

In addition to polymers, lipids and vitamins also have been incorporated into ocular lubricants. Retinyl, the alcohol form of vitamin A, is available as a solution for topical use on the eye. The formulation *Viva-Drops* contains vitamin A, polysorbate 80, and EDTA. Definitive data on the benefits of vitamin-containing formulations in dry eye disorders are not available and large-scale, well-controlled masked studies are lacking regarding efficacy of vitamin A or its derivatives in patients with ocular surface disease. A topical cyclosporine 0.05% formulation is available as *Restasis*. It is a prescription product and is indicated in patients with moderate to severe dry eye.

Administer artificial tear solutions at dosage frequencies of 4 to 6 hours. However, depending on the severity of the clinical signs and symptoms, they may be used as often as hourly or only occasionally. It is highly recommended that the prescriber of the artificial tear product recommend a specific dosage schedule for the patient, particularly at the start of therapy.

OINTMENTS/GELS

Petrolatum, lanolin, and mineral oil ointments are the second most frequent approach for ocular lubrication. When placed on the eye, they dissolve at the temperature of the ocular tissue and disperse with the tear fluid. A major advantage is that ointments appear to be retained in the cul-de-sac longer than artificial tear solutions.

Ointments are usually applied directly to the inferior conjunctival sac as a 0.25- to 0.5-inch ribbon. An alternative method is to place the ointment on a cotton-tipped applicator and apply it to the lid margins and lashes. Blurring of vision and possible irritation are minimized with this method of instillation. Recently, manufacturers have begun to formulate preservative-free ointment preparations. These preparations are less toxic and less allergenic than those containing preservatives.

Ophthalmic lubricant ointments are generally preferred for bedtime use. Depending on the clinical signs and patient symptoms, they may also be used as often as necessary during the day. Because ointments may block access of solution to the ocular surface, solutions should be instilled prior to application.

Gels are often less "greasy," cause less blurry vision, and more amenable for patient use.

SOLID DEVICES

Another approach to relief of dry eye symptoms is use of a preservative-free, water-soluble, polymeric insert (*Lacrisert*). The cylindrical rod, which contains 5 mg hydroxypropylcellulose, is placed in the lower cul-de-sac. It then imbibes fluid and swells. As it dissolves, the polymer is released to the ocular surface for 12 to 24 hours.

The device can be beneficial in dry eye syndromes such as keratitis sicca. It is generally comfortable, but some disadvantages are associated with its use. Manual dexterity is required for placement in the cul-de-sac, and the cost to the patient is greater than use of solutions and ointments. A common patient complaint is blurred vision as the rod dissolves, causing the tear film to thicken. Adding fluid drops to the eye (eg, isotonic saline) following insertion of the pellet can reduce viscosity and minimize visual complaints. Because of low usage, the inserts may be difficult to obtain.

ANTIINFLAMMATORY THERAPY

A topical cyclosporine 0.05% formulation is available as *Restasis*. Recent studies have demonstrated that decreased tear production and secretion promote ocular surface inflammation. An increase in cytokines and proteases in the tear film, adhesion molecule expression, and T-cell infiltration of the conjunctiva contribute to the pathogenesis of dry eye disease. Ocular surface and lacrimal gland inflammation are believed to play a role in the pathogenesis of dry eye disease. Cyclosporine (*Restasis*) is the first anti-inflammatory medication approved for the treatment of dry eye or KCS.

$P2Y_2$ RECEPTOR AGONISTS

$P2Y_2$ receptors help to coordinate mucosal hydration and mucociliary clearance in the eyes, lungs, and sinuses. *Diquafosol* (INS365) is an ophthalmic preparation in development to stimulate the $P2Y_2$ on the ocular surface and eyelid to increase secretion of mucin, lipids, salt, and water. *Inspire* is currently awaiting approval from the FDA.

ORAL THERAPY

Pilocarpine hydrochloride (*Salagen*), an oral cholinergic agonist with muscarinic secretagogue effects has been used in the treatment of dry mouth secondary to radiation treatment for head and neck. The drug can decrease symptoms of dry mouth, eyes, skin, and nose. Secretive improvement in dry eye symptoms has been reported in the treatment of KCS in Sjogren Syndrome.

For More Information

Bartlett JD, Jaanus SD, eds. *Clinical Ocular Pharmacology*, 5th ed. St. Louis, MO: Elsevier; 2008.

Bernal DL, Ubels JL. Quantitative evaluation of the corneal epithelial barrier: Effect of artificial tears and preservatives. *Curr Eye Res.* 1991;10:645.

Fiscella RG, Jensen MK. Ophthalmic Disorders (28) in *Handbook of Nonprescription Drugs*, 15th ed. Washington DC: American Pharmacists Association; 2006.

Marquardt R. Therapy of the dry eye. In: Lemp MA, Marquardt R, eds. *The Dry Eye*. Berlin: Springer-Verlag, 1992.

Nelson JD, Friedlander M, Yeatts RP, et al. Oral pilocarpine for symptomatic relief of keratoconjunctivitis sicca in patients with Sjogren's Syndrome. The MGI PHARMA Sjogren's Syndrome Study Group.

Pflungfelder SC. Antiinflammatory therapy for dry eye. *Am J Ophthamol.* 2004;137:337-342.

Sterenson D, Tauber J, Reis BL. The Cyclosporin A Phase 2 Study Group: Efficacy and safety of cyclosporin A ophthalmic emulsion in the treatment of moderate-to-severe dry eye disease. *Ophthalmology.* 2000;107:967-974.

Tuberville AW, et al. Punctal occlusion in tear deficiency syndromes. *Ophthalmology.* 1982;89:1170.

Tabbara KF, Wagoner MD. Diagnosis and management of dry-eye syndrome. *Int Ophthalmol Clin.* 1996;36:61-75.

ARTIFICIAL TEAR SOLUTIONS

Actions:

Pharmacology: These products contain the following: Balanced amounts of salts to maintain ocular tonicity (0.9% NaCl equivalent); buffers to adjust pH; viscosity agents to prolong eye contact time; preservatives for sterility. See the Dosage Forms and Routes of Administration chapter for a description and listing of these ingredients.

Indications:

Ophthalmic lubricants: These products offer tear-like lubrication for the relief of dry eyes and eye irritation associated with deficient tear production and exposure to wind, sun, or other irritants. Also used as ocular lubricants for artificial eyes.

Contraindications:

Hypersensitivity to any component of the product.

Patient Information:

To avoid contamination, do not touch the tip of the container or dropper to any surface. Close container immediately after use.

If headache, eye pain, vision changes, or irritation occurs, if redness continues, or if the condition worsens or persists for more than 3 days, discontinue use and consult a health care provider.

May cause mild stinging or temporary blurred vision.

Some of these products should not be used with soft contact lenses. Check package label.

Administration and Dosage:

Instill 1 to 2 drops into eye(s) 3 or 4 times daily, as needed.

otc	**20/20 Tears** (S.S.S. Company)	**Solution:** PVA 1.4%, benzalkonium Cl 0.01%, EDTA 0.05%, KCl, NaCl	Thimerosal free. In 15 mL.
otc	**Akwa Tears** (Akorn)	**Solution:** PVA 1.4%, benzalkonium Cl 0.005%, EDTA, NaCl, sodium phosphate	In 15 mL.
otc	**Artificial Tears** (Various, eg, Rugby, United)	**Solution:** PVA 1.4%, NaCl, EDTA, benzalkonium Cl 0.01%, KCl	In 15 mL.
otc	**Bion Tears** (Alcon)	**Solution:** dextran 70 (0.1%), hydroxypropyl methylcellulose 2910 (0.3%), carbon dioxide, hydrochloric acid, sodium hydroxide	Preservative free. In 0.45 mL (UD 28s).
otc	**Celluvisc** (Allergan)	**Solution:** carboxymethylcellulose 1%, calcium chloride, KCl, NaCl, sodium lactate	Preservative free. In 0.1 mL (UD 30s).
otc	**Dry Eye Therapy** (Bausch & Lomb)	**Solution:** glycerin 0.3%, KCl, NaCl, sodium citrate, sodium phosphate	Preservative free. In 3 mL.

otc	**FreshKote** (Focus Laboratories)	**Solution:** PVP 2%, PVA 0.9% and 1.8%, Amisol clear, NaCl, KCl, boric acid, EDTA, polixetonium	In 3.5 and 15 mL.
otc	**GenTeal Mild** (Novartis Ophthalmics)	**Solution:** hydroxypropyl methylcellulose 0.2%, boric acid, NaCl, KCl, phosphoric acid, sodium perborate, calcium chloride dihydrate	In 15 and 25 mL.
otc	**HypoTears** (Novartis Ophthalmics)	**Solution:** PVA 1%, PEG-400 1%, benzalkonium Cl 0.01%, dextrose, EDTA	In 15 and 30 mL.
otc	**Isopto Tears** (Alcon)	**Solution:** hydroxypropyl methylcellulose 2910 (0.5%), benzalkonium Cl 0.01%, NaCl, sodium citrate, sodium phosphate	In 15 mL.
otc	**Moisture Eyes** (Bausch & Lomb)	**Solution:** propylene glycol 1%, glycerin 0.3%, benzalkonium Cl 0.01%, boric acid, NaCl, KCl, sodium borate, edetate disodium	In 15 and 30 mL.
otc	**Moisture Eyes Preservative Free** (Bausch & Lomb)	**Solution:** propylene glycol 1%	In 0.6 mL (UD 32s).
otc	**Moisture Eyes Liquid Gel** (Bausch & Lomb)	**Solution:** dextran 70 (0.1%), hypromellos 0.8%	In 10 mL.
otc	**Moisture Eyes Liquid Gel Preservative Free** (Bausch & Lomb)	**Solution:** dextran 70 (0.1%), hypromellos 0.8%	In 0.5 mL (UD 28s).
otc	**Murine Tears for Dry Eyes** (Prestige/Medtech)	**Solution:** PVP 0.6%, PVA 0.5%, benzalkonium Cl, dextrose, EDTA, KCl, NaCl, sodium bicarbonate, sodium citrate, sodium phosphate	In 15 and 30 mL.
otc	**Murocel** (Bausch & Lomb)	**Solution:** methylcellulose 1%, propylene glycol, methylparaben 0.028%, propylparaben 0.012%, boric acid, NaCl, sodium borate	In 15 mL.
otc	**Optive** (Allergan)	**Solution:** CMC 0.5%, glycerin 0.9%, in *Purite*	In 15 and 30 mL.
otc	**Puralube Tears** (Fougera)	**Solution:** PVA 1%, PEG-400 1%, benzalkonium Cl, dextrose, EDTA	In 15 mL.
otc	**Refresh** (Allergan)	**Solution:** PVA 1.4%, PVP 0.6%, NaCl	Preservative free. In 0.3 mL (UD 30s and 50s).
otc	**Refresh Endura** (Allergan)	**Solution:** glycerin 1%, polysorbate 80 (1%)	Preservative free. In 0.4 mL single-use containers (20s).
otc	**Refresh Plus** (Allergan)	**Solution:** carboxymethylcellulose sodium 0.5%, calcium chloride, KCl, magnesium chloride, NaCl, sodium lactate	Preservative free. In 0.3 mL (UD 30s, 50s, and 70s).
otc	**Refresh Tears** (Allergan)	**Solution:** carboxymethylcellulose sodium 0.5%, boric acid, calcium chloride, KCl, magnesium chloride, NaCl, *Purite* (stabilized oxychloro complex)	In 3, 15, and 30 mL and 30 mL twin pack.
otc	**Soothe** (Alimera Sciences)	**Solution:** *Restoryl* (*Drakeol*-15 1% and *Drakeol*-35 4.5%), polysorbate 80 (0.4%), octoxynol 40, NaCl, sodium phosphate, EDTA, polyhexamethylene biguanide preservative	In 15 mL.

otc	**Systane** (Alcon)	**Solution:** PEG-400 (0.4%), propylene glycol 0.3%, boric acid, calcium chloride, hydroxypropyl guar, magnesium chloride, polyquaternium preservative, KCl, NaCl, zinc chloride	In 15 and 30 mL.
otc	**Teargen II** (Zenith-Goldline)	**Solution:** hydroxypropyl methylcellulose 2910 (0.4%), benzalkonium Cl 0.01%, EDTA, KCl, NaCl, sodium phosphate	In 15 mL.
otc	**Tears Again Eye Drops** (OCuSOFT)	**Solution:** PVA 1.4%, sodium phosphate, edetate disodium, sodium phosphate, NaCl, phosphoric acid, benzalkonium chloride 0.01%	In 15 mL.
otc	**Tears Again Gel Drops** (OCuSOFT)	**Solution:** carboxymethyl cellulose 0.7%, boric acid, phosphoric acid, NaCl, KCl, carbopol 940, dissipate preservative (stabilized peroxy-complex)	In 15 mL.
otc	**Tears Again MC** (OCuSOFT)	**Solution:** hydroxypropyl methylcellulose 0.3%, boric acid, phosphoric acid, KCl, NaCl	Preservative free. In 15 mL.
otc	**Tears Naturale II** (Alcon)	**Solution:** hydroxypropyl methylcellulose 2910 (0.3%), dextran 70 (0.1%), polyquaternium-1 (0.001%), KCl, NaCl, sodium borate	In 15 and 30 mL *Drop-Tainers.*
otc	**Tears Naturale Forte** (Alcon)	**Solution:** dextran 70 (0.1%), hydroxypropyl methylcellulose 0.3%, glycerin 0.2%, polyquaternium-1 (0.001%), NaCl, KCl, sodium borate	In 15 and 30 mL.
otc	**Tears Naturale Free** (Alcon)	**Solution:** hydroxypropyl methylcellulose 2910 (0.3%), dextran 70 (0.1%)	Preservative free. In 0.6 mL (UD 36s and 60s).
otc	**Tears Plus** (Allergan)	**Solution:** PVA 1.4%, PVP 0.6%, chlorobutanol 0.5%, NaCl	In 15 and 30 mL.
otc	**Tears Renewed** (Akorn)	**Solution:** hydroxypropyl methylcellulose 2906 (0.3%), dextran 70 (0.1%), benzalkonium Cl 0.01%, EDTA, hydrochloric acid, KCl, NaCl, sodium hydroxide	In 15 mL.
otc	**TheraTears** (Advanced Vision)	**Solution:** sodium carboxymethylcellulose 0.25%, borate buffers, calcium chloride, KCl, magnesium chloride, NaCl, sodium bicarbonate, sodium phosphate	Preservative free. In 15 and 30 mL.
otc	**Visine Tears** (Pfizer)	**Solution:** PEG-400 1%, hydroxypropyl methylcellulose 0.2%, glycerin 0.2%, ascorbic acid, benzalkonium Cl, boric acid, dextrose, disodium phosphate, glycine, KCl, magnesium chloride, NaCl, sodium borate, sodium citrate, sodium lactate	In 15 mL.
otc	**Visine Pure Tears** (Pfizer)	**Solution:** PEG-400 1%, hydroxypropyl methylcellulose 0.2%, glycerin 0.2%	In 9.5 mL single-drop dispenser.
otc	**Viva-Drops** (Vision Pharm)	**Solution:** polysorbate 80, citric acid, EDTA, mannitol, NaCl, pyruvate, retinyl palmitate, sodium citrate	Preservative free. In 10 and 15 mL.
otc	**Zi** (Rohto)	**Solution:** PVP 1.8%, alcohol 0.1%, benzalkonium chloride, boric acid, NaCl, KCl, poloxamer 407, polysorbate 80, sodium borate	In 13 mL.

OCULAR LUBRICANTS (Ointments and Gels)

Actions:

Pharmacology: These products serve as lubricants and emollients.

Indications:

Ophthalmic lubrication: Protection and lubrication of the eye.

Contraindications:

Hypersensitivity to any component of the products.

Patient Information:

To avoid contamination, do not touch tube tip to any surface.

Do not use with contact lenses.

If eye pain, vision changes, or irritation occurs, if redness continues, or if the condition worsens or persists for longer than 72 hours, discontinue use and contact a health care provider.

Refer to the Dosage Forms and Routes of Administration for more complete information.

Administration and Dosage:

Pull down the lower lid of affected eye(s) and apply a small amount (0.25 inch) of ointment to the inside of the eyelid.

Storage/Stability: Store at room temperature 15° to 30°C (59° to 86°F). Store away from heat.

otc	**GenTeal Gel** (Novartis Ophthalmics)	**Gel:** hydroxypropyl methylcellulose 0.3%, sodium perborate 0.028%, carbopol 980, phosphoric acid, sorbitol	In 10 mL.
otc	**Refresh Liquigel** (Allergan)	**Gel:** carboxymethylcellulose sodium 1%; **Purite** (stabilized oxychloro complex)	In 30 mL.
otc	**Tears Again Night & Day** (Altaire)	**Gel:** carboxymethylcellulose sodium 1.5%, PVP 0.1% (polyvinylpyrrolidone)	In 3.5 g.
otc	**Tears Again Preservative Free** (Altaire)	**Gel:** carboxymethylcellulose 1.5%	Preservative free. In 3.5 g.
otc	**TheraTears** (Advanced Vision)	**Gel:** sodium carboxymethylcellulose 1%, borate buffers, calcium chloride, magnesium chloride, KCl, sodium bicarbonate, NaCl, sodium phosphate	In 17 mL.
otc	**Akwa Tears** (Akorn)	**Ointment:** white petrolatum, mineral oil, lanolin	Preservative free. In 3.5 g.

otc	**Artificial Tears** (Rugby)	**Ointment:** white petrolatum 83%, mineral oil 15%, lanolin oil	In 3.5 g.
otc	**Lacri-Lube S.O.P.** (Allergan)	**Ointment:** white petrolatum 56.8%, mineral oil 42.5%, chlorobutanol, lanolin alcohols	In 3.5 and 7 g.
otc	**Moisture Eyes PM** (Bausch & Lomb)	**Ointment:** white petrolatum 80%, mineral oil 20%	Preservative free. In 3.5 mg.
otc	**Puralube** (Fougera)	**Ointment:** white petrolatum, light mineral oil	In 3.5 g.
otc	**Refresh PM** (Allergan)	**Ointment:** white petrolatum 56.8%, mineral oil 41.5%, lanolin alcohols, NaCl	Preservative free. In 3.5 g.
otc	**Stye** (Del Pharm)	**Ointment:** white petrolatum 57.7%, mineral oil 31.9%, stearic acid, wheat germ oil, microcrystalline wax	In 3.5 g.
otc	**Tears Again Ointment** (Altaire)	**Ointment:** white petrolatum, mineral oil	In 3.5 g.
otc	**Tears Naturale P.M.** (Alcon)	**Ointment:** white petrolatum, anhydrous liquid lanolin, mineral oil	Preservative free. In 3.5 g.
otc	**Tears Renewed** (Akorn)	**Ointment:** white petrolatum, light mineral oil, lanolin oil	Preservative free. In 3.5 g.
otc	**Natures Tears** (Allscripts)	**Spray:** benzalkonium chloride 0.1%, edetic acid 0.5%, hydroxypropyl methylcellulose 0.3%, dextran 70	In 15 mL.
otc	**Tears Again Liposome Spray** (OCuSOFT)	**Spray:** purified water, lecithin, ethanol 1%, vitamin A, vitamin E, NaCl, phenoxyethanol 0.5%	In 10 mL.

ARTIFICIAL TEAR INSERT

Actions:

Pharmacology: The hydroxypropyl cellulose insert acts to stabilize and thicken the precorneal tear film and prolong tear film breakup time, which is usually accelerated in patients with dry eye states. The insert also acts to lubricate and protect the eye.

Signs and symptoms resulting from moderate to severe dry eye syndromes, such as conjunctival hyperemia, corneal and conjunctival staining with rose bengal, exudation, itching, burning, foreign body sensation, smarting, photophobia, dryness, and blurred or cloudy vision are reduced. Progressive visual deterioration may be retarded, halted, or sometimes reversed.

Pharmacokinetics: Hydroxypropyl cellulose is a physiologically inert substance. Dissolution studies in rabbits showed that the inserts became softer within 1 hour after they were placed in the conjunctival sac. Most dissolved completely in 14 to 18 hours; with a single exception, all had disappeared by 24 hours after insertion. Similar dissolution of inserts was observed during prolonged use (no more than 54 weeks).

Clinical Trials: In a multicenter crossover study, the 5 mg insert administered into the inferior cul-de-sac once a day during the waking hours was compared with artificial tears used at least 4 times daily. There was a prolongation of tear film breakup time and a decrease in foreign body sensation associated with dry eye syndrome in patients during treatment with inserts as compared with artificial tears. Improvement was greater in most patients who used the inserts.

Indications:

Dry eye syndromes, moderate to severe: Keratoconjunctivitis sicca (especially in patients who remain symptomatic after an adequate trial of artificial tear solutions); exposure keratitis; decreased corneal sensitivity; recurrent corneal erosions.

Contraindications:

Hypersensitivity to hydroxypropyl cellulose.

Adverse Reactions:

The following have occurred, but in most instances were mild and transient: Transient blurring of vision; ocular discomfort or irritation; matting or stickiness of eyelashes; photophobia; hypersensitivity; edema of the eyelids; hyperemia.

Patient Information:

May produce transient blurring of vision; exercise caution while operating hazardous machinery or driving a motor vehicle.

If improperly placed in the inferior cul-de-sac, corneal abrasion may result. Patient should practice insertion and removal in health care provider's office until proficiency is achieved.

Illustrated instructions are included in each package.

If symptoms worsen, remove insert and notify health care provider.

Administration and Dosage:

Once daily, inserted into inferior cul-de-sac beneath the base of the tarsus, not in apposition to the cornea nor beneath the eyelid at the level of the tarsal plate. Individual patients may require twice-daily use for optimal results.

If not properly positioned, the insert will be expelled into the interpalpebral fissure, and may cause symptoms of a foreign body.

Occasionally, the insert is inadvertently expelled from the eye, especially in patients with shallow conjunctival fornices. Caution the patient against rubbing the eye(s), especially upon awakening, so as not to dislodge or expel the insert. If required, another insert may be used. If transient blurred vision develops, the patient may want to remove the insert a few hours after insertion.

Rx	**Lacrisert** (Aton Pharma)	**Insert:** hydroxypropyl cellulose 5 mg	Preservative free. In 60s with applicator.

COLLAGEN IMPLANTS

Actions:

Pharmacology: These absorbable implants partially block the punctum and horizontal canaliculus, eliminating tear loss.

Indications:

Dry eyes: For the relief of dry eyes and secondary abnormalities such as conjunctivitis, corneal ulcer, pterygium, blepharitis, keratitis, red lid margins, recurrent chalazion, recurrent corneal erosion, filamentary keratitis, and other noninfectious external eye diseases; to enhance the effect of ocular medications; treatment of symptoms of dry eye (eg, redness, burning, reflex tearing, itching, foreign body sensation); after eye surgery to prevent complications; for patients experiencing dry eye-related contact lens problems.

Contraindications:

Tearing secondary to chronic dacryocystitis with mucopurulent discharge; allergy to bovine collagen; inflammation of eyelid; epiphora.

Patient Information:

Relief may not occur immediately after insertion.

No removal is necessary; implants dissolve within 7 to 10 days.

Reexamination is usually required within 14 days.

Successful treatment may indicate a need for permanent treatment (eg, nondissolvable silicone plugs).

Administration and Dosage:

Implants must be inserted by a health care provider or doctor of optometry. Placement of implants in all 4 canaliculi is recommended to prevent a false-negative response.

Rx	**Collagen Implant** (Lacrimedics)	**Implant:** collagen implant	In 0.3, 0.4, and 0.5 mm sizes (72s).
Rx	**TearSaver** (Ciba Vision)		In 0.2, 0.3, and 0.4 mm sizes.
Rx	**Temporary Punctal/Canalicular Collagen Implant** (Eagle Vision)		In 0.2, 0.3, and 0.4 mm sizes (60s).

TYLOXAPOL (CLEANING/LUBRICANT FOR ARTIFICIAL EYES)

Actions:

Pharmacology: The cleaning/lubricant solution is a sterile, buffered isotonic solution formulated especially for artificial eye wearers. It contains the antibacterial agent benzalkonium chloride to kill most germs that are commonly found in the eye socket of artificial eye wearers. Tyloxapol, a detergent, liquifies the solid matter so that it is less irritating. Benzalkonium chloride, in addition to its germ-killing action, aids tyloxapol in wetting the artificial eye so that it is completely covered.

Indications:

Cleaner/Lubricant: To lubricate, clean, and wet artificial eyes to increase wearing comfort.

Contraindications:

Hypersensitivity to any component of the formulation.

Patient Information:

If irritation persists or increases, discontinue use and consult a health care provider. Keep container tightly closed. Keep out of the reach of children.

To avoid contamination, do not touch dropper tip to any surface. Replace cap after using.

Administration and Dosage:

Use drops as ordinary eyedrops are used. With the artificial eye in place, apply 1 or 2 drops 3 or 4 times daily. The artificial eye may be removed periodically if advised by a health care provider, and 2 or 3 drops applied to remove oily or mucous materials. The artificial eye is then rubbed between the fingers and rinsed with tap water. Then 1 or 2 drops may be applied to the artificial eye, either prior to or after reinsertion.

Storage/Stability: Store at 8° to 27°C (46° to 80°F).

otc	**Enuclene** (Alcon)	**Solution:** 0.25%[1]	In 15 mL *Drop-Tainers.*

[1] 0.02% benzalkonium Cl.

Anti-Infective Agents

ANTIBIOTIC AGENTS

Topical systemic antibiotics may be utilized in the treatment of ocular infections. The most common ocular infections include blepharitis, conjunctivitis, dacryoadenitis, dacryocystitis, keratitis, orbital cellulitis, endophthalmitis, attendant sinusitis, and superficial erysipelas of the skin. Intravitreal antibiotics are often the treatment of choice for endophthalmitis.

The indigenous flora of the eyelids and conjunctiva are primarily *Staphylococcus aureus* and *Staphylococcus epidermidis*, which can overwhelm the ocular defenses and produce infection. Staphylococcal species are most commonly associated with acute papillary conjunctivitis, chronic blepharitis, dacryocystitis, impetigo, blepharoconjunctivitis, superficial keratitis, and endophthalmitis. Corneal ulcers are associated with gram-positive bacteria approximately 75% of the time and gram-negative organisms 25% of the time. Broad spectrum coverage is now available from the fluoroquinolones for single antibiotic coverage of corneal ulcers obviating cultures if the infection responds promptly. Beware of the emerging prevalence of methicillin-resistant *S. aureus* strains (MRSA), which may now require vancomycin. Fungal organisms may be seen in up to 10% of corneal ulcers in Florida.

A purulent discharge and papillary conjunctivitis are associated with a bacterial infection. A serous discharge with conjunctival chemosis and itching is more frequently associated with conjunctival allergy. Conjunctival hemorrhages are associated with more virulent organisms such as streptococcus, haemophilus, or adenovirus. Infiltrative keratitis in the visual axis, decreased vision, hazing of the anterior chamber, or hypopyon are harbingers of imminent visual loss and require prompt microbiologic studies for organism identification and proper antibiotic selection. Similar fastidious cultures of the lids or conjunctiva are important for any chronic conjunctivitis.

ANTIFUNGAL AGENT

Natamycin (*Natacyn*) is the only topical ophthalmic antifungal agent available commercially. It is a tetraene polyene antibiotic derived from *Streptomyces natalensis*. It possesses in vitro activity against a variety of yeasts and filamentous fungi, including *Candida, Aspergillus, Cephalosporium, Fusarium*, and *Penicillium*.

Miconazole IV may be used topically if natamycin is not available. Amphotericin B 0.5% to 1% topical is a valuable alternative. Fluconazole IV may also be used topically in a 0.2% solution if the fungal keratitis is *Candida* species.

ANTIVIRAL AGENTS

The topical ophthalmic antiviral preparations appear to interfere with viral reproduction by altering DNA synthesis. Trifluridine is effective treatment for herpes simplex infections of the conjunctiva and cornea.

Ganciclovir ophthalmic gel (*Virgan*) by Sirion Therapeutics, Inc. is expected to be approved in *2008*. Virgan is a formulation of ganciclovir that will be indicated for the treatment of herpes simplex keratitis. Virgan has been available in Europe for over 10 years and is expected to have a superior safety profile over trifluridine.

Antiviral Agents for Ophthalmic Conditions			
Generic name	Trade name (manufacturer)	Preparations	Indications
Trifluridine	*Viroptic* (Monarch)	Solution 1%	Herpes simplex types 1 and 2; vidarabine-resistant keratitis

Viral infection, especially epidemic keratoconjunctivitis (EKC), is more often associated with a follicular conjunctivitis, a serous conjunctival discharge, and preauricular lymphadenopathy. The exceptionally contagious organism causing EKC is not susceptible to antiviral therapy at this time. Pustular lesions of the nose and face, and spade-shaped fascicular keratitis in association with chronic blepharitis, suggesting acne rosacea, warrants a trial of systemic tetracycline (eg, *Achromycin V*) or doxycycline (eg, *Vibramycin*) as both an antibiotic and potentially anti-inflammatory regimen (MMP = Matrix Metalloproteinase Inhibitor)

For More Information

Bartlett JD, Jaanus SD, eds. *Clinical Ocular Pharmacology*, 5th ed. St. Louis, MO: Elsevier; 2008.

Duane TD, ed. *Clinical Ophthalmology*. Philadelphia, PA: Lippincott-Raven; 1997.

Kucers A, Bennett NM. *The Use of Antibiotics*, 4th ed. Philadelphia, PA: J.B. Lippincott Company; 1987.

ANTIBIOTICS

Indications:

Ocular infections: Treatment of superficial ocular infections involving the conjunctiva or cornea (eg, conjunctivitis, keratitis, keratoconjunctivitis, corneal ulcers, blepharitis, blepharoconjunctivitis, acute meibomitis, dacryocystitis) caused by susceptible strains of microorganisms.

Erythromycin: Prophylaxis of ophthalmia neonatorum caused by *Neisseria gonorrhoeae* or *Chlamydia trachomatis.*

Azithromycin 1% ophthalmic solution (*AzaSite*) by InSite Vision, is indicated for the treatment of bacterial keratitis and is expected to be approved by end of 2007. *AzaSite* is a long-acting formulation of azithromycin, a macrolide antibiotic similar to erythromycin but with an larger spectrum of activity. *AzaSite* will be administered twice daily for the first first 2 days of treatment, then once daily on days 3 through 5 for bacterial conjunctivitis. In terms of clinical resolution and bacterial eradication, results from an active controlled phase 3 study found azithromycin 1% ophthalmic solution comparable to tobramycin 0.3% solution given 4 times daily.

Fourth Generation Fluoroquinolones: The advantages of fourth generation quinolones (gatifloxacin and moxifloxacin) include better gram positive activity than the older generation of quinolones (ciprofloxacin, ofloxacin, levofloxacin) and activity against some anaerobes, *Mycobacterium* or *Norcardia.* The fourth generation quinolones have improved MIC_{90} for gram positive organisms while maintaining essential gram negative coverage. Improved activity of fourth generation fluoroquinolones against gram positive pathogens is believed to be because of the 8-methoxy group (-OCH3), not present in the third generation fluoroquinolones.

There is less resistance with fourth generation quinolones because these drugs bind to both DNA gyrase and topoisomerase IV in bacterial chromosome and cause lethal breaks. The third generation quinolones target only one of those 2 enzymes, gyrase in gram negative and topoisomerase IV in gram positive, and may exhibit activity against fluoroquinolone resistant strains.

The table below lists common ocular conditions along with the antibiotics used most often to treat them. These antibiotics are preferred choices before cultures are available. Ofloxacin and ciprofloxacin have approved indications for the treatment of bacterial keratitis. However, other antibiotics commonly used for bacterial keratitis have been used prior to the release of the fluoroquinolones. The caveat to the use of aminoglycosides (gentamicin, tobramycin, amikacin), ceftazidime, and vancomycin in bacterial keratitis is that they must be extemporaneously compounded. The commercial strengths of gentamicin and tobramycin are "fortified" with injectable agents to increase their concentrations in the range of 10 to 15 mg/mL. Although study data are lacking, gatifloxacin and moxifloxacin may also become drugs of choice for bacterial keratitis because of improved MIC90's and increased spectrum of activity.

Antibiotic Treatment for Common Ocular Conditions			
	Blepharitis	Conjunctivitis	Keratitis
Bacitracin	X		
Polymyxin B	X		
Sodium sulfacetamide	X		
Trimethoprim		X	
Vancomycin			X

Antibiotic Treatment for Common Ocular Conditions			
	Blepharitis	Conjunctivitis	Keratitis
Ciprofloxacin		X	X
Gentamicin			X
Tobramycin		X	
Amikacin		X	
Ofloxacin		X	X
Ceftazidime			X
Gatifloxacin		X	
Moxifloxacin		X	

Contraindications:

Hypersensitivity to any component of these products; history of hypersensitivity to other quinolones; epithelial herpes simplex keratitis (dendritic keratitis); vaccinia; varicella; mycobacterial infections of the eye; fungal diseases of the ocular structure; use of steroid combinations after uncomplicated removal of a corneal foreign body.

Warnings:

Ciprofloxacin, gatifloxacin, moxifloxacin, and ofloxacin hypersensitivity reactions: Serious and occasionally fatal hypersensitivity (anaphylactic) reactions, some following the first dose, have been reported in patients receiving systemic quinolones, including ofloxacin. Some reactions were accompanied by cardiovascular collapse, loss of consciousness, angioedema (including laryngeal, pharyngeal, or facial edema), airway obstruction, dyspnea, urticaria, and itching. An occurrence of Stevens-Johnson syndrome, which progressed to toxic epidermal necrolysis, has been reported in a patient who was receiving topical ophthalmic ofloxacin. Discontinue drug if an allergic reaction occurs. Serious acute hypersensitivity reactions may require immediate emergency treatment. Administer oxygen and airway management, including intubation, as clinically indicated.

Sensitization: Topical use of an antibiotic may contraindicate the drug's later systemic use in serious infections. For this reason, topical preparations containing antibiotics not ordinarily administered systemically are preferable. Products with neomycin sulfate may cause cutaneous/conjunctival sensitization.

Cross-sensitivity: Allergic cross-reactions may occur that could prevent future use of any or all of the following antibiotics: kanamycin, neomycin, paromomycin, streptomycin, and, possibly, gentamicin.

Corneal healing: Ophthalmic ointments may retard corneal epithelial healing. Ciprofloxacin also has been reported to precipitate in 15% of patients treated for bacterial keratitis and slow epithelialization by 55%.

Pregnancy: Category B (erythromycin, tobramycin). *Category C* (gentamicin, ciprofloxacin, gatifloxacin, moxifloxacin, norfloxacin, ofloxacin, polymyxin B). Safety for use during pregnancy has not been established. Use only when clearly needed and when the potential benefits to the mother outweigh the potential hazards to the fetus.

Lactation: It is not known whether ciprofloxacin, norfloxacin, or ofloxacin appears in breast milk following ophthalmic use. Exercise caution when administering ciprofloxacin to a nursing mother. Because of the potential for adverse reactions in nursing infants from norfloxacin, ofloxacin, and tobramycin, decide whether to discontinue nursing or discontinue the drug, taking into account the importance of the drug to the mother.

Children: Tobramycin is safe and effective in children. Safety and efficacy of fluoroquinolones in infants younger than 1 year of age, and of polymyxin B/trimethoprim in infants younger than 2 months of age have not been established.

Precautions:

Monitoring: Perform culture and susceptibility testing during treatment.

Systemic antibiotics: In all, except very superficial infections, supplement the topical use of antibiotics with appropriate systemic medication. Systemic aminoglycoside antibiotics require monitoring the total serum concentration (peak and trough). Recent studies suggest that intracameral antibiotics may be effective, for the treatment of endophthalmitis with minimally virulent organisms, with visual acuity more than 20/400.

Crystalline precipitate: A white crystalline precipitate located in the superficial portion of the corneal defect was observed in approximately 17% of patients on ciprofloxacin. Onset was within 1 to 7 days after starting therapy. The precipitate resolved in most patients within 2 weeks, and did not preclude continued use nor adversely affect the clinical course or outcome. Streptococcal corneal ulcers are often resistant to ciprofloxacin.

Superinfection: Do not use topical antibiotics in deep-seated ocular infections or in those that are likely to become systemic. Use of antibiotics (especially prolonged or repeated therapy) may result in bacterial or fungal overgrowth of nonsusceptible organisms. Such overgrowth may lead to a secondary infection. Take appropriate measures if superinfection occurs.

Sulfite sensitivity: Some of these products contain sulfites, which may cause allergic-type reactions (eg, hives, itching, wheezing, anaphylaxis) in certain susceptible people. Although the overall prevalence of sulfite sensitivity in the general population is probably low, it is seen more frequently in asthmatics or in atopic nonasthmatic people. Specific products containing sulfites are identified in the product listings.

Adverse Reactions:

Sensitivity reactions such as transient irritation, burning, discomfort, redness, stinging, itching, inflammation, angioneurotic edema, urticaria, and vesicular and maculopapular dermatitis have occurred in some patients.

Fluoroquinolones:

Miscellaneous – White crystalline precipitates; lid margin crusting; crystals/scales; foreign body sensation; conjunctival hyperemia; bad/bitter taste in mouth; corneal staining; chemical conjunctivitis; keratopathy/keratitis; allergic reactions; lid and facial edema; tearing; photophobia; corneal infiltrates; nausea; decreased or blurred vision; chemosis; dryness; eye pain; conjunctival irritation; increased lacrimation; papillary conjunctivitis; chemosis; conjunctival hemorrhage; headache; ocular pruritus; subconjunctival hemorrhage; fever; increased cough; infection; otitis media; pharyngitis; rash; rhinitis; dizziness (rarely).

Aminoglycosides:

Local – Localized ocular toxicity and hypersensitivity, lid itching, lid swelling, and conjunctival erythema (less than 3% with tobramycin); bacterial/fungal corneal ulcers; nonspecific conjunctivitis; conjunctival epithelial defects; conjunctival hyperemia (gentamicin). Similar reactions may occur with the topical use of other aminoglycoside antibiotics.

Overdosage:

Symptoms: Symptoms of tobramycin toxicity include punctate keratitis, erythema, increased lacrimation, edema, and lid itching. These may be similar to adverse reactions.

Treatment: A topical overdose of ciprofloxacin may be flushed from the eyes with warm tap water.

Patient Information:

Tilt head back, place medication in conjunctival sac holding the dropper 1 inch from the eye, and close eyes. Apply light finger pressure on lacrimal sac for 1 minute following instillation.

May cause temporary blurring of vision or stinging following administration. Notify health care provider if stinging, burning, or itching becomes pronounced or if redness, irritation, swelling, decreasing vision, or pain persists or worsens.

To avoid contamination, do not touch tip of container to any surface. Replace cap after using.

In general, patients being treated for bacterial conjunctivitis should not wear contact lenses; however, if the health care provider considers contact lens use appropriate, wait at least 15 minutes after using any solutions containing benzalkonium chloride before inserting the lens, because benzalkonium chloride may be absorbed by the lens.

Quinolones: Discontinue use and notify health care provider at the first sign of a skin rash or other allergic reaction.

Administration and Dosage:

Administration and dosage varies for the individual products. Refer to the individual manufacturer inserts for complete information.

Individual drug monographs are on the following pages.

BACITRACIN

Complete prescribing information is found in the Ophthalmic Antibiotics group monograph.

Administration and Dosage:

Apply directly to conjunctival sac(s) 1 to 3 times daily.

Blepharitis: Carefully remove all scales and crusts and then spread ointment uniformly over lid margins.

Storage/Stability: Store at room temperature 15° to 30°C (59° to 86°F).

Rx	**Bacitracin** (Various, eg, Fougera)	**Ointment:** 500 units/g	In 3.5 and 3.75 g.

CIPROFLOXACIN

Complete prescribing information is found in the Ophthalmic Antibiotics group monograph.

Administration and Dosage:

Not for injection into the eye.

Remove contact lenses before using.

For the treatment of corneal ulcers: Instill 2 drops into the affected eye(s) every 15 minutes for the first 6 hours and then 2 drops every 30 minutes for the remainder of the first day. On the second day, instill 2 drops every hour. On the third through the fourteenth day, instill 2 drops every 4 hours. Treatment may be continued after 14 days if corneal re-epithelialization has not occurred.

For the treatment of bacterial conjunctivitis: Instill 1 or 2 drops into the conjunctival sac(s) every 2 hours while awake for 2 days, and 1 or 2 drops every 4 hours while awake for the next 5 days.

Storage/Stability: Store at 2° to 30°C (36° to 86°F). Protect from light.

Rx	**Ciprofloxacin** (Various, eg, Falcon)	**Solution:** 0.3% (equivalent to 3 mg base)	In 2.5, 5, and 10 mL bottles.
Rx	**Ciloxan** (Alcon)		In 5 and 10 mL *Drop-Tainers.*[1]
Rx	**Ciloxan** (Alcon)	**Ointment:** 0.3% (equivalent to 3 mg base)	In 3.5 g tube.[2]

[1] With benzalkonium chloride 0.006%, mannitol 4.6%, EDTA 0.05%.
[2] With mineral oil, white petrolatum.

ERYTHROMYCIN

Complete prescribing information is found in the Ophthalmic Antibiotics group monograph.

Indications:

For the treatment of superficial ocular infections involving the conjunctiva or cornea caused by organisms susceptible to erythromycin.

For prophylaxis of ophthalmia neonatorum caused by *Neisseria gonorrhoeae*. The Centers for Disease Control and the Committee on Drugs, the Committee on Infectious Diseases of the American Academy of Pediatrics, and the Committee on Fetus and Newborn recommend silver nitrate solution 1% in single-use ampules or single-use tubes of an ophthalmic ointment containing erythromycin 0.5% or tetracycline 1% as "effective and acceptable regimens for prophylaxis of gonococcal ophthalmia neonatorum." (For infants born to mothers with clinically apparent gonorrhea, give IV or IM injections of aqueous crystalline penicillin G: A single dose of 50,000 units for term infants or 20,000 units for infants of low birth weight. Topical prophylaxis alone is inadequate for these infants.)

For the prevention of neonatal conjunctivitis caused by *chlamydia trachomatis*, condition that may develop one to several weeks after delivery in infants of mothers whose birth canals harbor the organism.

Administration and Dosage:

External ocular infections: Apply directly to the infected area at least 1 times daily, depending on the severity of the infection.

Prophylaxis of neonatal gonococcal or chlamydial conjunctivitis: Instill a thin line of ointment approximately 0.5 to 1 cm in length into each conjunctival sac. Do not flush the ointment from the eye following application. Use a new tube for each infant. Administer to infants born by cesarian section and those delivered vaginally.

Storage/Stability: Store at room temperature 15° to 30°C (59° to 86°F).

Rx	**Erythromycin** (Various, eg, Akorn)	**Ointment:** 5 mg/g	In 3.5 g.
Rx	**Romycin** (OCuSOFT)		In 3.5 g.[1]

[1] With white petrolatum, mineral oil.

GATIFLOXACIN

Complete prescribing information is found in the Ophthalmic Antibiotics group monograph.

Administration and Dosage:

Not for injection into the eye(s).

Bacterial conjunctivitis: Days 1 and 2 instill 1 drop into the affected eye(s) every 2 hours while awake, up to 8 times per day. Days 3 through 7 instill 1 drop into the affected eye(s) while awake, up to 4 times per day.

Storage/Stability: Store at 15° to 25°C (59° to 77°F). Protect from freezing.

Rx	**Zymar** (Allergan)	**Solution:** 0.3% (3 mg/mL)	In 5 mL bottle.[1]

[1] With benzalkonium chloride 0.005%, EDTA, and NaCl. May contain hydrochloric acid and/or sodium hydroxide.

GENTAMICIN SULFATE

Complete prescribing information is found in the Ophthalmic Antibiotics group monograph.

Administration and Dosage:

Solution: Instill 1 or 2 drops into the affected eye(s) every 4 hours. In severe infections, dosage may be increased to 2 drops once every hour.

This solution is not for injection. Do not inject subconjunctivally. Do not directly introduce into the anterior chamber.

Ointment: Apply a small amount to affected eye(s) 2 to 3 times daily.

Storage/Stability: Store at 2° to 30°C (36° to 86°F). Store away from heat.

Rx	**Gentamicin Ophthalmic** (Various, eg, Bausch & Lomb, Rugby, Schein, Zenith Goldline)	**Solution:** 0.3%	In 5 and 15 mL.
Rx	**Gentak** (Akorn)		In 5 and 15 mL dropper bottles.[1]
Rx	**Gentamicin Ophthalmic** (Various, eg, Akorn)	**Ointment:** 0.3%	In 3.5 g.
Rx	**Gentak** (Akorn)		In 3.5 g.[2]

[1] With benzalkonium chloride 0.1 mg/mL, disodium phosphate, NaCl, monosodium phosphate.
[2] With white petrolatum, parabens.

LEVOFLOXACIN

Complete prescribing information is found in the Ophthalmic Antibiotics group monograph.

Administration and Dosage:

Gram-positive or gram-negative bacterial conjunctivitis: Days 1 and 2 instill 1 to 2 drops in the affected eye(s) every 2 hours while awake, up to 8 times per day. Days 3 through 7 instill 1 to 2 drops in the affected eye(s) every 4 hours while awake, up to 4 times per day.

Storage/Stability: Store at 15° to 25°C (59° to 77°F).

Rx	**Quixin** (Santen/J&J Vistakon)	**Solution:** 0.5%	In 5 mL.[1]

[1] With sodium chloride and benzalkonium chloride 0.005%. May contain hydrochloric acid and/or sodium hydroxide.

MOXIFLOXACIN

Complete prescribing information is found in the Ophthalmic Antibiotics group monograph.

Administration and Dosage:

Not for injection into the eye(s).

Bacterial conjunctivitis: Instill 1 drop in the affected eye(s) 3 times per day for 7 days.

Storage/Stability: Store at 2° to 25°C (36° to 77°F).

Rx	**Vigamox** (Alcon)	**Solution:** 0.5%	Preservative free. In 3 mL *Drop-Tainers.*

OFLOXACIN

Complete prescribing information is found in the Ophthalmic Antibiotics group monograph.

Administration and Dosage:

Not for injection into the eye(s).

Bacterial conjunctivitis: Instill 1 to 2 drops every 2 to 4 hours for the first 2 days and then 4 times daily into the affected eye for up to 5 additional days.

Bacterial corneal ulcer: Instill 1 to 2 drops every 30 minutes while awake; awaken approximately 4 and 6 hours after retiring and instill 1 to 2 drops for 2 days. Instill 1 to 2 drops while awake for the next 5 to 7 days. Instill 1 to 2 drops 4 times daily through treatment completion.

Storage/Stability: Store at 15° to 25°C (59° to 77°F).

Rx	**Ofloxacin** (Various, eg, Alcon, Bausch and Lomb, Pacific Pharma)	**Solution:** 0.3%	In 5 and 10 mL.
Rx	**Ocuflox** (Allergan)		In 5 mL.[1]

[1] With benzalkonium chloride 0.005%, NaCl.

TOBRAMYCIN

Complete prescribing information is found in the Ophthalmic Antibiotics group monograph.

Administration and Dosage:

Solution:

> *Mild to moderate disease* – Instill 1 or 2 drops into the affected eye(s) every 4 hours. Not for injection into the eye.

Severe infections – Instill 2 drops into the eye(s) hourly until improvement. Reduce treatment prior to discontinuation.

Ointment:

Mild to moderate disease – Apply 0.5-inch ribbon into the affected eye(s) 2 or 3 times daily.

Severe infections – Instill 0.5-inch ribbon into the affected eye(s) every 3 to 4 hours until improvement. Reduce treatment prior to discontinuation.

Storage/Stability: Store at 8° to 27°C (46° to 80°F).

Rx	**Tobramycin** (Various, eg, Bausch & Lomb)	**Solution**: 0.3%	In 5 mL bottle.
Rx	**AKTob** (Akorn)		In 5 mL.[1]
Rx	**Tobrasol** (OCuSOFT)		In 5 mL.[1]
Rx	**Tobrex** (Alcon)		In 5 mL *Drop-Tainers*.[2]
Rx	**Tobrex** (Alcon)	**Ointment**: 3 mg/g	In 3.5 g.[3]

[1] With benzalkonium chloride 0.01%, boric acid, sodium sulfate, NaCl, tyloxapol.
[2] With benzalkonium chloride 0.01%, tyloxapol, boric acid, NaCl.
[3] With white petrolatum, mineral oil, chlorobutanol 0.5%.

COMBINATION ANTIBIOTIC PRODUCTS

Complete prescribing information is found in the Ophthalmic Antibiotics group monograph.

	Product and distributor	Polymyxin B Sulfate (units/g or mL)	Neomycin Sulfate (mg/g or mL)	Bacitracin Zinc (units/g)	Other antibiotics	How supplied
Rx	**Bacitracin Zinc-Neomycin-Polymyxin B Ointment** (Various, eg, Bausch and Lomb)	10,000	3.5	400		In 3.5 g.
Rx	**Neomycin Sulfate-Polymyxin B Sulfate-Gramicidin Solution** (Various, eg, Bausch and Lomb, URL, Zenith Goldline)	10,000	1.75		gramicidin 0.025 mg/mL	In 2 and 10 mL.
Rx	**Neosporin Ophthalmic Solution** (Monarch)					In 10 mL *Drop Dose.*[1]
Rx	**Bacitracin Zinc and Polymyxin B Ointment** (Bausch & Lomb)	10,000		500		White petrolatum and mineral oil. In 3.5 g.
Rx	**AK-Poly-Bac Ointment** (Akorn)					Preservative free. White petrolatum, mineral oil. In 3.5 g.
Rx	**Terramycin w/Polymyxin B Ointment** (Roerig)	10,000			oxytetracycline hydrochloride 5 mg/g	White and liquid petrolatum. In 3.5 g.
Rx	**Trimethoprim Sulfate and Polymyxin B Sulfate Ophthalmic Solution** (Various, eg, Bausch & Lomb, Falcon)	10,000			trimethoprim 1 mg/mL	In 10 mL.
Rx	**Polytrim Ophthalmic Solution** (Allergan)	10,000			trimethoprim 1 mg/mL	In 5 and 10 mL.[2]

[1] With thimerosal 0.001%, alcohol 0.5%, propylene glycol.
[2] With benzalkonium chloride 0.004%, NaCl, sodium hydroxide.

STEROID AND ANTIBIOTIC SOLUTIONS AND SUSPENSIONS

Indications:

Inflammatory conditions: For steroid-responsive inflammatory ocular conditions where a corticosteroid is indicated and bacterial infection or risk of infection exists.

For inflammatory conditions of the palpebral and bulbar conjunctiva, cornea, and anterior segment of the globe in which the inherent risk of steroid use in certain infective conjunctivitis is accepted to obtain a diminution in edema and inflammation. For chronic anterior uveitis and corneal injury from chemical, radiation or thermal burns, or penetration of foreign bodies.

Administration and Dosage:

Store suspensions upright and shake well before using.

Instill 1 or 2 drops into the affected eye(s) every 3 or 4 hours, or more frequently as required. Taper to discontinuation as inflammation subsides.

Do not prescribe more than 20 mL initially; do not refill without further evaluation. For complete dosage instructions, see individual manufacturer inserts.

	Product and distributor	Steroid (per mL)	Antibiotic (per mL)	Other content	How supplied
Rx	**Neomycin/Polymyxin B Sulfate/Hydrocortisone** (Various, eg, Falcon, Bausch & Lomb)	hydrocortisone 1%	neomycin sulfate equivalent to neomycin base 0.35% and polymyxin B sulfate 10,000 units		In 7.5 mL.
Rx	**AK-Spore H.C. Ophthalmic Suspension** (Akorn)			thimerosal 0.001%, cetyl alcohol, glyceryl monostearate, polyoxyl 40 stearate, propylene glycol, mineral oil, NaCl	In 7.5 mL.
Rx	**Cortisporin Suspension** (Monarch)				In 7.5 mL *Drop Dose.*
Rx	**Poly-Pred Suspension** (Allergan)	prednisolone acetate 0.5%	neomycin sulfate equivalent to neomycin base 0.35%, polymyxin B sulfate 10,000 units	polyvinyl alcohol 1.4%, thimerosal 0.001%, polysorbate 80, propylene glycol	In 5 mL.

	Product and distributor	Steroid (per mL)	Antibiotic (per mL)	Other content	How supplied
Rx	**Pred-G Suspension** (Allergan)	prednisolone acetate 1%	gentamicin sulfate equivalent to gentamicin base 0.3%	polyvinyl alcohol 1.4%, benzalkonium chloride 0.005%, EDTA, hydroxypropyl methylcellulose, polysorbate 80, NaCl	In 5 and 10 mL.
Rx	**Neomycin Sulfate/ Dexamethasone Sodium Phosphate Solution** (Various, eg, Ivax, Zenith Goldline)	dexamethasone phosphate 0.1% (as sodium phosphate)	neomycin sulfate equivalent to neomycin base 0.35%		In 5 mL.
Rx	**TobraDex Suspension** (Alcon)	dexamethasone 0.1%	tobramycin 0.3%	benzalkonium chloride 0.01%, tyloxapol, EDTA, hydroxyethylcellulose, sodium sulfate, NaCl	In 2.5, 5, and 10 mL *Drop-Tainers.*
Rx	**Neomycin/Polymyxin B Sulfate/Dexamethasone Suspension** (Various, eg, Fougera, Falcon)	dexamethasone 0.1%	neomycin sulfate equivalent to neomycin base 0.35% and polymyxin B sulfate 10,000 units		In 5 mL.
Rx	**AK-Trol Suspension** (Akorn)			benzalkonium chloride 0.004%, polysorbate 20, hydroxypropyl methylcellulose 0.5%, NaCl	In 5 mL.
Rx	**Maxitrol Suspension** (Alcon)			hydroxypropyl methylcellulose 0.5%, polysorbate 20, benzalkonium chloride 0.004%, NaCl[1]	In 5 mL *Drop-Tainers.*
Rx	**Poly-Dex Suspension** (OCuSOFT)			hydroxypropyl methylcellulose, benzalkonium chloride 0.004%	In 5 mL *Drop-Tainers.*
Rx	**Zylet** (Bausch and Lomb)	loteprednol etabonate 0.5%	tobramycin 0.3%	edetate disodium, glycerin, povidone, tyloxapol, benzalkonium chloride 0.01%	In 2.5, 5, and 10 mL bottles.

[1] May contain hydrochloric acid and/or sodium hydroxide.

STEROID AND ANTIBIOTIC OINTMENTS

Administration and Dosage:

Apply ointment to the affected eye(s) every 3 or 4 hours, depending on the severity of the condition.

Do not prescribe more than 8 g initially, and do not refill the prescription until further evaluation. For complete dosage instructions, see individual manufacturer inserts.

	Product & Distributor	Steroid (per g)	Antibiotic (per g)	Other Content	How Supplied
Rx	**Bacitracin Zinc/ Neomycin Sulfate/ Polymyxin B Sulfate/ Hydrocortisone** (Various, eg, Fougera)	hydrocortisone 1%	neomycin sulfate equivalent to neomycin base 0.35%, bacitracin zinc 400 units, polymyxin B sulfate 10,000 units		In 3.5 g.
Rx	**Cortisporin** (Monarch)			White petrolatum	In 3.5 g.
Rx	**Cortomycin** (Major)			White petrolatum, mineral oil	In 3.5 g.
Rx	**Pred-G S.O.P.** (Allergan)	prednisolone acetate 0.6%	gentamicin sulfate equivalent to gentamicin base 0.3%	chlorobutanol 0.5%, white petrolatum, mineral oil, petrolatum, lanolin alcohol	In 3.5 g.
Rx	**Neomycin/Polymyxin B Sulfate/ Dexamethasone** (Various, eg, Bausch & Lomb)	dexamethasone 0.1%	neomycin sulfate equivalent to neomycin base 0.35%, polymyxin B sulfate 10,000 units		In 3.5 g.
Rx	**AK-Trol** (Akorn)			White petrolatum, lanolin oil, mineral oil, parabens	In 3.5 g.
Rx	**Maxitrol** (Alcon)			Parabens, white petrolatum, lanolin	In 3.5 g.

SULFONAMIDES

Actions:

Pharmacology: Sulfonamides are bacteriostatic against a wide range of susceptible gram-positive and gram-negative microorganisms. Through competition with para-aminobenzoic acid (PABA), they restrict synthesis of folic acid that bacteria require for growth.

Pharmacokinetics: Sulfonamides do not appear to be appreciably absorbed from mucous membranes.

Microbiology: Topically applied sulfonamides are considered active against susceptible strains of the following common bacterial eye pathogens: *Escherichia coli, Staphylococcus aureus, Streptococcus pneumoniae, Streptococcus* (viridans group), *Haemophilus influenzae, Klebsiella* sp, and *Enterobacter* sp.

Topically applied sulfonamides do not provide adequate coverage against *Neisseria* sp, *Serratia marcescens,* and *Pseudomonas aeruginosa.* A significant percentage of staphylococcal isolates are completely resistant to sulfa drugs.

Indications:

Ocular infections: For conjunctivitis, corneal ulcer, and other superficial ocular infections caused by susceptible microorganisms.

Trachoma: As an adjunct to systemic sulfonamide therapy in the treatment of trachoma.

Contraindications:

Hypersensitivity to sulfonamides or any component of the product; infants younger than 2 months of age; in epithelial herpes simplex keratitis (dendritic keratitis), vaccinia, varicella, and many other viral diseases of the cornea and conjunctiva; mycobacterial infection or fungal diseases of the ocular structures; after uncomplicated removal of a corneal foreign body (steroid combinations).

Warnings:

Staphylococcus species: A significant percentage of isolates are resistant to sulfa drugs.

Hypersensitivity: Severe sensitivity reactions have been identified in individuals with no prior history of sulfonamide hypersensitivity (see Adverse Reactions).

Pregnancy: Category C. Safety for use during pregnancy has not been established. Use only when clearly needed and when potential benefits to the mother outweigh potential hazards to the fetus.

Lactation: Systemic sulfonamides are excreted in breast milk.

Children: Safety and efficacy not established. Contraindicated in infants younger than 2 months of age.

Precautions:

For topical ophthalmic use only: Not for injection.

Epithelial healing: Ophthalmic ointments may retard corneal wound healing.

Sensitization: Sensitization may occur when a sulfonamide is readministered, regardless of route. Cross-sensitivity between different sulfonamides may occur. If signs of sensitivity or other untoward reactions occur, discontinue use of the preparation.

PABA: PABA present in purulent exudates inactivates sulfonamides.

Dry eye: Use with caution in patients with severe dry eye.

Superinfection: Use of antibiotics (especially prolonged or repeated therapy) may result in bacterial or fungal overgrowth of nonsusceptible organisms. Such overgrowth may lead to a secondary infection. Take appropriate measures if this occurs.

Sulfite sensitivity: May cause allergic-type reactions (eg, hives, itching, wheezing, anaphylaxis) in certain susceptible persons. Although overall prevalence in the general population is probably low, it is more common in asthmatics or in atopic nonasthmatics. Specific products containing sulfites are identified in product listings.

Drug Interactions:

Silver preparations are incompatible with these solutions.

Adverse Reactions:

Headache; local irritation; itching; periorbital edema, burning, and transient stinging; bacterial and fungal corneal ulcers. As with all sulfonamide preparations, severe sensitivity reactions include rare occurrences of Stevens-Johnson syndrome, exfoliative dermatitis, toxic epidermal necrolysis, photosensitivity, fever, skin rash, GI disturbance, and bone marrow depression; fatalities have occurred.

Patient Information:

For topical use only.

To avoid contamination, do not touch tip of container to any surface.

Keep bottle tightly closed when not in use. Do not use if solution has darkened.

Notify health care provider if improvement is not seen after several days, if condition worsens, or if pain, increased redness, itching, or swelling of the eye occurs or persists for longer than 48 hours. Do not discontinue use without consulting health care provider.

Administration and Dosage:

Usual duration of treatment is 7 to 10 days.

Solutions:

Conjunctivitis or other superficial ocular infections – Instill 1 to 2 drops into the lower conjunctival sac(s) every 1 to 4 hours initially according to severity of infection. Dosages may be tapered by increasing the time interval between doses as the condition responds.

Trachoma – Instill 2 drops every 2 hours. Concomitant systemic sulfonamide therapy is indicated.

Ointments: Apply a small amount (approximately 0.25 inch) into the lower conjunctival sac(s) 3 to 4 times daily and at bedtime. Dosages may be tapered by increasing the time interval between doses as the condition responds. Or apply 0.5 to 1 inch into the conjunctival sac(s) at night in conjunction with the use of drops during the day, or before an eye is patched.

Storage/Stability:

Solutions – Protect from light. On long standing, solutions will darken in color and should be discarded.

Ointments – Store away from heat.

SULFACETAMIDE SODIUM

Complete prescribing information is found in the Sulfonamides group monograph.

Rx	**Sulster** (Akorn)	**Solution:** 1%	In 5 and 10 mL.
Rx	**Sulfacetamide Sodium** (Various, eg, Bausch & Lomb)	**Solution:** 10%	In 15 mL.
Rx	**AK-Sulf** (Akorn)		In 2, 5, and 15 mL.[1]
Rx	**Bleph-10** (Allergan)		In 5 mL.[2]
Rx	**Sulfacetamide Sodium** (Various, eg, Fougera)	**Ointment:** 10%	In 3.5 g
Rx	**AK-Sulf** (Akorn)		In 3.5 g.[3]
Rx	**Bleph-10** (Allergan)		In 3.5 g.[4]

[1] With sodium thiosulfate pentahydrate 3.1 mg, methylcellulose 5 mg, methylparaben 0.5 mg, propylparaben 0.1 mg per mL.
[2] With polyvinyl alcohol 1.4%, benzalkonium Cl 0.005%, polysorbate 80, sodium thiosulfate, EDTA.
[3] With methylparaben 0.5 mg, propylparaben 0.1 mg, benzalkonium Cl 0.25 mg, petrolatum base per g.
[4] With phenylmercuric acetate 0.0008%, white petrolatum, mineral oil, petrolatum, lanolin alcohol.

STEROID AND SULFONAMIDE COMBINATIONS

The information for steroid preparations and sulfonamide preparations must be considered when using these products. See individual monographs.

Indications:

Inflammation/Infection: For corticosteroid-responsive inflammatory ocular conditions where a corticosteroid is indicated and superficial bacterial ocular infection or a risk of infection exists.

Administration and Dosage:

Solutions/Suspensions: Instill 1 to 3 drops into the conjunctival sac(s) every 1 to 4 hours during the day and at bedtime until a favorable response is obtained.

Do not prescribe more than 20 mL initially. Do not refill the prescription without further evaluation for steroid-induced glaucoma.

For complete dosage instructions, see individual manufacturer inserts.

Ointments: Apply a small amount (approximately 0.25-inch ribbon) into the conjunctival sac(s) 3 or 4 times daily and once at bedtime (or once or twice at night) until a favorable response is obtained.

Do not prescribe more than 8 g initially. Do not refill the prescription without further evaluation for steroid-induced glaucoma.

For complete dosage instructions, see individual manufacturer inserts.

Storage/Stability:

Solutions/Suspensions – Protect from light. Do not freeze. Shake suspensions well before using. Do not use if solution or suspension has darkened. Clumping may occur on long standing at high temperatures.

Ointments – Keep tightly closed. Store away from heat.

STEROID AND SULFONAMIDE COMBINATIONS, SUSPENSIONS AND SOLUTIONS

	Product and distributor	Steroid	Sulfonamide	Other content	How supplied
Rx	**FML-S Suspension** (Allergan)	fluorometholone 0.1%	sodium sulfacetamide 10%	EDTA, polyvinyl alcohol 1.4%, benzalkonium chloride 0.006%, polysorbate 80, povidone, sodium thiosulfate, NaCl	In 5 and 10 mL.
Rx	**Blephamide Suspension** (Allergan)	prednisolone acetate 0.2%	sodium sulfacetamide 10%	EDTA, polyvinyl alcohol 1.4%, polysorbate 80, sodium thiosulfate	In 5 and 10 mL.
Rx	**AK-Cide Suspension** (Akorn)	prednisolone acetate 0.5%	sodium sulfacetamide 10%	phenethyl alcohol 0.5%, tyloxapol, sodium thiosulfate, benzalkonium chloride 0.025%, EDTA	In 5 mL dropper bottle.
Rx	**Sulfacetamide Sodium and Prednisolone Sodium Phosphate** (Various, eg, Alcon)	prednisolone sodium phosphate 0.25%	sodium sulfacetamide 10%		In 5 and 10 mL.
Rx	**Sulster Solution** (Akorn)			thimerosal 0.01%, EDTA	In 5 and 10 mL.

STEROID AND SULFONAMIDE COMBINATIONS, OINTMENTS

	Product and distributor	Steroid	Sulfonamide	Other content	How supplied
Rx	**Blephamide S.O.P.** (Allergan)	prednisolone acetate 0.2%	sodium sulfacetamide 10%	phenylmercuric acetate 0.0008%, mineral oil, white petrolatum, lanolin alcohol	In 3.5 g.
Rx	**AK-Cide** (Akorn)	prednisolone acetate 0.5%	sodium sulfacetamide 10%	methylparaben 0.05%, propylparaben 0.01%, mineral oil, white petrolatum	In 3.5 g applicator tube.
Rx	**Vasocine** (Novartis)			mineral oil, white petrolatum, methylparaben 0.05%, propylparaben 0.01%	In 3.5 g applicator tube.

NATAMYCIN

Actions:

Pharmacology: Natamycin, a tetraene polyene antibiotic, is derived from *Streptomyces natalensis*. It possesses in vitro activity against a variety of yeast and filamentous fungi, including *Candida, Aspergillus, Cephalosporium, Fusarium,* and *Penicillium*. The mechanism of action appears to be through binding of the molecule to the fungal cell membrane. The polyenesterol complex alters membrane permeability, depleting essential cellular constituents. Although activity against fungi is dose-related, natamycin is predominantly fungicidal. It is not effective in vitro against gram-negative or gram-positive bacteria.

Pharmacokinetics: Topical administration appears to produce effective concentrations within the corneal stroma, but not in intraocular fluid. Absorption from the GI tract is very poor. Systemic absorption should not occur after topical administration.

Indications:

Fungal blepharitis, conjunctivitis, and keratitis: Caused by susceptible organisms. Natamycin is the initial drug of choice in *Fusarium solani* keratitis.

Contraindications:

Hypersensitivity to any component of the formulation.

Warnings:

Pregnancy: Category C. Safety for use during pregnancy has not been established. Use only when clearly needed and when potential benefits to the mother outweigh potential hazards to the fetus.

Lactation: It is not known if natamycin is excreted in breast milk. Use with caution in nursing women.

Children: Safety and efficacy have not been established

Precautions:

For topical use only: Not for injection. Conjunctival necrosis occurs if injected.

Fungal endophthalmitis: The effectiveness of topical natamycin as a single agent in fungal endophthalmitis has not been established.

Resistance: Failure of keratitis to improve following 7 to 10 days of administration suggests that the infection may be caused by a microorganism not susceptible to natamycin. Base continuation of therapy on clinical reevaluation and additional laboratory studies.

Toxicity: Adherence of the suspension to areas of epithelial ulceration or retention in the fornices occurs regularly. Should suspicion of drug toxicity occur, discontinue the drug.

Diagnosis/Monitoring: Determine initial and sustained therapy of fungal keratitis by the clinical diagnosis (laboratory diagnosis by smear and culture of corneal scrapings) and by response to the drug. Whenever possible, determine the in vitro activity of natamycin against the responsible fungus. Monitor tolerance to natamycin at least twice weekly.

Adverse Reactions:

One case of conjunctival chemosis and hyperemia, thought to be allergic in nature, was reported.

Patient Information:

Refer to the Dosage Forms and Routes of Administration chapter for more complete information.

Administration and Dosage:

Fungal keratitis: Instill 1 drop into the conjunctival sac(s) at 1- or 2-hour intervals. The frequency of application can usually be reduced to 1 drop 6 to 8 times daily after the first 3 to 4 days. Generally, continue therapy for 14 to 21 days, or until there is resolution of active fungal keratitis. In many cases, it may help to reduce the dosage gradually at 4- to 7-day intervals to ensure that the organism has been eliminated.

Fungal blepharitis and conjunctivitis: 4 to 6 daily applications may be sufficient.

Shake well before each use.

Storage/Stability: Store at room temperature 8° to 24°C (46° to 75°F) or refrigerate at 2° to 8°C (36° to 46°F). Do not freeze. Avoid exposure to light and excessive heat.

Rx	**Natacyn** (Alcon)	**Suspension:** 5%	With 0.02% benzalkonium chloride. In 15 mL.

TRIFLURIDINE (Trifluorothymidine)

Actions:

Pharmacology: A fluorinated pyrimidine nucleoside with in vitro and in vivo activity against herpes simplex virus types 1 and 2, and vaccinia virus. Some strains of adenovirus are also inhibited in vitro. Trifluridine interferes with DNA synthesis in cultured mammalian cells. However, its antiviral mechanism of action is not completely known.

Pharmacokinetics:

Absorption – Intraocular penetration occurs after topical instillation. Decreased corneal integrity or stromal or uveal inflammation may enhance the penetration into the aqueous humor. Systemic absorption following therapeutic dosing appears negligible.

Indications:

Primary keratoconjunctivitis and recurrent epithelial keratitis: Caused by herpes simplex virus types 1 and 2 in patients at least 6 years of age.

Epithelial keratitis: Epithelial keratitis when ocular toxicity has occurred. In a smaller number of patients resistant to topical vidarabine, trifluridine was effective.

Contraindications:

Hypersensitivity reactions or chemical intolerance to trifluridine.

Warnings:

Efficacy in other conditions: The clinical efficacy in the treatment of stromal keratitis and uveitis because of herpes simplex or ophthalmic infections caused by vaccinia virus and adenovirus, or in the prophylaxis of herpes simplex virus keratoconjunctivitis and epithelial keratitis has not been established by well-controlled clinical trials. Not effective against bacterial, fungal, or chlamydial infections of the cornea or trophic lesions.

Dosage/Frequency: Do not exceed the recommended dosage or frequency of administration.

Mutagenesis: Trifluridine has exerted mutagenic, DNA-damaging, and cell-transforming activities in various standard in vitro test systems. Although the significance of these test results is not clear or fully understood, it is possible that mutagenic agents may cause genetic damage in humans.

Pregnancy: Category C. Fetal toxicity consisting of delayed ossification of portions of the skeleton occurred at dose levels of 2.5 and 5 mg/kg/day in rats and rabbits. In addition, both 2.5 and 5 mg/kg/day produced fetal death and resorption in rabbits. There are no adequate and well-controlled studies in pregnant women. Use during pregnancy only if the potential benefit to the mother justifies the risk to the fetus.

Lactation: It is unlikely that trifluridine is excreted in breast milk after ophthalmic instillation because of the relatively small dosage (no more than 5 mg/day), its dilution in body fluids, and its extremely short half-life (about 12 minutes). However, do not prescribe for nursing mothers unless the potential benefits outweigh the potential risks.

Children: Safety and effectiveness in pediatric patients younger than 6 years of age have not been established.

Precautions:

Viral resistance: Although documented in vitro, viral resistance has not been reported following multiple exposure to trifluridine; this possibility may exist.

Adverse Reactions:

The most frequent adverse reactions reported are mild, transient burning or stinging upon instillation (4.6%), and palpebral edema (2.8%). Other adverse reactions in decreasing order of reported frequency were: superficial punctate keratopathy; epithelial keratopathy; hypersensitivity reaction; stromal edema; irritation; keratitis sicca; hyperemia and increased intraocular pressure.

Overdosage:

Local: Overdosage by ocular instillation is unlikely because any excess solution is quickly expelled from the conjunctival sac.

Systemic: No untoward effects are likely to result from ingestion of the entire contents of a bottle. Single IV doses of 1.5 to 30 mg/kg/day in children and adults with neoplastic disease produce reversible bone marrow depression as the only potentially serious toxic effect and only after 3 to 5 courses of therapy.

Patient Information:

Transient stinging may occur upon instillation.

Notify health care provider if improvement is not seen after 7 days, if condition worsens, or if irritation occurs. Do not discontinue use without consulting health care provider.

Refer to the Dosage Forms and Routes of Administration chapter for more complete information.

Administration and Dosage:

Instill 1 drop onto the cornea of the affected eye(s) every 2 hours while awake, for a maximum daily dosage of 9 drops until the corneal ulcer has completely re-epithelialized. Following re-epithelialization, treat for an additional 7 days with 1 drop every 4 hours while awake, for a minimum daily dosage of 5 drops.

If there are no signs of improvement after 7 days, or if complete re-epithelialization has not occurred after 14 days, consider other forms of therapy. Avoid continuous administration for periods longer than 21 days because of potential ocular toxicity.

Storage/Stability: Store under refrigeration, 2° to 8°C (36° to 46°F).

Rx	**Viroptic** (Monarch)	**Solution:** 1%	In aqueous solution with NaCl and 0.001% thimerosal. In 7.5 mL *Drop-Dose.*

ZINC SULFATE SOLUTION

Indications:

Astringent: A mild astringent for temporary relief of minor eye irritation.

Warnings:

Irritation/Eye pain: If irritation persists or increases, or if eye pain or a change in vision occurs, discontinue use and consult health care provider.

Administration and Dosage:

Instill 1 to 2 drops into eye(s) up to 4 times daily. If solution discolors or becomes cloudy, do not use.

otc	**20/20 Eye Drops** (S. S. S.)	**Solution:** 0.25%	In 15 mL.[1]
otc	**Clear Eyes ACR Eye Drops** (Prestige/Medtech)		In 15 and 30 mL.[2]
otc	**Visine A.C.** (Pfizer)		In 15 mL.[3]

[1] With glycerin 0.4%, naphazoline hydrochloride 0.012%, EDTA, KCl, and camphor.
[2] With glycerin 0.2%, naphazoline hydrochloride 0.012%, benzalkonium chloride, boric acid, EDTA, NaCl, and sodium citrate.
[3] With tetrahydrozoline hydrochloride 0.05%, EDTA, boric acid, NaCl and EDTA.

Ocular Hypotensive Agents

Glaucoma is a condition of the eye in which there is progressive cupping and atrophy of the optic nerve head, and deterioration of the visual fields. *Primary open-angle glaucoma* is the most common type of glaucoma. *Angle-closure glaucoma* and *congenital glaucoma* are treated primarily by surgical methods, although short-term drug therapy is used to decrease intraocular pressure (IOP) prior to surgery.

Drugs used in the therapy of primary open-angle glaucoma include a variety of agents with different mechanisms of action. The therapeutic goal in treating glaucoma is reducing the IOP, a major risk factor in the pathogenesis of glaucomatous visual field loss. The higher the level of IOP, the greater the likelihood of optic nerve damage and glaucomatous visual field loss. Reduction of IOP may be accomplished by: 1) decreasing the rate of production of aqueous humor or 2) increasing the rate of outflow (drainage) of aqueous humor from the eye.

The seven groups of agents used in the therapy of primary open-angle glaucoma are listed in Table 1: Agents for Glaucoma, which summarizes their mechanism of decreasing IOP, effects on pupil size and ciliary muscle, and duration of action.

EPINEPHRINES

Epinephrine (eg, *Epifrin*) and dipivefrin (*Propine*) have alpha and beta activity. They lower IOP mainly by increasing aqueous outflow. Epinephrine, usually used as an adjunct to miotic or beta-blocker therapy, may also be used as primary therapy. The combination of a miotic and a sympathomimetic (eg, epinephrine) will have additive effects in lowering IOP. However, epinephrine is no longer commercially available.

Dipivefrin hydrochloride is a prodrug metabolized to epinephrine in vivo. The IOP-lowering and intraocular effects are qualitatively and quantitatively similar to epinephrine; however, dipivefrin may be better tolerated and have a lower incidence of adverse effects because of its lower concentration.

Table 1: Agents for Glaucoma

Drug	Strength	Duration (hrs)	Decrease aqueous production	Increase aqueous outflow	Effect on pupil	Effect on ciliary muscle
Epinephrines						
Dipivefrin	0.1%	12	+	++	mydriasis	NR
Alpha-2 Adrenergic Agonists						
Apraclonidine	0.5%-1%	7-12	+++	NR	NR	NR
Brimonidine	0.15%	6-8	++	++	NR	NR
Beta-Blockers						
Betaxolol	0.25%	12	+++	NR	NR	NR
Carteolol	1%	12	+++	nd	NR	NR
Levobunolol	0.25%-0.5%	12-24	+++	NR	NR	NR
Metipranolol	0.3%	12-24	+++	NR	NR	NR
Timolol	0.25%-0.5%	12-24	+++	NR	NR	NR
Miotics, Direct-Acting						
Carbachol[1]	0.75%-3%	6-8	NR	+++	miosis	accommodation
Pilocarpine[2]	0.25%-10%	4-8	NR	+++	miosis	accommodation
Miotics, Cholinesterase Inhibitors						
Physostigmine	0.25%-0.5%	12-36	NR	+++	miosis	accommodation

Table 1: Agents for Glaucoma						
Drug	Strength	Duration (hrs)	Decrease aqueous production	Increase aqueous outflow	Effect on pupil	Effect on ciliary muscle
Echothiophate	0.125%	days/wks	NR	+++	miosis	accommodation
Carbonic Anhydrase Inhibitors						
Acetazolamide[3]	125-500 mg	8-12	+++	NR	NR	NR
Brinzolamide[4]	1%	≈ 8	+++	NR	NR	NR
Dorzolamide[4]	2%	≈ 8	+++	NR	NR	NR
Methazolamide[3]	25-50 mg	10-18	+++	NR	NR	NR
Prostaglandins and Prostamides						
Latanoprost	0.005%	24	NR	+++	NR	NR
Bimatoprost	0.03%	24	NR	+++	NR	NR
Travoprost	0.004%	24	NR	+++	NR	NR
Unoprostone	0.15%	12	NR	++	NR	NR

+++ = Significant activity.
++ = Moderate activity.
\+ = Some activity.
NR = No activity reported.
nd = No data available.
[1] Available as intraocular administration during surgery; carbachol also available as a topical agent.
[2] Also available as a gel and an insert; the duration of these dosage forms is longer (18 to 24 hours and 1 week, respectively) than the solution.
[3] Systemic agents.
[4] Topical ophthalmic agent.

ALPHA-2 ADRENERGIC AGONISTS

Alpha-2 adrenergic agonists (apraclonidine [*Iopidine*] and brimonidine [*Alphagan*]) are relatively new to the treatment of glaucoma. Apraclonidine is used primarily before or after laser surgery to control or prevent postsurgical elevations of IOP and as short-term adjunctive therapy for patients requiring additional IOP reduction. Approximately 30% of patients on apraclonidine developed an allergic response. Also, the drug loses its effectiveness in approximately 40% of patients after 2 to 3 months of chronic use. Brimonidine, the newer alpha-2 agonist, seems to have a much lower allergic response associated with it and is much more successful as chronic therapy for most patients. Brimonidine-P 0.15% in a lower concentration and neutral pH contains a different preservative (*Purite*) and has similar IOP lowering efficacy to 0.2%, but with less incidence of allergy.

BETA-ADRENERGIC BLOCKING AGENTS

Beta-adrenergic blocking agents (eg, betaxolol [*Betoptic*], carteolol [*Ocupress*], levobunolol [eg, *Betagan*], metipranolol [*OptiPranolol*], timolol [eg, *Betimol, Timoptic*]) may be used alone or in conjunction with other agents. They may be more effective than either pilocarpine or epinephrine alone and have the advantage of not affecting either pupil size or accommodation. They lower IOP by decreasing the rate of aqueous production.

DIRECT-ACTING MIOTICS

Direct-acting miotics, (eg, carbachol [eg, *Isopto Carbachol*], pilocarpine [eg, *Isopto Carpine*]) were considered the first step in glaucoma therapy. They have now yielded to the prostaglandin analog latanoprost. They are useful adjunctive agents that are additive to beta-blockers, carbonic anhydrase inhibitors, or sympathomimetics. Dosage and frequency of administration must be individualized. Study data indicate pilocarpine 2% and carbachol 1.5% every 12 hours with nasolacrimal occlusion (NLO) provide maximum effect. Increasing the concentration and dosage intervals may correct an inadequate response. Concentrations greater than pilocarpine 4% or carbachol 3% are occasionally required in patients with darkly pigmented irides.

CHOLINESTERASE INHIBITOR MIOTICS

Cholinesterase inhibitor miotics include both reversible/short-acting (physostigmine, demecarium [*Humorsol*]), and irreversible/long-acting (echothiophate [*Phospholine Iodide*]) agents, which enhance the effects of endogenous acetylcholine by inactivation of the enzyme acetylcholinesterase. These agents are more potent and longer acting than the direct-acting cholinergic agents. Side effects and systemic toxicity are more common and of greater significance. Using a direct-acting cholinergic and a cholinesterase inhibitor provides no improvement in response.

CARBONIC ANHYDRASE INHIBITORS

Carbonic anhydrase inhibitors (eg, acetazolamide [eg, *Diamox*], dichlorphenamide [*Daranide*], methazolamide) are administered systemically. Dorzolamide (*Trusopt*) and brinzolamide (*Azopt*) are administered topically. IOP is lowered by a direct action on the ciliary epithelium to suppress the secretion of aqueous humor (inflow). Carbonic anhydrase inhibitors are often used as adjunctive therapy.

HYPEROSMOTIC AGENTS

Hyperosmotic agents (eg, mannitol [eg, *Osmitrol*]), glycerin [*Osmoglyn*], isosorbide [eg, *Ismotic*]) are useful in lowering IOP in acute situations (see the Hyperosmotic Agents chapter). These agents lower IOP by creating an osmotic gradient between the ocular fluids and plasma. These agents are not for chronic use.

PROSTAGLANDINS

Although it has been long recognized that prostaglandins have IOP-lowering effects, side effects such as ocular redness, stinging, and burning discouraged use of this drug class as chronic treatment for glaucoma. The prostaglandin analog latanoprost (*Xalatan*) is very well tolerated with a similar side effect profile of timolol in regard to ocular redness, stinging, and burning. However, latanoprost does change the iris color in some patients after chronic use, but after 5 years of study, this appears to be only cosmetic. Yellow-blue, yellow-green, and blue-gray irises appear to be most susceptible to color change.

Xalatan is currently approved as first–line therapy and is the most used glaucoma drug worldwide. It is as effective or more effective than the beta-blockers for lowering IOP and is additive with most ocular hypotensive agents. Latanoprost is considered by many to have replaced timolol as the new "gold standard" because of its superior therapeutic index. Travoprost and bimatoprost have similar effects as latanoprost, but more hyperemia. Recently, a formulation of travoprost (*Travatan Z*) was introduced using a new ocular drop preservative instead of the more common BAK (benzalkonium chloride). The therapeutic profile of *Travatan Z* is similar to *Travatan*, and can be used in patients who are sensitive to BAK. Unoprostone is similar to the other prostaglandin analogs, but with significantly less efficacy.

For More Information

Bartlett JD, Jaanus SD, eds. *Clinical Ocular Pharmacology*, 4th ed. Boston, MA: Butterworth-Heinemann; 2001.

Becker B, Shaffer RN. *Diagnosis and Therapy of the Glaucomas*, 4th ed. St. Louis, MO: C.V. Mosby Co.; 1987.

Duane TD, ed. *Clinical Ophthalmology*. Philadelphia, PA: Lippincott-Raven; 1997.

Zimmerman TJ, ed. *Textbook of Ocular Pharmacology*. Philadelphia, PA: Lippincott-Raven; 1997.

DIPIVEFRIN HYDROCHLORIDE (Dipivalyl epinephrine)

Refer to the Agents for Glaucoma introduction for a general discussion of these products.

Actions:

Pharmacology: Dipivefrin is a prodrug of epinephrine formed by diesterification of epinephrine and pivalic acid, enhancing its lipophilic character and, consequently, penetrating the anterior chamber. Corneal penetration is about 17 times that of epinephrine. Dipivefrin, converted to epinephrine in the eye by enzymatic hydrolysis, appears to act by enhancing outflow facility. It has the same therapeutic effects as epinephrine with fewer local and systemic side effects.

Dipivefrin does not produce the miosis or accommodative spasm that cholinergic agents produce. The blurred vision and night blindness often associated with miotic agents do not occur with dipivefrin. In patients with cataracts, the inability to see around lenticular opacities caused by constricted pupil is avoided.

Pharmacokinetics: The onset of action with 1 drop occurs approximately 30 minutes after treatment, with maximum effect seen at about 1 hour.

Clinical Trials: In patients with a history of epinephrine intolerance, only 3% of dipivefrin-treated patients exhibited intolerance, while 55% treated with epinephrine again developed an intolerance. Response to dipivefrin twice daily is less than that to 2% epinephrine twice daily and comparable to 2% pilocarpine 4 times daily. Patients using dipivefrin twice daily had mean IOP reductions ranging from 20% to 24%.

Indications:

Glaucoma: Initial therapy or as an adjunct with other antiglaucoma agents for the control of IOP in chronic open-angle glaucoma.

Contraindications:

Hypersensitivity to dipivefrin or any formulation component; narrow-angles (any dilation of pupil may predispose patient to an attack of angle-closure glaucoma).

Warnings:

Pregnancy: Category B. There are no adequate and well-controlled studies in pregnant women. Use only when clearly needed.

Lactation: It is not known whether this drug is excreted in breast milk. Use caution in nursing mothers.

Children: Safety and efficacy for use in children have not been established.

Precautions:

Aphakic patients: Macular edema occurs in up to 30% of aphakic patients treated with epinephrine. Discontinuation generally results in reversal of the maculopathy.

Adverse Reactions:

Cardiovascular: Tachycardia; arrhythmias; hypertension (reported with epinephrine).

Local: Burning and stinging (6%); conjunctival injection (6.5%); follicular conjunctivitis; mydriasis; allergic reactions (infrequent). Epinephrine therapy can lead to adrenochrome deposits in the conjunctiva and cornea.

Dipivefrin 0.1% is less irritating than 1% epinephrine hydrochloride. Only 1.8% of dipivefrin patients reported discomfort from photophobia, glare, or light sensitivity.

Patient Information:

Slight stinging or burning on initial instillation may occur.

Do not try to "catch up" on missed doses by applying more than 1 dose at a time.

Administration and Dosage:

Initial glaucoma therapy: Instill 1 drop into the eye(s) every 12 hours.

Concomitant therapy: When patients receiving other antiglaucoma agents require additional therapy, add 1 drop of dipivefrin every 12 hours.

Rx	**Dipivefrin hydrochloride** (Falcon)	**Solution:** 0.1%	In 5, 10, and 15 mL.
Rx	**Propine** (Allergan)		In 10 and 15 mL.[1]

[1] With 0.005% benzalkonium chloride, sodium chloride, EDTA, hydrochloric acid.

ALPHA-2 ADRENERGIC AGONISTS

APRACLONIDINE HYDROCHLORIDE

Actions:

Pharmacology: Apraclonidine has the action of reducing elevated, as well as normal, IOP whether accompanied by glaucoma or not. Apraclonidine is a relatively selective alpha-2 adrenergic agonist that does not have significant membrane stabilizing (local anesthetic) activity. Topical application of apraclonidine reduces IOP and has minimal effect on cardiovascular parameters.

Optic nerve head damage and visual field loss may result from an acute elevation in IOP that can occur after argon laser surgical procedures. The higher the peak or spike of IOP, the greater the likelihood of visual field loss and optic nerve damage, especially in patients with previously compromised optic nerves. The onset of action is usually within 1 hour and the maximum IOP reduction occurs 3 to 5 hours after application of a single dose. Apraclonidine's mechanism of action is not completely established, although its predominant action may be related to a reduction of aqueous formation via stimulation of the alpha-adrenergic system.

Pharmacokinetics: Topical use of apraclonidine 0.5% leads to systemic absorption. Studies of apraclonidine ophthalmic solution 1 drop 3 times daily in both eyes for

10 days in healthy volunteers yielded mean peak and trough concentrations of 0.9 and 0.5 ng/mL, respectively. The half-life of apraclonidine 0.5% was calculated to be 8 hours.

Clinical Trials: The clinical utility of apraclonidine 0.5% is most apparent for those glaucoma patients on maximally tolerated medical therapy (ie, patients using combinations of a topical beta-blocker, sympathomimetics, parasympathomimetics, oral carbonic anhydrase inhibitors). Patients with advanced glaucoma and uncontrolled IOP scheduled to undergo laser trabeculoplasty or trabeculectomy surgery were enrolled in a study to determine whether apraclonidine dosed 3 times daily could delay the need for surgery for 3 months or less. Apraclonidine treatment resulted in a significantly greater percentage of treatment successes compared with patients treated with placebo.

Indications:

1%: Control or prevention of postsurgical elevations in IOP that occur in patients after argon laser trabeculoplasty or iridotomy.

0.5%: Short-term adjunctive therapy in patients on tolerated maximal medical therapy who require additional IOP reduction.

Contraindications:

Hypersensitivity to any component of this medication or to clonidine; concurrent monoamine oxidase (MAO) inhibitor therapy (see Drug Interactions).

Warnings:

Concomitant therapy: The addition of apraclonidine 0.5% to patients already using 2 aqueous-suppressing drugs (eg, beta-blocker plus carbonic anhydrase inhibitor) as part of their medical therapy may not provide additional benefit. This is because apraclonidine is an aqueous-suppressing drug and the addition of a third aqueous suppressant may not significantly reduce IOP.

Tachyphylaxis: The IOP-lowering efficacy of apraclonidine 0.5% diminishes over time in some patients. This loss of effect, or tachyphylaxis, appears to be an individual occurrence with a variable time of onset and should be closely monitored. The benefit for most patients is less than 3 months.

Hypersensitivity: Apraclonidine can lead to an allergic-like reaction characterized wholly or in part by the symptoms of hyperemia, pruritus, discomfort, tearing, foreign body sensation, and edema of the lids and conjunctiva. If ocular allergic-like symptoms occur, discontinue therapy.

Renal/Hepatic function impairment: Although the topical use of apraclonidine has not been studied in renal failure patients, structurally related clonidine undergoes a significant increase in half-life in patients with severe renal impairment. Close monitoring of cardiovascular parameters in patients with impaired renal function is advised if they are candidates for topical apraclonidine therapy. Close monitoring of cardiovascular parameters in patients with impaired liver function is also advised as the systemic dosage form of clonidine is partly metabolized in the liver.

Pregnancy: Category C. Apraclonidine has an embryocidal effect in rabbits when given in an oral dose of 3 mg/kg (60 times the maximum recommended human dose).

There are no adequate and well controlled studies in pregnant women. Use during pregnancy only if the potential benefit to the mother justifies the potential risk to the fetus.

Lactation: It is not known if topically applied apraclonidine is excreted in breast milk. Exercise caution when apraclonidine is administered to a nursing woman. Consider discontinuing nursing for the day(s) on which apraclonidine is used.

Children: Safety and efficacy for use in children have not been established.

Precautions:

Monitoring: Glaucoma patients on tolerated maximal medical therapy who are treated with apraclonidine 0.5% to delay surgery should have their visual fields monitored periodically. Discontinue treatment if IOP rises significantly or is not lowered.

IOP reduction: Apraclonidine is a potent depressor of IOP. An unpredictable decrease of IOP effect in some patients and incidence of ocular allergic responses and systemic side effects may limit the utility of apraclonidine 0.5%. However, patients on tolerated maximal medical therapy may still benefit from the additional IOP reduction provided by the short-term use of apraclonidine 0.5%.

Cardiovascular disease: Acute administration of apraclonidine has had minimal effect on heart rate or blood pressure; however, observe caution in treating patients with severe cardiovascular disease.

Use apraclonidine 0.5% with caution in patients with coronary insufficiency, recent myocardial infarction, cerebrovascular disease, chronic renal failure, Raynaud disease, or thromboangiitis obliterans.

Depression: Caution and monitor depressed patients; apraclonidine has been infrequently associated with causing depression or worsening existing depression.

Vasovagal attack: Consider the possibility of a vasovagal attack occurring during laser surgery; use caution in patients with a history of such episodes.

Corneal changes: Topical ocular administration of apraclonidine 1.5% to rabbits 3 times daily for 1 month resulted in sporadic and transient instances of minimal corneal cloudiness. No corneal changes were observed in humans given at least 1 dose of apraclonidine 1%.

Drug Interactions:

Apraclonidine Drug Interactions			
Precipitant drug	Object drug*		Description
Apraclonidine	Cardiovascular agents	⬇	Because apraclonidine may reduce pulse and blood pressure, caution in using cardiovascular drugs is advised. Patients using cardiovascular drugs concurrently with apraclonidine 0.5% should have pulse and blood pressures frequently monitored.
Apraclonidine	MAO inhibitors	⬆	Apraclonidine should not be used in patients receiving MAO inhibitors (see Contraindications).

* ⬆ = Object drug increased. ⬇ = Object drug decreased.

Adverse Reactions:

In clinical studies, the overall discontinuation rate related to apraclonidine was 15%. The most commonly reported events leading to discontinuation included (in decreasing order of frequency): Hyperemia; pruritus; tearing; discomfort; lid edema; dry mouth; foreign body sensation.

The following adverse effects were reported with the use of apraclonidine in laser surgery: Upper lid elevation (1.3%); conjunctival blanching (0.4%); mydriasis (0.4%).

The following additional adverse effects were reported (listed by solution strength):

Cardiovascular:

1% – Bradycardia; vasovagal attack; palpitations; orthostatic episode.

0.5% – Asthenia (less than 3%); peripheral edema, arrhythmia (less than 1%). Although there are no reports of bradycardia, consider the possibility.

CNS:

1% – Insomnia; dream disturbances; irritability; decreased libido; headache; paresthesia.

0.5% – Headache (less than 3%); somnolence, dizziness, nervousness, depression, insomnia, paresthesia (less than 1%).

Hypersensitivity: Use can lead to an allergic-like reaction (see Warnings).

GI:

1% – Abdominal pain; diarrhea; stomach discomfort; emesis; dry mouth.

0.5% – Dry mouth (2%); constipation, nausea (less than 1%).

Ophthalmic:

1% – Conjunctival blanching; upper lid elevation; mydriasis; burning; discomfort; foreign body sensation; dryness; itching; hypotony; blurred or dimmed vision; allergic response; conjunctival microhemorrhage.

0.5% – Hyperemia (13%); pruritus (10%); discomfort (6%); tearing (4%); lid edema, blurred vision, foreign body sensation, dry eye, conjunctivitis, discharge, blanching (less than 3%); lid margin crusting, conjunctival follicles, conjunctival edema, edema, abnormal vision, pain, lid disorder, keratitis, blepharitis, photophobia, corneal staining, lid erythema, blepharoconjunctivitis, irritation, corneal erosion, corneal infiltrate, keratopathy, lid scales, lid retraction (less than 1%).

Respiratory:

0.5% – Dry nose (2%); rhinitis, dyspnea, pharyngitis, asthma (less than 1%).

Miscellaneous:

1% – Taste abnormalities; nasal burning or dryness; head cold sensation; chest heaviness or burning; clammy or sweaty palms; body heat sensation; shortness of breath; increased pharyngeal secretion; extremity pain or numbness; fatigue; pruritus not associated with rash.

0.5% – Taste perversion (3%); contact dermatitis, dermatitis, chest pain, abnormal coordination, malaise, facial edema (less than 1%); myalgia, parosmia (0.2%).

Patient Information:

Do not touch dropper tip to any surface as this may contaminate the contents.

Apraclonidine can cause dizziness and somnolence. Patients who engage in hazardous activities requiring mental alertness should be warned of the potential for a decrease in mental alertness, physical dexterity, or coordination while using apraclonidine.

Administration and Dosage:

0.5%: Instill 1 to 2 drops in the affected eye(s) 3 times daily. Because apraclonidine 0.5% will be used with other ocular glaucoma therapies, use an approximate 5 minute interval between instillation of each medication to prevent washout of the previous dose. Not for injection into the eye.

1%: Instill 1 drop in scheduled operative eye 1 hour before initiating anterior segment laser surgery. Instill second drop into same eye immediately upon completion of surgery.

Storage/Stability: Store at room temperature. Protect from light and freezing (0.5%).

Rx	**Iopidine** (Alcon)	**Solution:** 0.5%	In 5 mL and 10 mL *Drop-Tainers.*[1]
		Solution: 1%	In 0.1 mL.[1]

[1] With 0.01% benzalkonium chloride.

BRIMONIDINE TARTRATE

Actions:

Pharmacology: Brimonidine tartrate is a relatively selective alpha-2 adrenergic agonist for ophthalmic use. It has a peak ocular hypotensive effect occurring at 2 hours post-dosing. Fluorophotometric studies in animals and humans suggest that brimonidine tartrate has a dual mechanism of action by reducing aqueous humor production and increasing uveoscleral outflow.

Pharmacokinetics: After ocular administration of a 0.2% solution, plasma concentration peaked within 1 to 4 hours and declined with a systemic half-life of approximately 3 hours. In humans it is systemically metabolized by the liver primarily, with urinary excretion as the major route of elimination of the drug and its metabolites. Brimonidine-P 0.15% contains the preservative *Purite* and is a more neutral pH than 0.2%. The clinical efficacy is similar for both strengths however the incidence of allergy is reduced.

Clinical Trials: Elevated IOP presents a major risk factor in glaucomatous field loss. The higher the level of IOP, the greater the likelihood of optic nerve damage and visual field loss. Brimonidine tartrate has the action of lowering IOP with minimal effect on cardiovascular and pulmonary parameters.

Indications:

To lower IOP in patients with open-angle glaucoma or ocular hypertension. The ability to lower IOP diminishes over time in some patients. This loss of effect appears with a variable time of onset in each patient, and should be closely monitored.

Contraindications:

Hypersensitivity to brimonidine tartrate or any component of this medication. It also is contraindicated in patients receiving monoamine oxidase (MAO) inhibitor therapy.

Warnings:

Pregnancy: Category B. Reproduction studies performed in rats revealed no evidence of impaired fertility or harm to the fetus caused by brimonidine tartrate. There are no studies of brimonidine tartrate in pregnant women; however, in animal studies, brimonidine crossed the placenta and entered into the fetal circulation to a limited extent. Brimonidine tartrate should be used during pregnancy only if the potential benefit to the mother justifies the potential risk to the fetus.

Lactation: It is not known whether brimonidine tartrate is excreted in human milk, although in animal studies brimonidine tartrate has been shown to be excreted in breast milk. A decision should be made whether to discontinue nursing or to discontinue the drug, taking into account the importance of the drug to the mother.

Children: Safety and efficacy in children have not been established. Agitation, apnea, bradycardia, convulsions, cyanosis, depression, dyspnea, emotional instability, hypotension, hypothermia, hypotonia, hypoventilation, irritability, lethargy, somnolence, and stupor have been reported in pediatric patients receiving brimonidine tartrate 0.2%.

Precautions:

Cardiovascular disease: Although in clinical studies, brimonidine tartrate had minimal effect on blood pressure, exercise caution in treating patients with severe cardiovascular disease.

Renal/Hepatic function impairment: Brimonidine tartrate has not been studied in patients with hepatic or renal impairment; use caution in treating such patients.

Depression: Use caution in patients with depression, cerebral or coronary insufficiency, Raynaud phenomenon, orthostatic hypotension, or thromboangiitis obliterans.

Hazardous tasks: Brimonidine tartrate may cause fatigue and drowsiness in some patients. Observe caution while driving, operating machinery, or performing other tasks requiring coordination or physical dexterity.

Drug Interactions:

CNS depressants: Consider the possibility of an additive or potentiating effect with CNS depressants (eg, alcohol, barbiturates, opiates, sedatives, anesthetics).

Concomitant therapy: Brimonidine tartrate did not have significant effects on pulse and blood pressure in clinical studies. However, caution is advised in using concomitant drugs such as beta-blockers (ophthalmic or systemic), antihypertensives, or cardiac glycosides.

Tricyclic antidepressants: Tricyclic antidepressants have been reported to blunt the hypotensive effect of systemic clonidine. It is not known whether the concurrent use of these agents with brimonidine tartrate can lead to an interference in IOP-lowering effect. No data on the level of circulating catecholamines after brimonidine tartrate is instilled are available. Caution is advised in patients taking tricyclic antidepressants, which can affect the metabolism and uptake of circulating amines.

Adverse Reactions:

The most commonly reported adverse events include the following: oral dryness, ocular hyperemia, burning and stinging, headache, blurring, foreign body sensation, fatigue/ drowsiness, conjunctival follicles, ocular allergic reactions, ocular pruritus, corneal staining/erosion, photophobia, eyelid erythema, ocular ache/pain, ocular dryness, tearing, upper respiratory symptoms, eyelid edema, conjunctival edema, dizziness, blepharitis, ocular irritation, gastrointestinal symptoms, asthenia, conjunctival blanching, abnormal vision, muscular pain, lid crusting, conjunctival hemorrhage, abnormal taste, insomnia, conjunctival discharge, depression, hypertension, anxiety, palpitations, nasal dryness, and syncope.

Patient Information:

Do not touch dropper tip to any surface as this may contaminate the contents.

The preservative in brimonidine tartrate 0.2%, benzalkonium chloride, may be absorbed by soft contact lenses. Instruct patients wearing soft contact lenses to wait at least 15 minutes after instilling brimonidine tartrate to insert soft contact lenses.

Brimonidine tartrate may cause fatigue and drowsiness in some patients. Caution patients who engage in hazardous activities of the potential for a decrease in mental alertness.

Administration and Dosage:

Instill 1 drop of brimonidine tartrate in the affected eye(s) 3 times daily, about 8 hours apart. Brimonidine is often dosed 2 times daily in clinical practice based on clinical study data.

Storage/Stability: Store at 25°C (77°F) or colder.

Rx	**Alphagan P** (Allergan)	**Solution:** 0.15%	In 5, 10, and 15 mL dropper bottles.[1]
Rx	**Brimonidine Tartrate** (Bausch & Lomb, Falcon, Pacific Pharma)	**Solution:** 0.2%	In 5, 10, 15 mL bottles.

[1] With 0.005% Purite; boric acid; potassium chloride; sodium borate; sodium chloride; hydrochloric acid and/or sodium hydroxide to adjust pH.

BETA-ADRENERGIC BLOCKING AGENTS

Actions:

Pharmacology: Timolol, levobunolol, carteolol, and metipranolol are noncardioselective (beta-1 and beta-2) beta-blockers; betaxolol is a cardioselective (beta-1) beta-blocker. Topical beta-blockers generally do not have significant membrane-stabilizing (local anesthetic) actions or intrinsic sympathomimetic activity (ISA) except for carteolol, which does have ISA.

The exact mechanism of ocular hypotensive action is not established, but it appears to be a reduction of aqueous production. Some studies show a slight increase in outflow facility with timolol and metipranolol.

These agents reduce IOP with little or no effect on pupil size or accommodation. Blurred vision and night blindness often associated with miotics are not associated with these agents. In addition, in patients with cataracts, the inability to see around lenticular opacities when the pupil is constricted, is avoided. These agents, as well as all topically applied ocular agents, may be absorbed systemically (see Warnings).

Pharmacokinetics:

Pharmacokinetics of Ophthalmic Beta-Adrenergic Blocking Agents				
Drug	β-receptor selectivity	Onset (min)	Maximum effect (hr)	Duration (hr)
Carteolol	β_1 and β_2	nd	nd	12
Betaxolol	β_1	30	2	12
Levobunolol	β_1 and β_2	< 60	2 to 6	12 to 24
Metipranolol	β_1 and β_2	≤ 30	≈ 2	12 to 24
Timolol	β_1 and β_2	30	1 to 2	12 to 24

nd = No data

Clinical Trials:

Timolol – In controlled studies of untreated IOP of at least 22 mm Hg, timolol 0.25% or 0.5% twice daily caused greater IOP reduction than 4% pilocarpine solution 4 times daily or 2% epinephrine hydrochloride solution twice daily. In comparative studies, mean IOP reduction was 31% to 33% with timolol, 22% with pilocarpine, and 28% with epinephrine.

In ocular hypertension, effects of timolol and acetazolamide are additive. Timolol, generally well tolerated, produces fewer and less severe side effects than pilocarpine or epinephrine. Timolol has been well tolerated in patients wearing conventional (PMMA) hard contact lenses.

Betaxolol – Betaxolol ophthalmic was compared with ophthalmic timolol and placebo in patients with reactive airway disease. Betaxolol had no significant effect on pulmonary function as measured by Forced Expiratory Volume (FEV_1), Forced Vital Capacity (FVC), and FEV_1/VC. Also, action of isoproterenol was not inhibited. Timolol significantly decreased these pulmonary functions. No evidence of cardiovascular beta-blockade during exercise was observed with betaxolol. Mean arterial blood pressure was not affected by any treatment; however, timolol significantly decreased mean heart rate. Betaxolol reduces mean IOP 25% from baseline. In controlled studies, the magnitude and duration of the ocular hypotensive effects of betaxolol and timolol were clinically similar. Clinical observation of glaucoma patients treated with betaxolol solution for up to 3 years shows that the IOP-lowering effect is well maintained.

Betaxolol has been successfully used in glaucoma patients who have undergone laser trabeculoplasty and have needed long-term hypotensive therapy. The drug is well tolerated in glaucoma patients with hard or soft contact lenses and in aphakic patients.

Levobunolol – Levobunolol effectively reduced IOP in controlled clinical studies from 3 months to more than 1 year when given topically twice daily; IOP was well maintained. The mean IOP decrease is clinically similar to timolol.

Metipranolol – Metipranolol reduced the average IOP approximately 20% to 26% in controlled studies of patients with IOP greater than 24 mm Hg at baseline. Clinical studies in patients with glaucoma treated 2 years and less indicate that an IOP lowering effect is maintained.

Carteolol – Carteolol produced a median percent IOP reduction of 22% to 25% when given twice daily in clinical trials ranging from 1.5 to 3 months.

Indications:

Glaucoma: Lowering IOP in patients with chronic open-angle glaucoma.

For specific approved indications, refer to individual drug monographs.

Contraindications:

Bronchial asthma, a history of bronchial asthma, or severe chronic obstructive pulmonary disease; sinus bradycardia; second-degree and third-degree AV block; overt cardiac failure; cardiogenic shock; hypersensitivity to any component of the products.

Warnings:

Systemic absorption: These agents may be absorbed systemically. The same adverse reactions found with systemic beta-blockers may occur with topical use. For example, severe respiratory reactions and cardiac reactions, including death caused by bronchospasm in asthmatics, and rarely, death associated with cardiac failure, have been reported with topical beta-blockers. These agents may decrease heart rate and blood pressure, and betaxolol has had adverse effects on pulmonary and cardiovascular parameters. Exercise caution with all of these agents.

Cardiovascular: Timolol can decrease resting and maximal exercise heart rate even in healthy subjects.

Cardiac failure – Sympathetic stimulation may be essential for circulation support in diminished myocardial contractility; its inhibition by beta-receptor blockade may precipitate more severe failure.

In patients without history of cardiac failure – Continued depression of myocardium with beta-blockers may lead to cardiac failure. Discontinue at the first sign or symptom of cardiac failure.

Non-allergic bronchospasm: Use caution when administering beta-blaockers to patients with a history of chronic bronchitis or emphysema, as they may block bronchodilation produced by catecholamine stimulation of beta-2 receptors.

Major surgery: Withdrawing beta-blockers before major surgery is controversial. Beta-receptor blockade impairs the heart's ability to respond to beta-adrenergically mediated reflex stimuli. This may augment the risk of general anesthesia. Some patients on beta-blockers have had protracted severe hypotension during anesthesia. Difficulty restarting and maintaining heartbeat has been reported. In elective surgery, gradual withdrawal of beta-blockers may be appropriate.

The effects of beta-blocking agents may be reversed by beta-agonists such as isoproterenol, dopamine, dobutamine, or norepinephrine.

Diabetes mellitus: Administer with caution to patients subject to spontaneous hypoglycemia or to diabetic patients (especially labile diabetics). Beta-blocking agents may mask signs and symptoms of acute hypoglycemia.

Thyroid: Beta-adrenergic blocking agents may mask clinical signs of hyperthyroidism (eg, tachycardia). Manage patients suspected of developing thyrotoxicosis carefully to avoid abrupt withdrawal of beta-blockers, which might precipitate thyroid storm.

Cerebrovascular insufficiency: Because of potential effects of beta-blockers on blood pressure and pulse, use with caution in patients with cerebrovascular insufficiency. If signs or symptoms suggesting reduced cerebral blood flow develop, consider alternative therapy.

Carcinogenesis: In female mice receiving oral metipranolol doses of 5, 50, and 100 mg/kg/day, the low dose had an increased number of pulmonary adenomas.

Pregnancy: Category C. There have been no adequate and well controlled studies in pregnant women. Use during pregnancy only if the potential benefits to the mother outweigh potential hazards to the fetus.

Carteolol – Increased resorptions and decreased fetal weights occurred in rabbits and rats at maternal doses approximately 1,052 and 5,264 times the maximum human dose, respectively. A dose-related increase in wavy ribs was noted in the developing rat fetus when pregnant rats received doses about 212 times the maximum human dose.

Betaxolol – In oral studies with rats and rabbits, evidence of post-implantation loss was seen at dose levels above 12 mg/kg and 128 mg/kg, respectively. Betaxolol was not teratogenic; however, there were no other adverse effects on reproduction at subtoxic dose levels.

Levobetaxolol – There was evidence of drug-related post-implantation loss in rabbits with levobetaxolol at 12 mg/kg/day and sternebrae malformations at 4 mg/kg/day. No other adverse effects on reproduction were noted at subtoxic dose levels.

Levobunolol – Fetotoxicity was observed in rabbits at doses 200 and 700 times the glaucoma dose.

Metipranolol – Increased fetal resorption, fetal death, and delayed development occurred in rabbits receiving 50 mg/kg orally during organogenesis.

Timolol – Doses 1,000 times the maximum recommended human oral dose were maternotoxic in mice and resulted in increased fetal resorptions. Increased fetal resorptions were also seen in rabbits at 100 times the maximum recommended human oral dose.

Lactation: It is not known whether betaxolol, levobunolol, or metipranolol are excreted in breast milk. Systemic beta-blockers and topical timolol maleate are excreted in milk. **Carteolol** is excreted in breast milk of animals. Exercise caution when administering to a nursing mother.

Because of the potential for serious adverse reactions from timolol in nursing infants, decide whether to discontinue nursing or discontinue the drug taking into account the importance of the drug to the mother.

Children: Safety and efficacy for use in children have not been established.

Precautions:

Angle-closure glaucoma: The immediate objective is to reopen the angle, requiring constriction of the pupil with a miotic. These agents have little or no effect on the pupil. When they are used to reduce elevated IOP in angle-closure glaucoma, use with a miotic.

Muscle weakness: Beta-blockade may potentiate muscle weakness consistent with certain myasthenic symptoms (eg, diplopia, ptosis, generalized weakness). Timolol has increased muscle weakness in some patients with myasthenic symptoms.

Long-term therapy: Diminished responsiveness to betaxolol and timolol after prolonged therapy has occurred. However, in long-term studies (2 and 3 years), no significant differences in mean IOP were observed after initial stabilization.

Sulfite sensitivity: Some of these products contain sulfites, which may cause allergic-type reactions (eg, hives, itching, wheezing, anaphylaxis) in certain susceptible patients. Although the overall prevalence of sulfite sensitivity in the general population is probably low, it is seen more frequently in asthmatics or atopic nonasthmatics.

Drug Interactions:

Ophthalmic Beta-Blocker Drug Interactions			
Precipitant drug	Object drug*		Description
Beta-blockers, ophthalmic	Beta-blockers, oral	↑	Use topical beta-blockers with caution because of the potential for additive effects on systemic and ophthalmic beta-blockade.
Beta-blockers, ophthalmic	Calcium antagonists	↑	Possible cases of hypotension, left ventricular failure, and atrioventricular conduction disturbances may occur from coadministration of timolol maleate and calcium antagonists. Avoid use in patients with impaired cardiac function.
Beta-blockers, ophthalmic	Catecholamine-depleting drugs (eg, reserpine)	↑	Use of reserpine with ophthalmic beta-blockers can cause additive effects and the production of hypotension or marked bradycardia, which may result in syncope, vertigo, or postural hypotension. Close observation is recommended.
Catecholamine-depleting drugs (eg, reserpine)	Beta-blockers, ophthalmic		
Beta-blockers, ophthalmic	Digitalis	↑	Coadministration of ophthalmic beta-blockers with digitalis and calcium antagonists may have additive effects in prolonging atrioventricular conduction time.
Digitalis	Beta-blockers, ophthalmic		
Quinidine	Beta-blockers, ophthalmic	↑	Decreased heart rate has been reported during combined treatment with timolol maleate and quinidine, possibly because quinidine inhibits the metabolism of timolol maleate via the P450 enzyme, CYP2D6.
Beta-blockers	Phenothiazine compounds	↑	Potential additive hypotensive effects due to mutual inhibition of metabolism.

* ↑ = Object drug increased.

Other drugs that may interact with systemic beta-adrenergic blocking agents may also interact with ophthalmic agents. These agents are listed below.

Antithyroid agents	Insulin	Phenothiazines
Calcium channel blockers	Lidocaine	Prazosin
Cimetidine	Morphine	Rifampin
Clonidine	Neuromuscular blockers, nondepolarizing	Salicylates
Contraceptives, oral	Nicotine	Smoking
Digoxin	NSAIDs	Sympathomimetics
Disopyramide	Phenobarbital	Theophylline
Haloperidol		Thyroid hormones
Hydralazine		

Adverse Reactions:

The following have occurred with ophthalmic beta-1 and beta-2 (nonselective) blockers:

Cardiovascular: Arrhythmia; syncope; heart block; cerebral vascular accident; cerebral ischemia; congestive heart failure; palpitation.

CNS: Headache; depression.

Dermatologic: Hypersensitivity, including localized and generalized rash.

Endocrine: Masked symptoms of hypoglycemia in insulin-dependent diabetics (see Warnings).

GI: Nausea.

Ophthalmic: Keratitis; blepharoptosis; visual disturbances including refractive changes (caused by withdrawal of miotic therapy in some cases); diplopia; ptosis.

The following adverse reactions have occurred with the individual agent:

Respiratory: Bronchospasm (predominantly in patients with preexisting bronchospastic disease); respiratory failure.

Carteolol:

Ophthalmic – Transient irritation, burning, tearing, conjunctival hyperemia, edema (about 25%), blurred/cloudy vision; photophobia; decreased night vision; ptosis; blepharoconjunctivitis; abnormal corneal staining; corneal sensitivity.

Systemic – Bradycardia; decreased blood pressure; arrhythmia; heart palpitation; dyspnea; asthenia; headache; dizziness; insomnia; sinusitis; taste perversion.

Betaxolol:

Ophthalmic – Brief discomfort (more than 25%); occasional tearing (5%), decreased corneal sensitivity, erythema, itching, corneal punctate staining, keratitis, anisocoria; photophobia (rare).

Systemic – Insomnia; depressive neurosis (rare).

Levobetaxolol:

Cardiovascular – Bradycardia; heart block; hypertension; hypotension; tachycardia; vascular anomaly (less than 2%).

CNS – Anxiety; dizziness; hypertonia; vertigo (less than 2%).

Dermatologic – Alopecia; dermatitis; psoriasis (less than 2%).

Endocrine – Diabetes; hypothyroidism (less than 2%).

GI – Constipation; dyspepsia (less than 2%).

GU – Breast abscess; cystitis (less than 2%).

Metabolic/Nutritional – Gout; hypercholesteremia; hyperlipidemia (less than 2%).

Musculoskeletal – Arthritis; tendonitis (less than 2%).

Ophthalmic – Transient ocular discomfort upon instillation (11%); transient blurred vision (approximately 2%); cataracts, vitreous disorders (less than 2%).

Pulmonary – Pulmonary distress characterized by bronchitis, dyspnea, pharyngitis, pneumonia, rhinitis, and sinusitis (less than 2%).

Special Senses – Ear pain; otitis media; taste perversion; tinnitus (less than 2%).

Miscellaneous – Accidental injury; headache; infection (less than 2%).

Levobunolol:

Cardiovascular – Effects may resemble those of timolol.

CNS – Ataxia, dizziness, lethargy (rare).

Dermatologic – Urticaria, pruritus (rare).

Ophthalmic – Transient burning/stinging (25%); blepharoconjunctivitis (5%); iridocyclitis (rare); decreased corneal sensitivity.

Metipranolol:

Ophthalmic – Transient local discomfort; conjunctivitis; eyelid dermatitis; blepharitis; blurred vision; tearing; browache; abnormal vision; photophobia; edema.

Systemic – Allergic reaction; headache; asthenia; hypertension; myocardial infarction; atrial fibrillation; angina; palpitation; bradycardia; nausea; rhinitis; dyspnea; epistaxis; bronchitis; coughing; dizziness; anxiety; depression; somnolence; nervousness; arthritis; myalgia; rash.

Timolol:

CNS – Dizziness; depression; fatigue; lethargy; hallucinations; confusion.

Cardiovascular – Bradycardia; arrhythmia; hypotension; syncope; heart block; cerebral vascular accident; cerebral ischemia; heart failure; palpitation; cardiac arrest. These generally occur in the elderly or in patients with preexisting cardiovascular problems.

Ophthalmic – Ocular irritation including conjunctivitis; blepharitis; keratitis; blepharoptosis; decreased corneal sensitivity; visual disturbances including refractive changes (in some cases, caused by withdrawal of miotics); diplopia; ptosis.

Respiratory – Bronchospasm (mainly in patients with preexisting bronchospastic disease); respiratory failure; dyspnea.

Miscellaneous – Aggravation of myasthenia gravis; alopecia; nail pigmentary changes; nausea; hypersensitivity, including localized and generalized rash; urticaria; asthenia; sexual dysfunction, including impotence, decreased libido; decreased ejaculation; hyperkalemia; masked symptoms of hypoglycemia in insulin-dependent diabetics; diarrhea; paresthesia.

Causal relationship unknown: Hypertension; chest pain; dyspepsia; anorexia; dry mouth; behavioral changes (eg, anxiety, disorientation, nervousness, somnolence, psychic disturbance); aphakic cystoid macular edema; retroperitoneal fibrosis.

Systemic beta-adrenergic blocker-associated reactions: Consider potential effects with ophthalmic use (see Warnings).

Overdosage:

If ocular overdosage occurs, flush eye(s) with water or normal saline. If accidentally ingested, efforts to decrease further absorption may be appropriate (gastric lavage).

The most common signs and symptoms of overdosage from systemic beta-blockers are bradycardia, hypotension, bronchospasm, and acute cardiac failure. If these occur, discontinue therapy and initiate appropriate supportive therapy.

Patient Information:

Refer to the Dosage Forms and Routes of Administration chapter for more complete information.

Transient stinging/discomfort is relatively common; notify health care provider if severe.

Administration and Dosage:

Concomitant therapy: If IOP is not controlled with these agents, institute concomitant pilocarpine, other miotics, dipivefrin, or carbonic anhydrase inhibitors.

Use of epinephrine with topical beta-blockers is controversial. Some reports indicate that initial effectiveness of the combination decreases over time (see Drug Interactions).

Monitoring: The IOP-lowering response to betaxolol and timolol may require a few weeks to stabilize. Determine the IOP during the first month of treatment. Thereafter, determine IOP on an individual basis.

Because of diurnal IOP variations in individual patients, satisfactory response to twice-a-day therapy is best determined by measuring IOP at different times during the day. IOPs 22 mm Hg or less may not be optimal to control glaucoma in each patient; therefore, individualize therapy.

Individual drug monographs are on the following pages.

BETAXOLOL HYDROCHLORIDE

For complete prescribing information, refer to the Beta-Adrenergic Blocking Agents group monograph.

Indications:

Treatment of ocular hypertension and chronic open-angle glaucoma. Betaxolol may be used alone or in combination with other antiglaucoma drugs.

Administration and Dosage:

Usual dose: Instill 1 drop twice daily.

Replacement therapy (single agent): Continue the agent already used and add 1 drop of betaxolol twice daily. The following day, discontinue the previous agent and continue betaxolol. Monitor with tonometry.

Replacement therapy (multiple agents): When transferring from several concomitant antiglaucoma agents, individualize dosage. Adjust 1 agent at a time at intervals of at least 1 week. One may continue the agents being used and add 1 drop betaxolol twice daily. The next day, discontinue another agent. Decrease or discontinue remaining antiglaucoma agents according to patient response.

Storage/Stability: Store at room temperature 15° to 30°C (59° to 86°F). Shake suspension well.

Rx	**Betoptic S** (Alcon)	**Suspension:** 2.8 mg (equiv. to 2.5 mg base) per mL (0.25%)	In 2,5, 5, 10, and 15 mL *Drop-Tainer* bottles.[1]

[1] With 0.01% benzalkonium chloride, mannitol, poly sulfonic acid, hydrochloric acid or sodium hydroxide, EDTA.

CARTEOLOL HYDROCHLORIDE

For complete prescribing information, refer to the Beta-Adrenergic Blocking Agents group monograph.

Indications:

Treatment of chronic open-angle glaucoma and ocular hypertension. It may be used alone or in combination with other IOP lowering drugs.

Administration and Dosage:

Usual dose: Instill 1 drop in affected eye(s) twice daily. If the patient's IOP is not at a satisfactory level on this regimen, concomitant therapy can be instituted.

Rx	**Ocupress** (Novartis)	**Solution:** 1%	In 5, 10, and 15 mL dropper bottles.[1]

[1] With 0.005% benzalkonium chloride, NaCl, sodium phosphate.

LEVOBUNOLOL HYDROCHLORIDE

For complete prescribing information, refer to the Beta-Adrenergic Blocking Agents group monograph.

Indications:

Lower IOP in chronic open-angle glaucoma or ocular hypertension.

Administration and Dosage:

Usual dose: Instill 1 drop in the affected eye(s) once or twice daily.

Rx	**Levobunolol** (Various, eg, Bausch & Lomb)	**Solution**: 0.25%	In 5 and 10 mL.
Rx	**Betagan Liquifilm** (Allergan)		In 5 and 10 mL dropper bottles with BID *C Cap.*[1]
Rx	**Levobunolol** (Various, eg, Bausch & Lomb)	**Solution**: 0.5%	In 5, 10, and 15 mL.
Rx	**Betagan Liquifilm** (Allergan)		In 2, 5, 10 and 15 mL bottles with BID and QD*C Cap.*[1]

[1] With 1.4% polyvinyl alcohol, 0.004% benzalkonium chloride, sodium metabisulfite, EDTA.

METIPRANOLOL HYDROCHLORIDE

For complete prescribing information, refer to the Beta-Adrenergic Blocking Agents group monograph.

Indications:

Treatment of ocular conditions in which lowering IOP is likely to be of therapeutic benefit, including ocular hypertension and chronic open-angle glaucoma.

Administration and Dosage:

Usual dose: Instill 1 drop in the affected eye(s) twice a day. If the patient's IOP is not at a satisfactory level on this regimen, more frequent administration or a larger dose is of benefit. Concomitant therapy to lower IOP can be instituted.

Rx	**Metipranolol** (Various, eg, Falcon)	**Solution**: 0.3%	In 5 or 10 mL dropper bottles.[1]
Rx	**OptiPranolol** (Bausch & Lomb)	**Solution**: 0.3%	In 5 or 10 mL dropper bottles.[1]

[1] With 0.004% benzalkonium chloride, EDTA, NaCl.

TIMOLOL MALEATE

For complete prescribing information, refer to the Beta-Adrenergic Blocking Agents group monograph.

Indications:

Treatment of elevated IOP in chronic open-angle glaucoma, ocular hypertension, aphakic glaucoma patients, some patients with secondary glaucoma, and patients with elevated IOP who need ocular pressure lowering.

Administration and Dosage:

Solution:

Initial therapy – Instill 1 drop of 0.25% or 0.5% twice daily. Because the pressure-lowering response may require a few weeks to stabilize, evaluation should include a determination of IOP after approximately 4 weeks of treatment. The starting dose of *Istalol* is 1 drop of 0.5% solution in the affected eye(s) once daily in the morning.

Gel: Invert the closed container and shake once before each use; it is not necessary to shake it more than once. Administer other ophthalmics at least 10 minutes before the gel. Dose is 1 drop (0.25% or 0.5%) once daily. Consider concomitant therapy if IOP is not at a satisfactory level. When patients are switched from timolol solution twice daily to the gel once daily, the ocular hypotensive effect should remain constant.

Because the pressure-lowering response may require a few weeks to stabilize, determine IOP after about 4 weeks of treatment.

Rx	**Timolol Maleate** (Various, eg, Falcon)	**Solution**: 0.25%	In 5, 10, and 15 mL.
Rx	**Betimol**[1] (Johnson & Johnson Vision Care)		In 2.5, 5, 10, and 15 mL.[2]
Rx	**Timoptic**[3] (Merck)		Preservative free. In UD 60s *Ocudose*.[4]
Rx	**Timolol Maleate** (Various, eg, Falcon)	**Solution**: 0.5%	In 5, 10, and 15 mL.
Rx	**Betimol**[1] (Johnson & Johnson Vision Care)		In 2.5, 5, 10, and 15 mL.[2]
Rx	**Timoptic**[3] (Merck)		Preservative free. In UD 60s *Ocudose*.[4]
Rx	**Timoptic**[3] (Merck)		In 2.5 mL *Ocumeters*.[5]
Rx	**Istalol** (IstaPharma)		5 mL in 10 mL container.

Rx	**Timolol Maleate Ophthalmic** (Falcon)	**Solution, gel-forming:** 0.25%	In 5 mL.[5]
Rx	**Timoptic-XE**[3] (Merck)		In 2.5 and 5 mL *Ocumeters.*[6]
Rx	**Timolol Maleate Ophthalmic** (Falcon)	**Solution, gel-forming:** 0.5%	In 2.5 and 5 mL.[5]
Rx	**Timoptic-XE**[3] (Merck)		In 2.5 and 5 mL *Ocumeters.*[6]

[1] As hemihydrate.
[2] With 0.01% benzalkonium chloride and monosodium and disodium phosphate dihydrate.
[3] As maleate.
[4] Use immediately after opening; discard remaining contents. With monobasic and dibasic sodium phosphate and sodium hydroxide.
[5] With 0.01% benzalkonium chloride, sodium hydroxide, and monobasic and dibasic sodium phosphate.
[6] With 0.012% benzododecinium bromide.

MIOTICS, DIRECT-ACTING

Actions:

Pharmacology: The direct-acting miotics are parasympathomimetic (cholinergic) drugs that duplicate the muscarinic effects of acetylcholine. When applied topically, these drugs produce pupillary constriction, stimulate the ciliary muscles, and increase aqueous humor outflow facility. Miosis, produced through contraction of the iris sphincter, causes increased tension on the scleral spur (reducing outflow resistance) and opening of the trabecular meshwork spaces facilitating outflow. With the increase in outflow facility, there is a decrease in IOP. Topical ophthalmic instillation of acetylcholine causes no discernible response as cholinesterase destroys the molecule more rapidly than it can penetrate the cornea; therefore, acetylcholine is used only intraocularly.

Miosis Induction of Direct-Acting Miotics			
Topical Miotic	Onset	Peak	Duration
Carbachol	10 to 20 min	—	4 to 8 hours
Pilocarpine	10 to 30 min	—	4 to 8 hours

Indications:

Carbachol, topical; pilocarpine: To decrease elevated IOP in glaucoma.

Acetylcholine; carbachol, intraocular: To induce miosis during surgery.

See individual monographs for specific indications.

Contraindications:

Hypersensitivity to any component of the formulation; where constriction is undesirable (eg, acute iritis, acute or anterior uveitis, some forms of secondary glaucoma, pupillary block glaucoma, acute inflammatory disease of the anterior chamber).

Warnings:

Corneal abrasion: Use carbachol with caution in the presence of corneal abrasion to avoid excessive penetration.

Pregnancy: Category C (carbachol, pilocarpine). Safety for use during pregnancy has not been established. Use only when clearly needed.

Lactation: It is not known whether these drugs are excreted in breast milk; exercise caution when administering to a nursing woman.

Children: Safety and efficacy for use in children have not been established.

Precautions:

Systemic reactions: Caution is advised in patients with acute cardiac failure, bronchial asthma, peptic ulcer, hyperthyroidism, GI spasm, urinary tract obstruction, Parkinson disease, recent MI, hypertension, or hypotension.

Retinal detachment: Retinal detachment has been caused by miotics in susceptible individuals, in individuals with preexisting retinal disease, or in those who are predisposed to retinal tears. Fundus examination is advised for all patients prior to initiation of therapy.

Miosis: Miosis usually causes difficulty in dark adaptation. Advise patients to use caution while night driving or performing hazardous tasks in poor light.

Angle-closure: Although withdrawal of the peripheral iris from the anterior chamber angle by miosis may reduce the tendency for angle-closure, miotics can occasionally precipitate angle closure by increasing resistance to aqueous flow from posterior to anterior chamber.

Pilocarpine ocular system (Ocusert): Carefully consider and evaluate patients with acute infectious conjunctivitis or keratitis prior to use.

Drug Interactions:

Nonsteroidal anti-inflammatory agents, topical: Although studies with acetylcholine chloride or carbachol revealed no interference, and there is no known pharmacological basis for an interaction, there have been reports that both of these drugs have been ineffective when used in patients treated with topical nonsteroidal anti-inflammatory agents.

Adverse Reactions:

Acetylcholine:

Ophthalmic – Corneal edema; clouding; decompensation.

Systemic – Bradycardia; hypotension; flushing; breathing difficulties; sweating.

Carbachol:

Ophthalmic – Transient stinging and burning; corneal clouding; persistent bullous keratopathy; postoperative iritis following cataract extraction with intraocular use; retinal detachment; transient ciliary and conjunctival injection; ciliary spasm with resultant temporary decrease of visual acuity.

Systemic – Headache; salivation; GI cramps; vomiting; diarrhea; asthma; syncope; cardiac arrhythmia; flushing; sweating; epigastric distress; tightness in bladder; hypotension; frequent urge to urinate.

Pilocarpine:

Ophthalmic – Transient stinging and burning; tearing; ciliary spasm; conjunctival vascular congestion; temporal, peri- or supra-orbital headache; superficial keratitis; induced myopia (especially in younger individuals who have recently started administration); blurred vision; poor dark adaptation; reduced visual acuity in poor illumination in older individuals and in individuals with lens opacity. A subtle corneal granularity has occurred with pilocarpine gel. Lens opacity (prolonged use), retinal detachment (rare; see Precautions).

Systemic – Hypertension; tachycardia; bronchiolar spasm; pulmonary edema; salivation; sweating; nausea; vomiting; diarrhea (rare).

Overdosage:

Should accidental overdosage in the eye(s) occur, flush with water.

Treatment: Treatment includes usual supportive measures. Observe patients for signs of toxicity (eg, salivation, lacrimation, sweating, nausea, vomiting, diarrhea). If these occur, therapy with anticholinergics (atropine) may be necessary. Bronchial constriction may be a problem in asthmatic patients.

Patient Information:

May sting upon instillation, especially first few doses.

May cause headache, browache, and decreased night vision. Use caution while driving at night or performing hazardous tasks in poor light.

To avoid contamination, do not touch tip of container to any surface. Replace cap after using. Keep bottle tightly closed when not in use. Discard solution after expiration date. Wash hands immediately after use.

Individual drug monographs are on the following pages.

CARBACHOL, TOPICAL

For complete prescribing information, refer to the Miotics, Direct-Acting group monograph.

Indications:

Glaucoma: For lowering IOP in the treatment of glaucoma.

Administration and Dosage:

Instill 1 drop into eye(s) up to 3 times daily.

Storage/Stability: Store at 8° to 27°C (46° to 80°F).

Rx	**Isopto Carbachol** (Alcon)	**Solution:** 1.5%	In 15 mL *Drop-Tainers.*[1]
Rx	**Isopto Carbachol** (Alcon)	**Solution:** 3%	In 15 and 30 mL *Drop-Tainers.*[1]

[1] With 0.005% benzalkonium chloride, 1% hydroxypropyl methylcellulose, sodium chloride, boric acid, sodium borate.

PILOCARPINE HYDROCHLORIDE

For complete prescribing information, refer to the Miotics, Direct-Acting group monograph.

Indications:

To lower IOP in glaucoma.

Chronic angle-closure glaucoma.

Acute (angle-closure) glaucoma: Alone, or in combination with beta–adrenergic blocking agents, carbonic anhydrase inhibitors, apraclonidine, or hyperosmotic agents to decrease IOP and break the attack.

Pre- and postoperative elevated IOP.

Administration and Dosage:

Solution:

Initial – Instill 1 drop 3 to 4 times daily. The frequency of instillation and the concentration are determined by patient response. Individuals with heavily pigmented irides may require higher strengths.

Gel: Apply a 0.5-inch ribbon in the lower conjunctival sac of affected eye(s) once daily at bedtime. If other glaucoma medication is also used at bedtime, use drops at least 5 minutes before the gel.

Storage/Stability: Do not freeze. Store at room temperature; 2° to 26°C (36° to 80°F).

Rx	**Isopto Carpine** (PolyMedica)	**Solution:** 0.25%	In 15 mL.[1]
Rx	**Pilocarpine hydrochloride** (Various, eg, Bausch & Lomb)	**Solution:** 0.5%	In 15 mL.
Rx	**Isopto Carpine** (PolyMedica)		In 15 and 30 mL.[1]
Rx	**Pilocarpine hydrochloride** (Various, eg, Alcon)	**Solution:** 1%	In 2 and 15 mL.
Rx	**Akarpine** (Akorn)		In 15 mL.
Rx	**Isopto Carpine** (Alcon)		In 15 mL.[1]
Rx	**Pilocarpine hydrochloride** (Various, eg, Alcon)	**Solution:** 2%	In 2 and 15 mL.
Rx	**Akarpine** (Akorn)		In 15 mL dropper bottles.
Rx	**Isopto Carpine** (Alcon)		In 15 mL.[1]
Rx	**Pilostat** (Bausch & Lomb)		In 15 mL and twin-pack (2 × 15 mL).[2]
Rx	**Pilocarpine hydrochloride** (Various, eg, Bausch & Lomb)	**Solution:** 3%	In 15 mL.
Rx	**Pilocar** (Novartis)		In 15 mL and twin-pack (2 × 15 mL).[3]
Rx	**Pilocarpine hydrochloride** (Various, eg, Alcon)	**Solution:** 4%	In 2 and 15 mL.
Rx	**Akarpine** (Akorn)		In 15 mL dropper bottles.
Rx	**Isopto Carpine** (Alcon)		In 15 mL.[1]
Rx	**Pilocar** (Novartis)		In 15 mL, twin-pack (2 × 15 mL) and 1 mL dropperettes.[3]
Rx	**Pilocarpine hydrochloride** (Various, eg, Bausch & Lomb)	**Solution:** 6%	In 15 mL.
Rx	**Isopto Carpine** (PolyMedica)	**Solution:** 10%	In 15 mL.[1]
Rx	**Pilopine HS** (Alcon)	**Gel:** 4%	In 4 g.[4]

[1] With 0.5% hydroxypropyl methylcellulose, 0.01% benzalkonium chloride.
[2] With hydroxypropyl methylcellulose, 0.01% benzalkonium chloride, EDTA.
[3] With hydroxypropyl methylcellulose, benzalkonium chloride, EDTA.
[4] With 0.008% benzalkonium chloride, carbopol 940, EDTA.

CHOLINESTERASE INHIBITORS

Actions:

Pharmacology: These indirect-acting agents inhibit the enzyme cholinesterase, potentiating the action of acetylcholine on the parasympathomimetic end organs. Topical application to the eye produces intense miosis and ciliary muscle contraction. IOP is reduced by a decreased resistance to aqueous outflow.

Cholinesterase inhibitors are subdivided into reversible and irreversible agents. Reversible agents (eg, physostigmine, demecarium) quickly combine with cholinesterase; the resulting complex is slowly hydrolyzed and the inhibited enzyme is regenerated. The demecarium-enzyme complex is hydrolyzed more slowly than the physostigmine complex; therefore, its duration of action is longer.

Irreversible agents (eg, echothiophate) also bind to cholinesterase; however, the resulting covalent bond is not hydrolyzed. Therefore, cholinesterase is not regenerated. More cholinesterase must be synthesized or supplied from depots elsewhere in the body before ophthalmic action dependent on cholinesterase returns. Echothiophate will depress both plasma and erythrocyte cholinesterase levels in most patients after a few weeks of eyedrop therapy.

These effects are accompanied by increased permeability of the blood-aqueous barrier and vasodilation. Myopia may be induced or, if present, may be augmented by the increased refractive power of the lens that results from the accommodative effect of the drug. Demecarium indirectly produces some of the muscarinic and nicotinic effects of acetylcholine as quantities of the latter accumulate.

Cholinesterase-Inhibiting Miotics

	Miosis		IOP reduction		
Miotics	Onset (minutes)	Duration	Onset (hours)	Peak (hours)	Duration
Reversible					
Physostigmine	20 to 30	12 to 36 hrs	—	2 to 6	12 to 36 hrs
Irreversible					
Echothiophate	10 to 30	1 to 4 weeks	4 to 8	24	7 to 28 days

Indications:

Glaucoma: Therapy of open-angle glaucoma.

For other specific indications, refer to the individual monographs.

Contraindications:

Hypersensitivity to cholinesterase inhibitors or any component of the formulation; active uveal inflammation or any inflammatory disease of the iris or ciliary body; glaucoma associated with iridocyclitis.

Echothiophate: Most cases of angle-closure glaucoma (because of the possibility of increasing angle-block).

Warnings:

Myasthenia gravis: Because of possible additive adverse effects, only administer demecarium and echothiophate with extreme caution to patients with myasthenia gravis who are receiving systemic anticholinesterase therapy. Conversely, exercise extreme caution in the use of anticholinesterase drugs for the treatment of myasthenia gravis patients who are already undergoing topical therapy with cholinesterase inhibitors.

Surgery: In patients receiving cholinesterase inhibitors, administer succinylcholine with extreme caution before and during general anesthesia (see Drug Interactions). Stop these drugs 4 to 6 weeks prior to ophthalmic surgery to avoid a severe inflammatory response.

Pregnancy: Category C (physostigmine, echothiophate). Safety for use during pregnancy has not been established. Use only when clearly needed and when the potential benefits to the mother outweigh the potential hazards to the fetus.

Lactation: It is not known whether these drugs are excreted in breast milk. Exercise caution when administering to a nursing woman. Because of the potential for serious adverse reactions in nursing infants, decide whether to discontinue nursing or the drug, taking into account the importance of the drug to the mother.

Children: The occurrence of iris cysts is more frequent in children (see Precautions). Exercise extreme caution in children receiving demecarium who may require general anesthesia. Safety and efficacy for use of physostigmine have not been established.

Precautions:

Concomitant therapy: Cholinesterase inhibitors may be used in combination with adrenergic agents, beta-blockers, carbonic anhydrase inhibitors, or hyperosmotic agents.

Narrow angle glaucoma: Use with caution in patients with chronic angle-closure (narrow-angle) glaucoma or in patients with narrow angles, because of the possibility of producing pupillary block and increasing angle blockage.

Ophthalmic ointments: Ophthalmic ointments may retard corneal healing.

Miosis: Miosis usually causes difficulty in dark adaptation. Use caution while driving at night or performing hazardous tasks in poor light.

Gonioscopy: Use only when shorter-acting miotics have proved inadequate. Gonioscopy is recommended prior to use of these medications. Routine examination (eg, slit-lamp) to detect lens opacities should accompany therapy.

Concomitant ocular conditions: When an intraocular inflammatory process is present, breakdown of the blood-aqueous barrier from anticholinesterase therapy requires abstention from, or cautious use of, these drugs. Use with great caution where there is a history of quiescent uveitis. After long-term use, blood vessel dilation and resultant greater permeability increase the possibility of hyphema or a severe inflammatory response during or after ophthalmic surgery. Discontinue 4 to 6 weeks before surgery.

Systemic effects: Repeated administration may cause depression of the concentration of cholinesterase in the serum and erythrocytes, with resultant systemic effects. Discontinue if salivation, urinary incontinence, diarrhea, profuse sweating, muscle weakness, respiratory difficulties, shock, or cardiac irregularities occur.

Although systemic effects are infrequent, use digital compression of the nasolacrimal ducts immediately before and for 2 minutes after instillation to minimize systemic absorption.

Iris cysts: Iris cysts may form, enlarge, and obscure vision (more frequent in children). The iris cyst usually shrinks upon discontinuation of the miotic, or following reduction in strength of the drops or frequency of instillation. Rarely, the cyst may rupture or break free into the aqueous humor. Frequent examination for this occurrence is advised.

Use caution in patients with marked vagotonia, bronchial asthma, spastic GI disturbances, peptic ulcer, pronounced bradycardia/hypotension, recent MI, epilepsy, parkinsonism, and other disorders that may respond adversely to vagotonic effects. Temporarily discontinue if cardiac irregularities occur.

Sulfite sensitivity: Some of these products contain sulfites, which may cause allergic-type reactions (eg, hives, itching, wheezing, anaphylaxis) in certain susceptible persons. Although the overall prevalence of sulfite sensitivity in the general population is probably low, it is seen more frequently in asthmatics or atopic nonasthmatics.

Drug Interactions:

Ophthalmic Cholinesterase Inhibitor Drug Interactions			
Precipitant drug	Object drug*		Description
Carbamate/ Organophosphate insecticides, pesticides	Cholinesterase inhibitors	↑	Warn patients on cholinesterase inhibitors who are exposed to these substances (eg, gardeners, organophosphate plant or warehouse workers, farmers) of systemic effects possible from absorption through respiratory tract or skin. Advise use of respiratory masks, frequent washing, and clothing changes.
Succinylcholine	Cholinesterase inhibitors	↑	Use extreme caution before or during general anesthesia in patients on cholinesterase inhibitors because of possible respiratory and cardiovascular collapse.
Anticholinesterases, systemic	Cholinesterase inhibitors	↑	Additive effects are possible; coadminister topical cholinesterase inhibitors cautiously, regardless of which therapy is added (see Warnings).

* ↑ = Object drug increased.

Adverse Reactions:

Ophthalmic: Iris cysts (see Precautions); burning; lacrimation; lid muscle twitching; conjunctival and ciliary redness; browache; headache; activation of latent iritis or uveitis; induced myopia with visual blurring; retinal detachment; lens opacities (see Precautions); conjunctival thickening and destruction of nasolacrimal canals (prolonged use).

Paradoxical increase in IOP by pupillary block may follow instillation.

Systemic: Nausea; vomiting; abdominal cramps; diarrhea; urinary incontinence; fainting; sweating; salivation; difficulty in breathing; cardiac irregularities.

Overdosage:

Treatment: Systemic effects can be reversed with atropine sulfate.

Adults – 0.4 to 0.6 mg.

Infants and children up to 12 years – 0.01 mg/kg repeated every 2 hours as needed until the desired effect is obtained, or adverse effects of atropine preclude further usage. The maximum single dose should not exceed 0.4 mg.

Much larger atropine doses for anticholinesterase intoxication in adults have been used. Initially, 2 to 6 mg followed by 2 mg/hr or more often, as long as muscarinic effects continue. Consider the greater possibility of atropinization with large doses, particularly in sensitive individuals.

Pralidoxime chloride (see Antidotes) has been useful in treating systemic effects caused by cholinesterase inhibitors. However, use in addition to, not as a substitute for, atropine.

A short-acting barbiturate is indicated for convulsions not relieved by atropine. Promptly treat marked weakness or paralysis of respiratory muscles by maintaining a clear airway and by artificial respiration.

Patient Information:

Local irritation and headache may occur at initiation of therapy.

Notify health care provider if abdominal cramps, diarrhea, or excessive salivation occurs.

Wash hands immediately after administration.

Use caution while driving at night or performing hazardous tasks in poor light.

Refer to the Dosage Forms and Routes of Administration chapter for more complete information.

Individual drug monographs are on the following pages.

ECHOTHIOPHATE IODIDE

For complete prescribing information, refer to the Miotics, Cholinesterase Inhibitors group monograph. The following section is included here for completeness to show all of the clinical uses of this class of drug.

Indications:

Glaucoma: Chronic open-angle glaucoma; if therapeutic goal is not achieved with direct-acting miotics, usually not useful in angle-closure glaucoma and most secondary glaucomas.

Accommodative esotropia: Concomitant esotropias with a significant accommodative component.

Administration and Dosage:

Tolerance may develop after prolonged use.

Glaucoma: 1 drop to eye(s) once or twice daily. Less frequent dosing can also produce the desired effect. Individualize dosage.

Concomitant therapy: May be coadministered with other glaucomal medication classes.

Accommodative esotropia:

> *Diagnosis* – Instill 1 drop of 0.125% solution once a day into both eyes at bedtime for 2 or 3 weeks. If the esotropia is accommodative, a favorable response may begin within a few hours.
>
> *Treatment* – Use the lowest concentration and frequency that gives satisfactory results. After initial period of treatment for diagnostic purposes, reduce schedule to 0.125% every other day or 0.06% every day. Dosages can often be gradually lowered as treatment progresses. The 0.03% strength has proven effective in some cases. The maximum recommended dose is 0.125% once a day, although more intensive therapy has been used for short periods.
>
> *Duration of treatment* – In diagnosis, only a short period is required and little time will be lost in instituting other procedures if the esotropia proves to be unresponsive. In therapy, there is no definite limit if the drug is well tolerated. However, if the eyedrops, with or without eyeglasses, are gradually withdrawn after 1 to 2 years and deviation recurs, consider surgery.

Storage/Stability: Store at room temperature 15° to 30°C (59° to 86°F). After reconstitution, keep eyedrops in refrigerator to obtain maximum useful life of 6 months. Use within 1 month if stored at room temperature.

Rx	**Phospholine Iodide** (Wyeth)	6.25 mg to make 0.125%	With 5 mL diluent.[1]

[1] With potassium acetate, 0.55% chlorobutanol, 1.2% mannitol.

CARBONIC ANHYDRASE INHIBITORS

Actions:

Pharmacology: These agents are nonbacteriostatic sulfonamides that inhibit the enzyme carbonic anhydrase. This action reduces the rate of aqueous humor formation, resulting in decreased IOP.

Pharmacokinetics:

Pharmacokinetics of Oral Carbonic Anhydrase Inhibitors

Carbonic anhydrase inhibitor	IOP Lowering Effects			Relative inhibitor potency
	Onset (hours)	Peak effect (hours)	Duration (hours)	
Acetazolamide				
Tablets	1 to 1.5	1 to 4	8 to 12	1
Capsules, sustained-release	2	3 to 6	18 to 24	
Injection (IV)	2 min	15 min	4 to 5	
Methazolamide	2 to 4	6 to 8	10 to 18	*

* Quantitative data not available; reported to be more active than acetazolamide.

Methazolamide – Peak plasma concentrations for the 25, 50, and 100 mg twice daily regimens were 2.5, 5.1, and 10.7 mcg/mL, respectively. Approximately 55% is bound to plasma proteins. The mean steady-state plasma elimination half-life is approximately 14 hours. At steady state, about 25% of the dose is recovered unchanged in the urine. Renal clearance accounts for 20% to 25% of the total clearance of drug. After repeated dosing, methazolamide accumulates to steady-state concentrations in 7 days.

Dorzolamide – When topically applied, dorzolamide reaches the systemic circulation. It binds moderately to plasma proteins (about 33%). The drug is primarily excreted unchanged in the urine, and the metabolite is also excreted in the urine.

After dosing is stopped, dorzolamide washes out of red blood cells (RBCs) nonlinearly, resulting in a rapid decline of drug concentration initially, followed by a slower elimination phase with a half-life of approximately 4 months.

Indications:

The following section is included here for completeness to show all of the clinical uses of this class of drug.

Oral: For adjunctive treatment of glaucoma.

Ophthalmic: Treatment of elevated IOP in patients with ocular hypertension or open-angle glaucoma.

Dorzolamide: Only indicated to decrease IOP in patients with ocular hypertension or open-angle glaucoma.

Contraindications:

Hypersensitivity to these agents; depressed sodium or potassium serum levels; marked kidney and liver disease or dysfunction; suprarenal gland failure; hyperchloremic acidosis; adrenocortical insufficiency; severe pulmonary obstruction with inability to increase alveolar ventilation because acidosis may be increased (dichlorphenamide); cirrhosis (acetazolamide, methazolamide).

Warnings:

Renal function impairment: Dorzolamide has not been studied in patients with severe renal impairment (Ccr less than 30 mL/min). However, because dorzolamide and its metabolite are excreted predominantly by the kidney, dorzolamide is not recommended in such patients.

Hepatic function impairment: Use of methazolamide in this condition could precipitate hepatic coma. Dorzolamide has not been studied in patients with hepatic impairment and should be used with caution in such patients.

Carcinogenesis:

> *Dorzolamide* – In a 2-year study of dorzolamide administered orally to rats, urinary bladder papillomas were seen in male rats in the highest dosage group of 20 mg/kg/day (250 times the recommended human ophthalmic dose). The increased incidence of urinary bladder papillomas is a class effect of carbonic anhydrase inhibitors in rats.

Pregnancy: Category C. Animal studies with some of these drugs have demonstrated teratogenicity (skeletal anomalies). Do not use during pregnancy, especially during the first trimester, unless the potential benefits to the mother outweigh the potential hazards to the fetus.

Lactation: Safety for use in the nursing mother has not been established. It is not known whether all carbonic anhydrase inhibitors are excreted in breast milk. Acetazolamide appeared in breast milk of a patient taking 500 mg twice/day. However, the infant ingested only 0.06% of the dose, an amount unlikely to cause adverse effects.

Children: Safety and efficacy have not been established.

Precautions:

Monitoring: Monitor for hematologic reactions common to sulfonamides.

Hypokalemia: During concomitant use of steroids or ACTH, and with interference with adequate oral electrolyte intake, hypokalemia may develop when severe cirrhosis is present. Hypokalemia can sensitize or exaggerate the response of the heart to the toxic effects of digitalis (eg, increased ventricular irritability). Hypokalemia may be avoided or treated with potassium supplements or foods with a high potassium content.

Pulmonary conditions: Use dichlorphenamide with caution in patients with severe degrees of respiratory acidosis. These drugs may precipitate or aggravate acidosis. Use with caution in patients with pulmonary obstruction or emphysema when alveolar ventilation may be impaired.

Cross-sensitivity: Cross-sensitivity between antibacterial sulfonamides and sulfonamide derivative diuretics, including acetazolamide and various thiazides, has occurred.

Corneal endothelium effects: The effect of continued administration of dorzolamide on the corneal endothelium has not been fully evaluated.

Ocular effects: Local ocular adverse effects, primarily conjunctivitis and lid reactions, occurred with chronic administration of dorzolamide. Many of these reactions had the clinical appearance and course of an allergic-type reaction that resolved upon discontinuation of drug therapy. If such reactions are observed, discontinue dorzolamide and evaluate the patient before considering restarting the drug.

Concomitant oral CA inhibitors: The coadministration of dorzolamide and oral CA inhibitors is not recommended.

Contact lenses: The preservative in dorzolamide solution, benzalkonium chloride, may be absorbed by soft contact lenses. Administer dorzolamide with this in mind.

Hazardous tasks: Carbonic anhydrase inhibitors may cause drowsiness in some patients. Observe caution while driving, operating machinery, or performing other tasks requiring coordination or physical dexterity.

Drug Interactions:

Carbonic Anhydrase Inhibitor (CAI) Drug Interactions			
Precipitant drug	Object drug*		Description
Acetazolamide	Cyclosporine	↑	Increased trough cyclosporine levels with possible nephrotoxicity and neurotoxicity may occur.
Acetazolamide	Primidone	↓	Primidone serum and urine concentrations may be decreased.
CAIs	Salicylates	↑	Concurrent use may result in accumulation and toxicity of the CAI, including CNS depression and metabolic acidosis. Also, CAI-induced acidosis may allow increased CNS penetration by salicylates.
Salicylates	CAIs	↑	
Diflunisal	CAIs	↑	Concurrent use may result in a significant decrease in IOP; the effect may be less pronounced with methazolamide. Increased side effects may also occur.

* ↑ = Object drug increased. ↓ = Object drug decreased.

Adverse Reactions:

Sulfonamide-type adverse reactions may occur.

Dorzolamide:

Miscellaneous – Ocular burning, stinging, or discomfort immediately following administration (approximately 33%); bitter taste following administration (approximately 25%); superficial punctate keratitis (10% to 15%); signs and symptoms of ocular allergic reaction (approximately 10%); blurred vision, tearing, dryness, photophobia (approximately 1% to 5%); urolithiasis, iridocyclitis (rare).

CNS: Convulsions; weakness; malaise; fatigue; nervousness; drowsiness; depression; dizziness; disorientation; confusion; ataxia; tremor; tinnitus; headache; lassitude; flaccid paralysis; paresthesias of the extremities.

Dermatologic: Urticaria; pruritus; skin eruptions; rash (including erythema multiforme, Stevens-Johnson syndrome, toxic epidermal necrolysis); photosensitivity.

GI: Melena; anorexia; nausea; vomiting; constipation; taste alteration; diarrhea.

Hematologic: Bone marrow depression; thrombocytopenia; thrombocytopenic purpura; hemolytic anemia; leukopenia; pancytopenia; agranulocytosis.

Renal: Hematuria; glycosuria; urinary frequency; renal colic; renal calculi; crystalluria; polyuria; phosphaturia.

Miscellaneous: Weight loss; fever; acidosis (usually corrected with bicarbonate); decreased/absent libido; impotence; electrolyte imbalance; hepatic insufficiency; transient myopia.

Overdosage:

Symptoms: Symptoms of overdosage or toxicity may include drowsiness, anorexia, nausea, vomiting, dizziness, paresthesias, ataxia, tremor, and tinnitus.

Treatment: In the event of overdosage, induce emesis or perform gastric lavage. The electrolyte disturbance most likely to be encountered from overdosage is hyperchloremic acidosis, which may respond to bicarbonate administration. Potassium supplementation may be required. Observe carefully; give supportive treatment.

Patient Information:

Oral: If GI upset occurs, take with food.

Avoid prolonged exposure to sunlight or sunlamps; may cause photosensitivity.

May cause drowsiness; observe caution while driving or performing other tasks requiring alertness, coordination, or physical dexterity.

Notify health care provider if sore throat, fever, unusual bleeding or bruising, tingling or tremors in the hands or feet, flank or loin pain, skin rash, or eye irritation occurs.

> *Bioavailability* – Consult health care provider before switching brands of carbonic anhydrase inhibitors. Problems with bioavailability have been documented with products from different manufacturers.

Ophthalmic: To avoid contamination, do not touch tip of container to any surface. Replace cap after use.

Advise patients that if they develop an intercurrent ocular condition (eg, trauma, ocular surgery, infection), they should immediately seek their health care provider's advice concerning the continued use of the present multidose container.

If more than one topical ophthalmic drug is being used, administer the drugs at least 10 minutes apart.

Dorzolamide should not be administered while wearing soft contact lenses.

Individual drug monographs are on the following pages.

ACETAZOLAMIDE

For complete prescribing information, see the Carbonic Anhydrase Inhibitors group monograph. The following section is included here for completeness to show all of the clinical uses of this class of drug.

Administration and Dosage:

To lower IOP:

Adults – 250 mg to 1 g/day, in divided doses every 6 to 12 hours. Dosage greater than 1 g/day does not usually increase the effect.

Secondary glaucoma and preoperative treatment of acute congestive (closed-angle) glaucoma:

Adults –

Short-term therapy: 250 mg every 4 hours or 250 mg twice daily.

Acute cases: 500 mg followed by 125 or 250 mg every 4 hours.

IV therapy may be used for rapid decreases of IOP. A complementary effect occurs when used with miotics or beta-blockers.

Children:

Parenteral – 5 to 10 mg/kg/dose, IM or IV, every 6 hours.

Oral – 10 to 15 mg/kg/day in divided doses, every 6 to 8 hours.

Sustained release: 500 mg twice daily.

Parenteral: Direct IV administration is preferred; IM administration is painful because of the alkaline pH of the solution.

Preparation and storage of parenteral solution: Reconstitute each 500 mg vial with at least 5 mL of sterile water for injection. Reconstituted solutions retain potency for 1 week if refrigerated. However, because this product contains no preservative, use within 24 hours of reconstitution.

Oral liquid dose form: If required, acetazolamide tablets may be crushed and suspended in a cherry, chocolate, raspberry, or other sweet syrup. Do not use a vehicle with alcohol or glycerin. Alternatively, 1 tablet can be submerged in 10 mL of hot water and added to 10 mL of honey or syrup. When prepared in a 70% sorbitol solution with a pH of 4 to 5 and stored in amber glass bottles, the suspension is stable for at least 2 to 3 months at temperatures colder than 30°C (86°F).

Rx	**Acetazolamide** (Various, eg, Mutual, URL)	**Tablets:** 125 mg	In 50s, 100s, 250s, 500s, and 1,000s.
Rx	**Diamox**		In 100s.
Rx	**Diamox**	**Tablets:** 250 mg	In 100s.
Rx	**Diamox Sequels** (Barr)	**Capsules, sustained release:** 500 mg	In 100s.

Rx	**Acetazolamide** (Various, eg, Bedford Labs)	**Powder for injection, lyophilized:** 500 mg (as sodium)	In 10 mL vials.
Rx	**Diamox** (Barr)		

BRINZOLAMIDE

Actions:

Pharmacology: Brinzolamide is an inhibitor of carbonic anhydrase II (CA-II); an enzyme found in many tissues of the body including the eye. It catalyzes the reversible reaction involving the hydration of carbon dioxide and the dehydration of carbonic acid. Inhibition of carbonic anhydrase in the ciliary processes of the eye decreases aqueous humor secretion, presumably by slowing the formation of bicarbonate ions with subsequent reduction in sodium and fluid transport. The result is a reduction in IOP.

Pharmacokinetics: Elevated IOP is a major risk factor in the pathogenesis of optic nerve damage and glaucomatous visual field loss. Following topical ocular administration, brinzolamide is absorbed into the systemic circulation.

Clinical Trials: In two, 3-month studies, brinzolamide 1% dosed 3 times per day in patients with elevated IOP, produced significant reductions in IOPs (4 to 5 mm Hg). These IOP reductions are equivalent to the reductions observed with dorzolamide hydrochloride ophthalmic solution 2% dosed 3 times daily in the same studies.

In 2 clinical studies with elevated IOP, brinzolamide was associated with less stinging and burning upon instillation than dorzolamide hydrochloride.

Indications:

For the treatment of elevated IOP in patients with ocular hypertension or open-angle glaucoma.

Contraindications:

Hypersensitivity to any component of this product.

Warnings:

Systemic effects: Brinzolamide is a sulfonamide and, although administered topically, it is absorbed systemically. Therefore, the same types of adverse reactions that are attributed to sulfonamides may occur with the topical administration of brinzolamide. Fatalities have occurred, although rarely, because of severe reactions to sulfonamides including Stevens-Johnson syndrome, toxic epidermal necrolysis, fulminant hepatic necrosis, agranulocytosis, aplastic anemia, and other blood dyscrasias. Sensitization may occur when a sulfonamide is readministered irrespective of the route of administration. If signs of serious reactions or hypersensitivity occur, discontinue the use of this preparation.

Carcinogenesis: Carcinogenicity data on brinzolamide is not available.

Mutagenesis: The following tests for mutagenic potential were negative: (1) in vivo mouse micronucleus assay; (2) in vivo sister chromatid exchange assay; and (3) Ames

E. coli test. The in vitro mouse lymphoma forward mutation assay was negative in the absence of activation, but positive in the presence of microsomal activation.

Fertility impairment: In reproductive studies of brinzolamide in rats, there were no adverse effects on the fertility or reproductive capacity of males or females at doses up to 18 mg/kg/day (375 times the recommended human ophthalmic dose).

Pregnancy: Category C. Developmental toxicity studies with brinzolamide in rabbits at oral doses of 1, 3, and 6 mg/kg/day (20, 62, and 125 times the recommended human ophthalmic dose) produced maternal toxicity at 6 mg/kg/day and a significant increase in the number of fetal variations, such as skull bones, which was only slightly higher than the historic value at 1 and 6 mg/kg. There are no adequate and well-controlled studies in pregnant women. Brinzolamide should be used during pregnancy only if the potential benefit to the mother justifies the potential risk to the fetus.

Lactation: It is not known whether this drug is excreted in breast milk. Because of the potential for serious adverse reactions to the nursing infant, a decision should be made whether to discontinue the nursing or discontinue the drug, taking into account the importance of the drug to the mother.

Children: Safety and efficacy have not been established.

Precautions:

Corneal endothelium effects: Carbonic anhydrase activity has been observed in the cytoplasm and around the plasma membranes of the corneal endothelium. The effects of continued administration of brinzolamide on the corneal endothelium has not been fully evaluated.

Acute angle-closure glaucoma: The management of acute angle-closure glaucoma requires therapeutic interventions in addition to ocular hypotensive agents. Brinzolamide has not been studied in patients with acute-closure glaucoma.

Severe renal impairment: Brinzolamide has not been studied in patients with severe renal impairment. Because brinzolamide and its metabolite are excreted predominantly by the kidney, it is not recommended in these patients.

Oral carbonic anhydrase inhibitors: There is potential for an additive effect on the known systemic effects of carbonic anhydrase inhibitors and brinzolamide. The concomitant administration of brinzolamide and oral carbonic anhydrase inhibitors is not recommended.

Drug Interactions:

Although brinzolamide 1% is a carbonic anhydrase inhibitor, acid-base and electrolyte alterations were not reported in the clinical trials. However, in patients treated with oral carbonic anhydrase inhibitors, rare instances of drug interactions have occurred with high-dose salicylate therapy. Therefore, consider the potential for such drug interactions.

Adverse Reactions:

The most frequently reported adverse events associated with brinzolamide were blurred vision and bitter, sour, or unusual taste. These events occurred in about 5% to 10% of patients. Blepharitis, dermatitis, dry eye, foreign body sensation, headache, hyperemia, ocular discharge, keratitis, ocular pain, ocular pruritus, and rhinitis were reported at an incidence of 1% to 5%. The following adverse reactions were reported at an incidence of less than 1%: allergic reactions; alopecia; chest pain; conjunctivitis; diarrhea; diplopia; dizziness; dry mouth; dyspepsia; eye fatigue; hypertonia; keratoconjunctivitis; keratopathy; kidney pain; lid margin crusting or sticky sensation; nausea; pharyngitis; tearing; and urticaria.

Overdosage:

Symptoms: Although there is no human data available, electrolyte imbalance, development of an acidotic state, and possible nervous system effects may occur following oral administration of an overdose. Serum electrolyte levels (particularly potassium) and blood pH levels should be monitored.

Patient Information:

Vision may be temporarily blurred following dosing with brinzolamide. Exercise care in operating machinery or driving a motor vehicle.

Instruct patients to avoid allowing the tip of the dispensing container to contact the eye or surrounding structures or surfaces, because the product can become contaminated by common bacteria known to cause ocular infections.

Advise patients to immediately seek their health care provider's advice concerning the continued use of the present multidose container if they have ocular surgery or develop an intercurrent ocular condition (eg, trauma, infection).

Administration and Dosage:

Shake well before use. Instill 1 drop in the affected eye(s) 3 times daily.

Concurrent therapy: Brinzolamide may be used concurrently with other ophthalmic drug products to lower IOP. If more than one topical ophthalmic drug is being used, the drugs should be administered at least 10 minutes apart.

Rx	**Azopt** (Alcon)	**Suspension:** 1%	In 2.5, 5, 10, and 15 mL plastic *Drop-Tainer* bottles with controlled dispensing tip.

DORZOLAMIDE HYDROCHLORIDE

Actions:

Pharmacology: Dorzolamide is a carbonic anhydrase inhibitor formulated for topical ophthalmic use. Carbonic anhydrase (CA) is an enzyme found in many tissues of the body, including the eye. It catalyzes the reversible reaction involving the hydration of carbon dioxide and the dehydration of carbonic acid. In humans, carbonic anhydrase exists as a number of isoenzymes, the most active being carbonic anhydrase II (CA-II), found primarily in RBCs, but also in other tissues. Inhibition of CA in the ciliary processes of the eye decreases aqueous humor secretion, presumably by slowing the formation of bicarbonate ions with subsequent reduction in sodium and fluid transport. The result is a reduction in IOP. Dorzolamide, by inhibiting CA-II, reduces elevated IOP. Elevated IOP is a major risk factor in the pathogenesis of optic nerve damage and glaucomatous visual field loss.

Pharmacokinetics: When topically applied, dorzolamide reaches the systemic circulation. To assess the potential for systemic CA inhibition following topical administration, drug and metabolite concentrations in RBCs and plasma and CA inhibition in RBCs were measured. Dorzolamide accumulates in RBCs, during chronic dosing as a result of binding to CA-II. The parent drug forms a single N-desethyl metabolite that inhibits CA-II less potently than the parent drug but also inhibits CA-I. The metabolite also accumulates in RBCs, where it binds primarily to CA-I. Plasma concentrations of parent and metabolite are generally below the assay limit of quantitation. Dorzolamide binds moderately to plasma proteins (approximately 33%). The drug is primarily excreted unchanged in the urine, and the metabolite is also excreted in urine. After dosing is stopped, dorzolamide washes out of RBCs nonlinearly, resulting in a rapid decline of drug concentration initially, followed by a slower elimination phase with a half-life of approximately 4 months.

To simulate the systemic exposure after long-term topical ocular administration, dorzolamide was given orally to 8 healthy subjects for up to 20 weeks. The oral dose of 2 mg twice daily closely approximates the amount of drug delivered by topical ocular administration of 2% three times daily. Steady-state was reached within 8 weeks. The inhibition of CA-II and total CA activities was below the degree of inhibition anticipated to be necessary for a pharmacological effect on renal function and respiration in healthy individuals.

Clinical Trials: The efficacy of dorzolamide was demonstrated in clinical studies in the treatment of elevated IOP in patients with glaucoma or ocular hypertension (baseline IOP at least 23 mm Hg). The IOP-lowering effect of dorzolamide was approximately 3 to 5 mm Hg throughout the day, and this was consistent in clinical studies with durations of up to 1 year.

Indications:

Elevated IOP: Treatment of elevated IOP in patients with ocular hypertension or open-angle glaucoma.

Contraindications:

Hypersensitivity to any component of this product.

Warnings:

Systemic effects: Dorzolamide is a sulfonamide and, although administered topically, is absorbed systemically. Therefore, the same types of adverse reactions attributable to sulfonamides may occur with topical administration of dorzolamide. Fatalities have occurred, although rarely, because of severe reactions to sulfonamides including Stevens-Johnson syndrome, toxic epidermal necrolysis, fulminant hepatic necrosis, agranulocytosis, aplastic anemia, and other blood dyscrasias. Sensitization may recur when a sulfonamide is readministered, regardless of the route of administration. If signs of serious reactions or hypersensitivity occur, discontinue the use of this preparation.

Renal/Hepatic function impairment: Dorzolamide has not been studied in patients with severe renal impairment (Ccr less than 30 mL/min). However, because dorzolamide and its metabolite are excreted predominantly by the kidney, dorzolamide is not recommended in such patients.

Dorzolamide has not been studied in patients with hepatic impairment and should be used with caution in such patients.

Carcinogenesis: In a 2 year study of dorzolamide administered orally to male and female Sprague-Dawley rats, urinary bladder papillomas were seen in male rats in the highest dosage group of 20 mg/kg/day (250 times the recommended human ophthalmic dose); papillomas were not seen in rats given oral doses equivalent to approximately 12 times the recommended dose. The increased incidence of urinary bladder papillomas is a class effect of CA inhibitors in rats.

Elderly: Of all the patients in clinical studies, 44% were at least 65 years of age and 10% were at least 75 years of age. No overall differences in efficacy or safety were observed between these patients and younger patients, but greater sensitivity of some older individuals to the product cannot be ruled out.

Pregnancy: Category C. Studies in rabbits at oral doses of at least 2.5 mg/kg/day (31 times the recommended human ophthalmic dose) revealed malformations of the vertebral bodies. These malformations occurred at doses that caused metabolic acidosis with decreased body weight gain in dams and decreased fetal weights. There are no adequate and well-controlled studies in pregnant women. Use during pregnancy only if the potential benefit to the mother justifies the risk to the fetus.

Lactation: In lactating rats, decreases in body weight gain of 5% to 7% were seen in offspring at an oral dose of 7.5 mg/kg/day (94 times the recommended human ophthalmic dose). A slight delay in postnatal development (eg, incisor eruption, vaginal canalization, eye openings), secondary to lower fetal body weight, was noted.

It is not known whether this drug is excreted in breast milk. Because of the potential for serious adverse reactions in nursing infants, decide whether to discontinue nursing or to discontinue the drug, taking into account the importance of the drug to the mother.

Children: Safety and IOP-lowering effects of *Trusopt* have been demonstrated in pediatric patients in a 3-month, multi-center, double masked, active-treatment-controlled trial.

Precautions:

Corneal endothelium effects: The effect of continued administration of dorzolamide on the corneal endothelium has not been fully evaluated.

Ocular effects: Local ocular adverse effects, primarily conjunctivitis and lid reactions, were reported with chronic administration of dorzolamide. Many of these reactions had the clinical appearance and course of an allergic-type reaction that resolved upon discontinuation of drug therapy. If such reactions are observed, discontinue dorzolamide and evaluate the patient before considering restarting the drug.

Concomitant oral CA inhibitors: The concomitant administration of dorzolamide and oral CA inhibitors is not recommended.

Contact lenses: The preservative in dorzolamide solution, benzalkonium chloride, may be absorbed by soft contact lenses. Dorzolamide should not be administered while wearing soft contact lenses.

Corneal decompensation: Cases of corneal decompensation from dorzolamide have been reported in patients undergoing corneal transplants.

Drug Interactions:

Although acid-base and electrolyte disturbances were not reported in the clinical trials with dorzolamide, these disturbances have occurred with oral CA inhibitors and have, in some instances, resulted in drug interactions (eg, toxicity associated with high-dose salicylate therapy). Therefore, consider the potential for such drug interactions in patients receiving dorzolamide.

Adverse Reactions:

Ocular burning, stinging, or discomfort immediately following administration (approximately 33%); bitter taste following administration (approximately 25%); superficial punctate keratitis (10% to 15%); signs and symptoms of ocular allergic reaction (approximately 10%); blurred vision, tearing, dryness, photophobia (approximately 1% to 5%); headache, nausea, asthenia/fatigue (infrequent); skin rashes, urolithiasis, iridocyclitis (rare).

Overdosage:

Electrolyte imbalance, development of an acidotic state, and possible CNS effects may occur. Monitor serum electrolyte levels (particularly potassium) and blood pH levels. Significant lethality was observed in female rats and mice after single oral doses of 1,927 and 1,320 mg/kg, respectively.

Patient Information:

Dorzolamide is a sulfonamide and, although administered topically, it is absorbed systemically. Therefore, the same types of adverse reactions that are attributable to sulfonamides may occur with topical administration. Advise patients that if serious or unusual reactions or signs of hypersensitivity occur, they should discontinue use of the product.

Advise patients that if they develop any ocular reactions, particularly conjunctivitis and lid reactions, they should discontinue use and seek their health care provider's advice.

Instruct patients to avoid allowing the tip of the dispensing container to contact the eye or surrounding structures. Ocular solutions, if handled improperly or if the tip of the dispensing container contacts the eye or surrounding structures, can become contaminated by common bacteria known to cause ocular infections. Serious damage to the eye and subsequent loss of vision may result from using contaminated solutions.

Advise patients that if they develop an intercurrent ocular condition (eg, trauma, ocular surgery, infection), they should immediately seek their health care provider's advice concerning the continued use of the present multidose container.

If more than one topical ophthalmic drug is being used, administer the drugs 5 to 10 minutes apart with the drugs with sustained-release vehicles such as *Pilopine HS*, *Timoptic XE*, and *Betoptic S* administered last.

Administration and Dosage:

Dosage: Instill 1 drop in the affected eye(s) 3 times daily; twice daily when used concomitantly with a beta-blocker.

Concomitant therapy: Dorzolamide may be used concomitantly with other topical ophthalmic drug products to lower IOP. If more than 1 ophthalmic drug is being used, administer the drugs 5 minutes apart. Can be used twice daily with beta-blocker or other aqueous-secretion inhibitor.

Rx	**Trusopt** (Merck)	**Solution:** 2%	In 5 and 10 mL.[1]

[1] 0.0075% benzalkonium Cl.

METHAZOLAMIDE

For complete prescribing information, refer to the Carbonic Anhydrase Inhibitors group monograph.

Administration and Dosage:

Glaucoma: 25 to 100 mg 2 or 3 times daily. May be used with glaucoma agents from other classes.

Rx	**Methazolamide** (Various, eg, Teva)	**Tablets:** 25 mg	In 100s and 1,000s.
Rx	**GlaucTabs** (Akorn)		In 100s.
Rx	**Methazolamide** (Various, eg, Teva)	**Tablets:** 50 mg	In 100s and 1,000s.
Rx	**GlaucTabs** (Akorn)		In 100s.

PROSTAGLANDINS AND PROSTAMIDES

BIMATOPROST

Actions:

Pharmacology: Bimatoprost is a synthetic prostamide structural analog with ocular hypotensive activity. It selectively mimics the effects of naturally occurring substances, prostamides. Bimatoprost is believed to lower IOP in humans by increasing outflow of aqueous humor through the trabecular meshwork and uveoscleral routes.

Pharmacokinetics: Bimatoprost was administered once daily to both eyes of healthy subjects for 2 weeks with peak blood concentrations within 10 minutes and below the lower limit of detection (0.025 ng/mL) within 1.5 hours. Steady-state levels were reached during the first week of ocular dosing. There was no significant systemic drug accumulation over time.

Bimatoprost is moderately distributed into body tissues with a steady-state volume of distribution of 0.67 L/kg. In human blood, bimatoprost resides mainly in the plasma. Approximately 12% of bimatoprost remains unbound in human plasma.

Clinical Trials: In clinical studies of patients with open angle glaucoma or ocular hypertension, bimatoprost once daily at bedtime reduced a mean baseline IOP of 26 mm Hg by 7 to 8 mm Hg. Bimatoprost once daily at bedtime was compared with timolol 0.5% twice daily in 2 randomized, double-masked trials. Bimatoprost reduced IOP 33%

vs 23% for timolol and provided at least 2.5 mm Hg greater IOP reduction at all time points out to month 6. Of patients using bimatoprost, 64% reached a low IOP of at most 17 mm Hg vs 37% with timolol.

Indications:

For the reduction of elevated IOP in patients with open angle glaucoma or ocular hypertension who are intolerant of other IOP-lowering medications or insufficiently responsive (failed to achieve target IOP determined after multiple measurements over time) to another IOP-lowering medication. Bimatoprost has not been evaluated for the treatment of angle closure, inflammatory, or neovascular glaucoma.

Contraindications:

Hypersensitivity to bimatoprost or any other ingredient of this product.

Warnings:

Ocular changes: Bimatoprost has been reported to cause changes to pigmented tissues. The most frequently reported changes have been increased pigmentation of the iris and periorbital tissue (eyelid) and increased pigmentation and growth of eyelashes. These changes may be permanent.

Eyelid skin darkening has been reported in association with the use of bimatoprost.

Bimatoprost may gradually change eyelashes in the treated eye; these changes include increased length, thickness, pigmentation, or number of lashes.

Inform patients who are expected to receive treatment in only 1 eye about the potential for increased brown pigmentation of the iris, periorbital, or eyelid tissue, and eyelashes in the treated eye and thus heterochromia between the eyes. Advise them of the potential for a disparity between the eyes in length, thickness, or number of eyelashes.

Pregnancy: Category C. There are no adequate and well controlled studies of bimatoprost administration in pregnant women. Bimatoprost was not mutagenic or clastogenic in the Ames test in the mouse lymphoma test or in the in vivo mouse micronucleus tests.

Lactation: It is not known whether bimatoprost is excreted in human milk, although in animal studies, bimatoprost has been shown to be excreted in breast milk. Because many drugs are excreted in human milk, exercise caution when bimatoprost is administered to a nursing woman.

Children: Safety and efficacy not established.

Precautions:

Bacterial keratitis: There have been reports of bacterial keratitis associated with the use of multiple-dose containers of topical ophthalmic products. These containers had been inadvertently contaminated by patients who, in most cases, had a concurrent corneal disease or a disruption of the ocular epithelial surface.

Active intraocular inflammation: Use bimatoprost with caution in patients with active intraocular inflammation (eg, uveitis).

Macular edema: Macular edema, including cystoid macular edema, has been reported during treatment with bimatoprost ophthalmic solution. Use bimatoprost with caution in aphakic patients, in pseudophakic patients with a torn posterior lens capsule, or in patients with known risk factors for macular edema.

Contact lenses: Do not administer bimatoprost while wearing contact lenses. Remove contact lenses prior to instillation of bimatoprost; lenses may be reinserted 15 minutes after bimatoprost administration. Advise patients that bimatoprost contains benzalkonium chloride, which may be absorbed by soft contact lenses.

Adverse Reactions:

In clinical trials, the most frequent events associated with the use of bimatoprost occurring in approximately 15% to 45% of patients included conjunctival hyperemia, growth of eyelashes, and ocular pruritus. Approximately 3% of patients discontinued therapy caused by conjunctival hyperemia.

Ophthalmic: Adverse events that occurred in approximately 3% to 10% of patients included the following: Ocular dryness, visual disturbances, ocular burning, foreign body sensation, eye pain, pigmentation of the periocular skin, blepharitis, cataract, superficial punctate keratitis, eyelid erythema, ocular irritation, and eyelash darkening. The following ocular adverse events were reported in approximately 1% to 3% of patients: Eye discharge, tearing, photophobia, allergic conjunctivitis, asthenopia, increases in iris pigmentation, and conjunctival edema. In fewer than 1% of patients, intraocular inflammation was reported as iritis.

Systemic: Systemic adverse events reported in approximately 10% of patients were infectious (primarily colds and upper respiratory tract infections). The following systemic adverse events were reported in about 1% to 5% of patients included headaches, abnormal liver function tests, asthenia, and hirsutism.

Patient Information:

Inform patients that bimatoprost may cause increased growth and darkening of eyelashes and darkening of the skin around the eye in some patients. Some patients may slowly develop darkening of the iris. These changes may be permanent.

Remove contact lenses prior to instillation of bimatoprost; lenses may be reinserted 15 minutes after bimatoprost administration. Advise patients that bimatoprost contains benzalkonium chloride, which may be absorbed by soft contact lenses.

Administration and Dosage:

The recommended dosage is 1 drop in the affected eye(s) once daily in the evening. The dosage should not exceed once daily because it has been shown that more frequent administration does not increase the IOP-lowering effect.

Reduction of IOP starts approximately 4 hours after the first administration with maximum effect reached within about 8 to 12 hours.

Bimatoprost may be used concomitantly with other topical ophthalmic drug products to lower IOP. If more than 1 topical drug is being used, administer the drugs at least 5 minutes apart.

Storage/Stability: Store in the original container at 15° to 25°C (59° to 77°F).

Rx	**Lumigan** (Allergan)	**Solution:** 0.03%	In 2.5, 5, and 7.5 mL.[1]

[1] 0.05 mg benzalkonium chloride/mL.

LATANOPROST

Actions:

Pharmacology: Latanoprost is a prostanoid-selective FP receptor agonist for ophthalmic use. It is believed to reduce IOP by increasing the outflow of aqueous humor. Studies in animals and humans suggest that increased uveoscleral outflow is the main mechanism of action.

Pharmacokinetics: Latanoprost is absorbed through the cornea where the isopropyl ester prodrug is hydrolyzed to the acid form to become biologically active. Studies indicate that peak concentration in the aqueous humor is reached about 2 hours after topical administration. The distribution volume in humans is 0.16 ± 0.02 L/kg. The acid of latanoprost could be measured in aqueous humor during the first 4 hours, and in plasma only during the first hour after local administration. Latanoprost is primarily metabolized by the liver with excretion by renal pathway. Approximately 88% and 98% of the dose is recovered in the urine after topical and intravenous dosing, respectively.

> *Animal studies* – Latanoprost was shown to induce increased pigmentation of the iris in monkeys. The increased pigmentation is unlikely to be associated with proliferation of melanocytes and is believed to be caused by the stimulation of melanin production in melanocytes of the iris stroma. Doses of 4 times the daily human dose in cynomolgus monkeys demonstrated increased palpebral fissure. This effect has been reversible and occurred at doses above the standard clinical dose level.

Clinical Trials: Patients with a mean baseline IOP of 24 to 25 treated with *Xalatan* 0.005% for 6 months demonstrated 6 to 8 mm Hg reductions in IOP. This was equivalent to the effect of timolol 0.5% twice daily.

Indications:

To lower IOP in patients with open-angle glaucoma and ocular hypertension.

Contraindications:

Hypersensitivity to latanoprost, benzalkonium chloride, or any other ingredient in the product.

Warnings:

Eye color change: Latanoprost may gradually change eye color by increasing the amount of brown pigmentation in the iris. This is caused by increasing the number of melanosomes (pigment granules) in melanocytes. The long term effects of this are currently unknown.

The color change occurs slowly and over a long period of time. Inform patients of the possibility of an increasing brown color in the eye. In patients receiving treatment in only one eye, heterochromia may occur between the eyes. The change in pigmentation may be permanent.

Renal/Hepatic function impairment: Use with caution in patients with renal or hepatic impairment as this drug has not been studied in these patients.

Carcinogenesis: Latanoprost was not carcinogenic in bacteria, mouse lymphoma, or mouse micronucleus tests or when mice and rats were given doses up to 2,800 times the recommended human dose for 20 and 24 months, respectively.

Mutagenesis: Unscheduled DNA synthesis was negative in rats, both in vivo and in vitro.

Fertility impairment: Latanoprost was not found to have any effect on fertility in animal studies. Chromosome aberrations were observed in vitro with human lymphocytes.

Pregnancy: Category C. In rabbits receiving 80 times the maximum human dose, 4 of 16 females had no viable fetuses, with the highest nonembryocidal dose approximately 15 times the maximum human dose. There are no adequate and well-controlled studies in pregnant women. Use during pregnancy only if the potential benefit to the mother justifies the potential risk to the fetus.

Lactation: It is not known whether latanoprost or its metabolites is excreted in breast milk. Because many drugs are excreted in human milk, exercise caution when administering to a nursing woman.

Children: Safety and efficacy have not been established.

Precautions:

Cornea: Latanoprost is hydrolyzed in the cornea. The effect of continued administration of latanoprost on the corneal endothelium has not been fully evaluated.

Bacterial keratitis: There have been reports of bacterial keratitis with the use of multidose containers or topical ophthalmic products because of the contamination of the containers by patients with concurrent corneal disease or a disruption of the ocular epithelial surface.

Brown pigmentation: Patients may develop increased brown pigmentation in the iris over several months to years. Usually, the brown pigmentation spreads toward the periphery of the affected eye, but the entire iris or parts of it may also become more brownish. Examine patients regularly. Treatment may be stopped if increased pigmentation occurs, depending upon the clinical situation. The increase in brown iris pigment did not progress further upon stopping treatment in clinical trials; however, the color change may be permanent. Freckles and nevi of the iris did not appear to be affected by treatment.

Uveitis: Until further study, significant, previous bouts of uveitis are relative contraindications for the use of this drug.

Cystoid Macular Edema (CME): Previous bouts of CME are relative contraindications for the use of this drug.

Contact lenses: Do not administer latanoprost while wearing contact lenses.

Other conditions: There is no experience in the use of latanoprost for angle closure, inflammatory, or neovascular glaucoma, and only limited experience in pseudophakic patients.

Drug Interactions:

In vitro studies have shown that precipitation occurs when eyedrops containing thimerosal are mixed with latanoprost. If using these drugs concurrently, allow at least 5 minutes between applications.

Adverse Reactions:

Ophthalmic: Blurred vision, burning and stinging, conjunctival hyperemia, foreign body sensation, itching, increased pigmentation of iris, punctate epithelial keratopathy (5% to 15%); dry eye, excessive tearing, eye pain, lid crusting, lid edema, lid erythema, lid discomfort/pain, photophobia (1% to 4%); conjunctivitis, diplopia, discharge from eye (less than 1%). Eye lash changes (increased length, thickness, pigmentation, and number of lashes). The following events occurred extremely rarely: Retinal artery embolus, retinal detachment, and vitreous hemorrhage from diabetic retinopathy.

Local conjunctival hyperemia occurred; however, less than 1% of patients discontinued therapy because of intolerance.

Systemic: Upper respiratory tract infection, cold, flu (about 4%); muscle, joint, back, and chest pain, angina pectoris, rash, allergic skin reaction (1% to 2%).

Overdosage:

Symptoms: Ocular irritation and conjunctival or episcleral hyperemia are the only ocular side effects of a latanoprost overdose. Transient bronchoconstriction has occurred in monkeys receiving large doses intravenously. However, no bronchoconstriction was induced in 11 patients with bronchial asthma receiving latanoprost. No adverse reactions were observed in healthy volunteers receiving 3 mcg/kg infused intravenously, but mean plasma concentrations were 200 times higher than during clinical ocular topical treatment. IV dosages of 5.5 to 10 mcg/kg caused abdominal pain, dizziness, fatigue, hot flushes, nausea, and sweating.

Treatment: Treat latanoprost overdosage symptomatically.

Patient Information:

The color of the iris can change because of an increase of the brown pigment. If only one eye is treated, a cosmetically different eye coloration may occur. Iris pigmentation changes may be more noticeable in patients with green-brown, blue/gray-brown, or yellow-brown irises.

Do not allow the dispensing container to touch the eye or surrounding structures to avoid contracting an eye infection from the resultant contamination of common bacteria. Serious damage to the eye and subsequent loss of vision can occur from using contaminated containers.

Patients should contact their health care provider concerning the continued use of the multidose container if they experience any eye trauma or infection or have ocular surgery.

Patients should contact their health care provider if they experience any ocular side effects, especially conjunctivitis and lid reactions.

Latanoprost contains benzalkonium chloride, which may be absorbed by contact lenses. Remove contact lenses prior to administering the latanoprost solution. Lenses can be reinserted 15 minutes after latanoprost administration.

If using more than 1 topical ophthalmic drug, administer drugs at least 5 minutes apart.

Administration and Dosage:

Administer 1 drop in the affected eye(s) once daily. Do not administer this medicine more frequently than once daily.

Reduction of IOP begins approximately 3 to 4 hours after administration, with the maximum effect reached after 8 to 12 hours. Preliminary data suggest that maximal effect is not achieved in some patients for weeks or months.

Latanoprost may be used with other topical ophthalmic products to lower IOP. If using more than one topical ophthalmic drug, administer the drugs at least 5 minutes apart.

Storage/Stability: Protect from light. Refrigerate until dispensed. During shipment, may be maintained at temperatures up to 40°C (104°F) for no longer than 8 days. Opened container may be stored at room temperature up to 25°C (77°F) for 6 weeks.

Rx	**Xalatan** (Pharmacia)	**Solution:** 0.005%	In 2.5 mL plastic ophthalmic dispenser bottle with dropper tip and 2.5 mL Multi-pack (3 × 2.5 mL).[1]

[1] With 0.02% benzalkonium chloride, sodium chloride, sodium dihydrogen phosphate monohydrate, disodium hydrogen phosphate anhydrous.

TRAVOPROST

Actions:

Pharmacology: Travoprost free acid is a selective FP prostanoid receptor agonist, which is believed to reduce IOP by increasing uveoscleral outflow. The exact mechanism of action is unknown.

Pharmacokinetics: Travoprost is absorbed through the cornea as an isopropyl ester prodrug and is hydrolyzed by esterases in the cornea to its biologically active free acid. In humans, peak plasma concentrations of travoprost free acid (25 pg/mL or less) were reached within 30 minutes following topical ocular administration and were rapidly eliminated. Systemically, travoprost free acid is metabolized to inactive metabolites. Elimination as travoprost free acid from human plasma is rapid. Plasma levels are below the limit of quantitation (less than 10 pg/mL) within 1 hour following ocular instillation.

Clinical Trials: Glaucoma or ocular hypertension patients with baseline pressure IOP of 25 to 27 mm Hg were dosed once daily in the evening and demonstrated 7 to 8 mm Hg reductions in IOP. In subgroup analyses, mean IOP reduction in black patients was up to 1.8 mm Hg greater than in non-black patients. It is not known at this time whether this difference is attributed to race or to heavily pigmented irides. In a multi-center, randomized, controlled trial, patients with mean baseline IOP of 24 to

26 mm Hg on timolol 0.5% twice daily were treated with travoprost 0.004% dosed every day adjunctively to timolol 0.5% twice daily demonstrated 6 to 7 mm Hg reductions in IOP.

Indications:

For the reduction of IOP in patients with open-angle glaucoma or ocular hypertension who are intolerant of other IOP-lowering medications or insufficiently responsive (failed to achieve target IOP determined after multiple measurements over time) to another IOP-lowering medication. Travoprost has not been evaluated for the treatment of angle closure, inflammatory, or neovascular glaucoma.

Contraindications:

Known hypersensitivity to travoprost, benzalkonium chloride, or any other ingredients of the product. Travoprost may interfere with the maintenance of pregnancy and should not be used by women during pregnancy or by women attempting to become pregnant.

Warnings:

Ocular changes: Travoprost has been reported to cause changes to pigmented tissues. The most frequently reported changes have been increased pigmentation of the iris and periorbital tissue (eyelid) and increased pigmentation and growth of eyelashes. These changes may be permanent.

Mutagenesis: Travoprost was not mutagenic in the Ames test, mouse micronucleus test, and rat chromosome assay. A slight increase in the mutant frequency was observed in 1 of 2 mouse lymphoma assays in the presence of rat S-9 activation enzymes.

Fertility impairment: Travoprost did not affect mating or fertility indices in male or female rats at SC doses up to 10 mcg/kg/day (250 times the maximum recommended human ocular dose [MRHOD] of 0.04 mcg/kg/day on a mcg/kg basis). At 10 mcg/kg/day, the mean number of corpora lutea was reduced, and the post-implantation losses were increased. These effects were not observed at 3 mcg/kg/day (75 times the MRHOD).

Elderly: No overall differences in safety or effectiveness have been observed between elderly and other adult patients.

Pregnancy: Category C. Because prostaglandins are biologically active and may be absorbed through the skin, women who are pregnant or attempting to become pregnant should exercise appropriate precautions to avoid direct exposure to the contents of the bottle. In case of accidental contact with the contents of the bottle, thoroughly cleanse the exposed area with soap and water immediately.

Travoprost was teratogenic in rats, at an IV dose up to 10 mcg/kg/day (250 times the MRHOD), evidenced by an increase in the incidence of skeletal malformations as well as external and visceral malformations, such as fused sternebrae, domed head, and hydrocephaly. Travoprost was not teratogenic in rats at IV doses up to 3 mcg/kg/day (75 times the MRHOD), and in mice at SC doses up to 1 mcg/kg/day (25 times the MRHOD). Travoprost produced an increase in post-implantation losses and a decrease in fetal viability in rats at IV doses greater than 3 mcg/kg/day (75 times the MRHOD) and in mice at SC doses more than 0.3 mcg/kg/day (7.5 times the MRHOD). In the offspring of female rats that received travoprost SC from day 7 of pregnancy to lactation day 21 at doses of at least 0.12 mcg/kg/day (3 times the MRHOD), the incidence of postnatal mortality was increased, and neonatal body weight gain was decreased. Neonatal development was also affected, evidenced by delayed eye opening, pinna detachment, and preputial separation, and by decreased motor activity.

No adequate and well-controlled studies have been performed in pregnant women. Travoprost may interfere with the maintenance of pregnancy and should not be used by women during pregnancy or by women attempting to become pregnant.

Lactation: A study in lactating rats demonstrated that radiolabeled travoprost or its metabolites were excreted in milk. It is not known whether this drug or its metabolites are excreted in human milk. Because many drugs are excreted in human milk, exercise caution when travoprost is administered to a nursing woman.

Children: Safety and efficacy not established.

Precautions:

Cornea: Reports of bacterial keratitis have been associated with the use of multiple-dose containers of topical ophthalmic products. These containers had been inadvertently contaminated by patients, who, in most cases, had a concurrent corneal disease or a disruption of the epithelial surface.

Iris pigmentation: Patients may slowly develop increased brown pigmentation of the iris. This change may not be noticeable for months to years (see Warnings). Iris pigmentation changes may be more noticeable in patients with mixed colored irdies (ie, blue-brown, grey-brown, yellow-brown, green-brown); however, it has also been observed in patients with brown eyes. The color change is believed to be caused by increased melanin content in the stromal melanocytes of the iris. The exact mechanism of action is unknown at this time. Typically, the brown pigmentation around the pupil spreads concentrically towards the periphery in affected eyes, but the entire iris or parts of it may become more brownish. Until more information about increased brown pigmentation is available, examine patients regularly and, depending on the situation, treatment may be stopped if increased pigmentation ensues.

Iritis/Uveitis: Use with caution in patients with active intraocular inflammation.

Macular edema: Macular edema, including cystoid macular edema, has been reported during treatment with prostaglandin $F_{2\alpha}$ analogs. These reports have mainly occurred in aphakic patients, pseudophakic patients with a torn posterior lens capsule, or in patients with known risk factors for macular edema. Use travoprost with caution in these patients.

Contact lenses: Travoprost should not be administered while wearing contact lenses. Advise patients that travoprost contains benzalkonium chloride, which may be absorbed by the contact lenses. Remove contact lenses prior to the administration of the solution. Lenses may be reinserted 15 minutes following travoprost administration.

Adverse Reactions:

Ophthalmic: The most common ocular adverse event observed in controlled clinical studies with travoprost was ocular hyperemia, which was reported in 35% to 50% of patients. Approximately 3% of patients discontinued therapy because of conjunctival hyperemia.

Ocular adverse events reported at an incidence of 5% to 10% included decreased visual acuity, eye discomfort, foreign body sensation, pain, and pruritus.

Ocular adverse events reported at an incidence of 1% to 4% included abnormal vision, blepharitis, blurred vision, cataract, cells, conjunctivitis, dry eye, eye disorder, flare, iris discoloration, keratitis, lid margin crusting, photophobia, subconjunctival hemorrhage, and tearing.

Systemic: Nonocular adverse events reported at a rate of 1% to 5% were the following: Accidental injury, angina pectoris, anxiety, arthritis, back pain, bradycardia, bronchitis, chest pain, cold syndrome, depression, dyspepsia, GI disorder, headache, hypercholesterolemia, hypertension, hypotension, infection, pain, prostate disorder, sinusitis, urinary incontinence, and urinary tract infection.

Patient Information:

Patients should be advised concerning all the information contained in the Warnings and Precautions sections.

Instruct patients to avoid allowing the tip of the dispensing container to contact the eye or surrounding structures because this could cause the tip to become contaminated by common bacteria known to cause ocular infections. Serious damage to the eye and subsequent loss of vision may result from using contaminated solutions.

Advise patients that if they develop an intercurrent ocular condition (eg, trauma, infection) or have ocular surgery, they should immediately seek their health care provider's advice concerning the continued use of the multi-dose container.

Advise patients that if they develop any ocular reactions, particularly conjunctivitis and lid reactions, they should immediately seek their health care provider's advice.

If more than 1 topical ophthalmic drug is being used, administer the drugs at least 5 minutes apart.

Administration and Dosage:

The recommended dosage is 1 drop in the affected eye(s) once daily in the evening. The travoprost dosage should not exceed once daily.

Reduction of IOP starts approximately 2 hours after administration, and the maximum effect is reached after 12 hours.

Travoprost may be used concomitantly with other topical ophthalmic drugs to lower IOP. If more than 1 topical ophthalmic drugs is being used, the drugs should be administered at least 5 minutes apart.

Storage/Stability: Store between 2° to 25°C (36° to 77°F).

Rx	**Travatan** (Alcon)	**Solution:** 0.004%	In 2.5 mL *Drop-Tainers* and twin-pack (5 mL).[1]
Rx	**Travatan Z** (Alcon)		In 2.5 and 5 mL *Drop-Tainers.*[2]

[1] 0.015% benzalkonium chloride, EDTA.

[2] Polyoxyl 40 hydrogenated castor oil, *sofZia* (boric acid, propylene glycol, sorbitol, zinc chloride) as a preservative.

UNOPROSTONE ISOPROPYL

Actions:

Pharmacology: Unoprostone is a prostaglandin $F_{2\alpha}$ analog that is believed to reduce elevated IOP by increasing the outflow of aqueous humor, but the exact mechanism is unknown.

Pharmacokinetics:

Absorption – Unoprostone is absorbed through the cornea and conjunctival epithelium, where it is hydrolyzed by esterases to unoprostone-free acid. The systemic exposure of its metabolite unoprostone-free acid was minimal following the ocular administration.

Excretion – Elimination of unoprostone-free acid from human plasma is rapid, with a half-life of 14 minutes. Plasma levels of unoprostone-free acid dropped below the lower limit of quantitation (less than 0.25 ng/mL) 1 hour following ocular instillation. The metabolites are excreted predominantly in the urine.

Clinical Trials: In patients with mean baseline IOP of 23 mm Hg, unoprostone lowers IOP by approximately 3 to 4 mm Hg throughout the day. Unoprostone appears to lower IOP without affecting cardiovascular or pulmonary function.

Indications:

For the lowering of IOP in patients with open-angle glaucoma or ocular hypertension who are intolerant of other IOP-lowering medications or insufficiently responsive (failed to achieve target IOP determined after multiple measurements over time) to another IOP-lowering medication.

Contraindications:

Known hypersensitivity to unoprostone isopropyl, benzalkonium chloride, or any other ingredients of the product.

Warnings:

Ocular changes: Unoprostone has been reported to cause changes in pigmented tissue. These changes may be permanent.

It may gradually change eye color, increasing the amount of brown pigment in the iris. The long-term effects and consequences of potential injury to the eye are currently unknown. The change in iris color occurs slowly and may not be noticeable for months to several years. Inform patients of the possibility of iris color change.

Carcinogenesis: Unoprostone was not carcinogenic in rats administered oral doses up to 12 mg/kg/day for up to 2 years (approximately 580- and 240-fold the recommended human dose).

Pregnancy: Category C. There are no adequate and well-controlled studies in pregnant women. Because animal studies are not always predictive of human response, use unoprostone during pregnancy only if the potential benefit to the mother justifies the potential risk to the fetus.

Lactation: It is not known whether topical ocular administration could result in sufficient systemic absorption to produce detectable quantities in breast milk. Nevertheless, exercise caution when unoprostone is administered to a nursing mother.

Children: Safety and efficacy not established.

Precautions:

Bacterial keratitis: There have been reports of bacterial keratitis associated with the use of multiple-dose containers of topical ophthalmic products. These containers had been inadvertently contaminated by patients who, in most cases, had a concurrent corneal disease or a disruption of the ocular epithelial surface.

Active intraocular inflammation: Use unoprostone with caution in patients with active intraocular inflammation (eg, uveitis).

Contact lenses: Do not administer unoprostone to patients while they are wearing contact lenses. Advise patients that unoprostone contains benzalkonium chloride, which may be absorbed by contact lenses. Remove contact lenses prior to administration of the solution. Lenses may be reinserted 15 minutes following unoprostone administration.

Adverse Reactions:

Ophthalmic: The most common ocular adverse events were burning/stinging upon drug instillation, dry eyes, itching, increased length of eyelashes, and infection. These were reported in about 10% to 25% of patients. Approximately 10% to 14% of patients were observed to have an increase in the length of eyelashes (at least 1 mm) at 12 months, while 7% of patients were observed to have a decrease in the length of eyelashes.

Ocular adverse events occurring in approximately 5% to 10% of patients were abnormal vision, eyelid disorder, foreign body sensation, and lacrimation disorder.

Ocular adverse events occurring in about 1% to 5% of patients were blepharitis, cataract, conjunctivitis, corneal lesion, discharge from the eye, eye hemorrhage, eye pain, keratitis, irritation, photophobia, and vitreous disorder.

Other ocular adverse events reported in fewer than 1% of patients were acute elevated IOP, color blindness, corneal deposits, corneal edema, corneal opacity, diplopia, hyperpigmentation of the eyelid, increased number of eyelashes, iris hyperpigmentation, iritis, optic atrophy, ptosis, retinal hemorrhage, and visual field effect.

Systemic: Flu syndrome (approximately 6%); accidental injury, allergic reaction, back pain, bronchitis, cough increased, diabetes mellitus, dizziness, headache, hypertension, insomnia, pharyngitis, pain, rhinitis, sinusitis (1% to 5%).

Overdosage:

If overdosage occurs, treatment should be symptomatic.

There is no published information available regarding overdosage with unoprostone. The risk of adverse effects caused by accidental oral ingestion is very low because the amount of active ingredient in each bottle is limited (7.5 mg in a 5 mL vial). Accidental ingestion of a vial by a child with 30 kg body weight will amount to a 0.25 mg/kg body weight.

Patient Information:

Instruct patients to avoid allowing the tip of the dispensing container to contact the eye or surrounding structures because this could cause the tip to become contaminated by common bacteria known to cause ocular infections. Serious damage to the eye and subsequent loss of vision may result from using contaminated solutions.

Advise patients that if they develop an intercurrent ocular condition (eg, trauma, infection) or have ocular surgery, they should immediately seek their health care provider's advice concerning the continued use of the multidose container.

Advise patients that if they develop any ocular reactions, particularly conjunctivitis and eyelid reaction, they should immediately seek their health care provider's advise.

If more than 1 topical ophthalmic drug is being used, administer the drugs at least 5 minutes apart.

Administration and Dosage:

The recommended dosage is 1 drop in the affected eye(s) twice daily. Unoprostone may be used concomitantly with other topical ophthalmic drug products to lower IOP. If 2 drugs are used, administer at least 5 minutes apart.

Storage/Stability: Store between 2° to 25°C (36° to 77°F).

Rx	**Rescula** (Novartis)	**Solution:** 0.15%	In 5 mL.[1]

[1] 0.015% benzalkonium chloride, EDTA, sodium hydroxide, hydrochloric acid.

CARBONIC ANHYDRASE INHIBITOR/BETA-ADRENERGIC BLOCKING AGENT

DORZOLAMIDE HYDROCHLORIDE-TIMOLOL MALEATE

Actions:

Pharmacology: Comprised of 2 components, dorzolamide hydrochloride-timolol maleate decreases elevated IOP, whether associated with glaucoma, by reducing aqueous humor secretion. Elevated IOP is a major risk factor in the pathogenesis of optic nerve damage and glaucomatous visual field loss. The higher the level of IOP, the greater the likelihood glaucomatous field loss and optic nerve damage. Dorzolamide hydrochloride is an inhibitor of human carbonic anhydrase II. Timolol maleate is a beta-1/beta-2 (non-selective) adrenergic receptor blocking agent that does not have significant intrinsic sympathomimetic, direct myocardial depressant, or local anesthetic (membrane-stabilizing) activity. The combined effect of these 2 agents results in additional IOP reduction compared with either component administered alone, but the reduction is not as great when each are administered concomitantly.

Pharmacokinetics: Dorzolamide and timolol reach the systemic circulation when applied topically.

Dorzolamide accumulates in RBCs and is primarily excreted unchanged in the urine. Topical administration approximates an oral dose of 2 mg twice daily. Steady state is achieved in approximately 8 weeks.

Timolol topical administration attains a mean peak plasma concentration following morning dosing of 0.46 ng/mL.

Indications:

For the reduction of elevated IOP in patients with open-angle glaucoma or ocular hypertension who are insufficiently responsive to beta-blockers (failed to achieve target IOP determined after multiple measurements over time).

Contraindications:

Hypersensitivity to any component of this product; bronchial asthma or history of bronchial asthma; severe chronic obstructive pulmonary disease; sinus bradycardia; second or third degree atrioventricular block; overt cardiac failure; cardiogenic shock.

Warnings:

Systemic exposure: Although administered topically, dorzolamide hydrochloride-timolol maleate is absorbed systemically. Therefore, severe reactions could occur because of the sulfonamide, dorzolamide (eg, allergic, hematologic, hepatic). In addition, severe respiratory reactions and cardiac reactions, including death caused by bronchospasm in patients with asthma, and rarely death in association with cardiac failure, have been reported following systemic or ophthalmic administration of timolol maleate. Refer to complete monographs on these agents for thorough descriptions.

Cardiac failure: Sympathetic stimulation may be essential for support of the circulation in individuals with diminished myocardial contractility and its inhibition by beta adrenergic receptor blockade may precipitate more severe failure. Even in patients without a history of cardiac failure, continued myocardial depression with beta-blocking agents can, in some cases, lead to cardiac failure. At the first sign or symptom of cardiac failure, discontinue use.

Obstructive pulmonary disease: Patients with chronic obstructive pulmonary disease (eg, chronic bronchitis, emphysema) of mild to moderate severity, bronchospastic disease, or a history of bronchospastic disease should generally not receive beta-blocking agents.

Major surgery: Withdrawal of beta-adrenergic blocking agents prior to major surgery is controversial. Beta-adrenergic receptor blockade impairs the ability of the heart to respond to beta-adrenergically mediated reflex stimuli. This may augment the risk of general anesthesia in surgical procedures. Some patients receiving beta-adrenergic receptor blocking agents have experienced protracted severe hypotension during anesthesia. Difficulty in restarting and maintaining the heartbeat has also been reported. In patients undergoing elective surgery, some authorities recommend gradual withdrawal of beta-adrenergic receptor blocking agents. The anesthesiologist must be informed of this and any other drug therapy prior to surgery.

Diabetes mellitus: Administer beta-adrenergic blocking agents with caution in patients subject to spontaneous hypoglycemia or to diabetes (especially those with labile diabetes) who are receiving insulin or oral hypoglycemic agents. Beta-adrenergic receptor blocking agents may mask the signs and symptoms of acute hypoglycemia.

Thyrotoxicosis: Beta-adrenergic blocking agents may mask certain clinical signs (eg, tachycardia) of hyperthyroidism. Carefully manage patients suspected of developing thyrotoxicosis to avoid abrupt withdrawal of beta-adrenergic blocking agents that might precipitate a thyroid storm.

Pregnancy: Category C. This medication should only be used during pregnancy if the potential benefit to the mother justifies the potential risk to the fetus.

Lactation: It is not known if dorzolamide is excreted in human milk. Timolol maleate has been detected in human milk following oral and ophthalmic drug administration. Because of the potential for serious adverse reactions from this medicine in nursing infants, a decision should be made whether to discontinue nursing or to discontinue the drug, taking into account the importance of the drug to the mother.

Children: Safety and effectiveness have not been established.

Precautions:

Myasthenia gravis: Beta-adrenergic blockade has been reported to potentiate muscle weakness consistent with certain myasthenic symptoms (eg, diplopia, ptosis, generalized weakness). Timolol has been reported rarely to increase muscle weakness in some patients with myasthenia gravis or myasthenic symptoms.

Choroidal detachment: Choroidal detachment after filtration procedures has been reported with the administration of aqueous suppressant therapy (eg, timolol).

Bacterial keratitis: Bacterial keratitis is associated with the use of multidose containers of topical ophthalmic products. These containers have been inadvertently contaminated by patients who, in most cases, had a concurrent corneal disease or a disruption of the ocular epithelial surface.

Acid-based disturbances: Although acid-base and electrolyte disturbances were not reported in the clinical trials with dorzolamide hydrochloride ophthalmic solution, these disturbances have been reported with oral carbonic anhydrase inhibitors and have, in some instances, resulted in drug interactions (eg, toxicity associated with high-dose salicylate therapy). Consider the potential drug interactions in patients receiving this medicine.

Drug Interactions:

Ophthalmic Beta-Blocker Drug Interactions			
Precipitant drug	Object drug*		Description
Dorzolamide/ Timolol Maleate	Carbonic Anhydrase Inhibitors (oral)	↑	There is potential for an additive effect on the known systemic effects of carbonic anhydrase inhibition in patients receiving an oral carbonic anhydrase inhibitor and dorzolamide hydrochloride-timolol maleate. Concomitant administration is not recommended.
	Beta-adrenergic agents (oral)	↑	Observe patients who are receiving a beta-adrenergic blocking agent orally and dorzolamide hydrochloride-timolol maleate for potential additive effects of beta-blockade, both systemic and on IOP. Concomitant use is not recommended.
	Calcium antagonists	↔	Use caution in the coadministration of beta-adrenergic blocking agents and oral or intravenous calcium antagonists because of possible atrioventricular conduction disturbances, left ventricular failure, and hypotension. In patients with impaired cardiac function, avoid coadministration.
	Catecholamine-depleting drugs	↑	Close observation of the patient is recommended when a beta-blocker is administered to patients receiving catecholamine-depleting drugs, such as reserpine, because of possible additive effects, hypotension, or marked bradycardia, which may result in vertigo, syncope, or postural hypotension.
	Acid-base disturbances	↔	Although acid-base and electrolyte disturbances were not reported in the ophthalmic clinical trials, these disturbances have been reported with oral carbonic anhydrase inhibitors and have resulted in drug interactions (eg, toxicity associated with high-dose salicylate therapy). Consider potential drug interactions in patients receiving this medicine.

* ↑ = Object drug increased. ↔ = Undetermined effect.

Adverse Reactions:

Approximately 5% of 1035 patients discontinued therapy with this medicine because of adverse reactions. The most frequently reported adverse events were taste perversion (bitter, sour, unusual taste) or ocular burning or stinging in up to 30% of patients. Conjunctival hyperemia, blurred vision, superficial punctate keratitis, or eye itching were reported in 5% to 15% of patients.

The following adverse reactions were reported in 1% to 5% of patients:

CNS – Dizziness; headache.

GI – Abdominal pain; dyspepsia; nausea.

GU – Urinary tract infection.

Ophthalmic – Blepharitis; cloudy vision; conjunctival discharge; conjunctival edema; conjunctival follicles; conjunctival injection; conjunctivitis; corneal erosion; corneal staining; cortical lens opacity; dryness of eyes; eye debris; eye discharge; eye pain; eye tearing; eyelid edema; eyelid erythema; eyelid exudate/scales; eyelid pain or discomfort; foreign body sensation; glaucomatous cupping; lens nucleus coloration; lens opacity; nuclear lens opacity; post-subcapsular cataract; visual field defect; vitreous detachment.

Miscellaneous – Back pain; hypertension; influenza.

Respiratory – Bronchitis; cough; pharyngitis; sinusitis; upper respiratory tract infection.

Dorzolamide:

Dermatologic – Contact dermatitis.

Hypersensitivity – Signs and symptoms of systemic allergic reactions including angioedema; bronchospasm; pruritus; urticaria.

Special Senses – Signs and symptoms of ocular allergic reaction; transient myopia.

Miscellaneous – Asthenia/fatigue.

Timolol (ocular and oral administration):

Cardiovascular – Arrhythmia; syncope; heart block; cerebral ischemia; worsening of angina pectoris; palpitation; cardiac arrest; pulmonary edema; claudication; Raynaud's phenomenon; cold hands and feet; worsening of arterial insufficiency; vasodilation.

CNS – Increase in signs and symptoms of myasthenia gravis, somnolence, insomnia, nightmares, behavioral changes and psychic disturbances including confusion, hallucinations, anxiety, disorientation, nervousness, memory loss; vertigo; local weakness; diminished concentration; reversible mental depression progressing to catatonia, an acute reversible syndrome characterized by disorientation for time and place; emotional liability; slightly clouded sensorium; decreased performance on neuropsychometrics.

Dermatologic – Alopecia; psoriasiform rash or exacerbation of psoriasis; pruritus; skin irritation; increased pigmentation; sweating.

Endocrine – Hyperglycemia; hypoglycemia (masked symptoms of hypoglycemia in diabetic patients).

GI – Anorexia; gastrointestinal pain; hepatomegaly; mesenteric arterial thrombosis; ischemic colitis.

GU – Retroperitoneal fibrosis; decreased libido; impotence; Peyronie's disease; urination difficulties.

Hematologic – Nonthrombocytopenic purpura; thrombocytopenic purpura; agranulocytosis.

Hypersensitivity – Erythematous rash; fever combined with aching and sore throat; laryngospasm with respiratory distress; signs and symptoms of systemic allergic reactions including angioedema, urticaria, localized and generalized rash.

Immunologic – Systemic lupus erythematosus.

Musculoskeletal – Arthralgia.

Respiratory – Bronchial bronchospasm (predominantly in patients with preexisting bronchospastic disease); bronchial obstruction; rales; respiratory failure.

Special Senses – Ptosis; decreased corneal sensitivity; cystoid macular edema; visual disturbances including refractive changes and diplopia; pseudopemphigoid; choroidal detachment following filtration surgery; tinnitus.

Miscellaneous – Asthenia/fatigue; extremity pain; decreased exercise tolerance; weight loss.

Patient Information:

Advise patients with bronchial asthma, a history of bronchial asthma, severe chronic obstructive pulmonary disease, sinus bradycardia, second or third degree atrioventricular block, or cardiac failure not to take this product.

If any ocular reactions develop, particularly conjunctivitis and lid reaction, patients should discontinue use and seek their health care provider's advice.

Patients should inform their health care provider and anesthesiologist when undergoing surgery about this and any other drug therapy.

Avoid allowing the tip of the dispensing container to contact the eye or surrounding structures. If handled improperly or if the tip of the dispensing container contacts the eye or surrounding structures, it can become contaminated by common bacteria known to cause ocular infections. Serious damage to the eye and subsequent loss of vision may result from using contaminated solutions.

If patients have ocular surgery or develop an intercurrent ocular condition (eg, trauma, infection), they should immediately seek their health care provider's advice concerning the continued use of the present multidose container.

If more than 1 topical ophthalmic drug is being used, administer the drugs at least 10 minutes apart.

Dorzolamide hydrochloride-timolol maleate contains chloride, which may be absorbed by soft contact lenses. Contact lenses should be removed prior to administration of the solution. Lenses may be reinserted 15 minutes following administration.

Administration and Dosage:

Place 1 drop of dorzolamide hydrochloride-timolol maleate in the affected eye(s) 2 times daily.

If more than 1 topical ophthalmic drug is being used, administer the drugs at least 10 minutes apart.

Storage/Stability: Store between 15° and 25°C (59° to 77°F). Protect from light.

Rx	**Cosopt** (Merck)	**Solution**: 20 mg dorzolamide, 5 mg timolol per mL	In 5 and 10 mL dispenser with controlled drop tip.[1]

[1] With sodium citrate, hydroxyethyl cellulose, sodium hydroxide, mannitol. Benzalkonium chloride 0.0075% is added as a preservative.

Hyperosmotic Agents

Hyperosmotic agents (also referred to as osmotic agents) can be administered topically or intravenously to increase osmotic pressure of tears and plasma relative to that of the ocular structures. As a result of the osmotic gradient established, fluid moves from the eye to hyperosmotic tear fluid with topical instillation, or plasma of ocular blood vessels following intravenous administration.

TOPICAL AGENTS

The clinical objective of topical osmotherapy is to enhance the rate of fluid movement from the edematous cornea. When these agents are applied to the eye, water is drawn from the cornea to the hyperosmolal tear film and eliminated through the usual tear flow mechanisms.

Sodium chloride and glucose have proven useful for reducing corneal edema of various etiologies, including bullous keratopathy and Fuchs endothelial dystrophy.

Hypertonic solutions of sodium chloride or glucose can be useful for prolonged treatment of corneal edema. Sodium chloride appears less effective when the corneal epithelium is traumatized because of its increased ability to penetrate the epithelial barrier. Administer both sodium chloride and glucose at regular intervals for maximum clinical effect. Because vision is usually worse upon awakening, more frequent application during the first waking hours can be helpful.

SYSTEMIC AGENTS

Hyperosmotic agents administered intravenously are useful for initial management of acute angle-closure glaucoma and prior to intraocular surgery to reduce intraocular pressure (IOP).

Following intravenous administration, a relatively rapid increase in serum osmolarity can occur. Transfer of fluid from the eye to the circulation results in a decrease in IOP. Factors that determine the difference in osmotic pressure between the ocular fluids and plasma include the following:

- Molecular weight and concentration
- Dose administered
- Rate of absorption
- Distribution in body water
- Ocular penetration
- Rate of excretion
- Nature of diuresis

The integrity of the ocular tissues can also influence the osmotic effect. Inflammation may enhance ocular penetration and decrease the osmotic gradient, resulting in a reduction in the pressure-lowering effect of these agents.

Osmotic Diuretic Pharmacokinetics

Diuretic	Route	Onset (min)	Peak (hrs)	Duration (hrs)	Half-life	Metabolized (%)	Ocular penetration	Distribution
Mannitol	IV	30 to 60	1	6 to 8	15 to 100 minutes	7 to 10	very poor	E[1]
Urea	IV	30 to 45	1	5 to 6	N	N	good	TBW[2]

[1] E = extracellular water
[2] TBW = total body water

Mannitol (*Osmitrol*) is currently the hyperosmotic of choice for intravenous use. It is not absorbed from the gastrointestinal tract and is ineffective by the oral route. Intravenous administration can reduce IOP within 20 to 30 minutes. The effect can last 4 to 8 hours. Mannitol exhibits minimal cellular penetration, is not metabolized, and is excreted in the urine. Therefore, it can be used in diabetic patients, but administered with caution in patients with renal disease. Because mannitol is confined to the extracellular fluid, dehydration and a profound diuresis can result following administration.

For More Information

Bartlett JD, Jaanus SD, eds. *Clinical Ocular Pharmacology,* 5th ed. St. Louis, MO: Elsevier; 2008.

Becker B, et al. Hyperosmotic agents. In: Leopold IE, ed. *Symposium in Ocular Therapy.* St. Louis, MO: C.V. Mosby Co.; 1968.

Lambert DW. Topical hyperosmotic agents and secretory stimulants. *Am J Ophthalmol.* 1980;20:163.

Luxenberg MN, Green K. Reduction of corneal edema with topical hypertonic agents. *Am J Ophthalmol.* 1970;9:418.

GLUCOSE, TOPICAL

Indications:

Corneal edema: Topical osmotherapy for reducing corneal edema.

Contraindications:

Hypersensitivity to any component of the product.

Precautions:

Irritation: If irritation develops, discontinue use.

Administration and Dosage:

May be used 2 to 6 times daily.

Depress lower lid with index finger while looking upward. Introduce a small amount of ointment behind depressed eyelid into conjunctival sac. Close and open eyes 2 times. Wipe off excess ointment. If eyelids are sticky, clean them before each application with a pledget of cotton and lukewarm boiled water.

MANNITOL

Actions:

Pharmacology: Mannitol is a nonelectrolyte osmotic diuretic that is pharmacologically inert.

IV mannitol is confined to the extracellular space. Only small amounts are metabolized. Mannitol is readily diffused through the glomeruli. Approximately 80% of a 100 g dose will appear in the urine in 3 hours, with lesser amounts thereafter. Even at peak concentrations, mannitol will exhibit less than 10% of tubular reabsorption and is not secreted by tubular cells. Mannitol will hinder tubular reabsorption of water and enhance excretion of sodium and chloride by elevating the osmolarity of the glomerular filtrate.

This increase in extracellular osmolarity affected by the IV administration of mannitol will induce the movement of intracellular water to the extracellular and vascular spaces. This action underlies the role of mannitol in reducing intracranial pressure, intracranial edema, and elevated IOP.

Indications:

Reduction of elevated IOP when the pressure cannot be lowered by other means.

Contraindications:

Anuria caused by severe renal disease; severe pulmonary congestion or frank pulmonary edema; active intracranial bleeding except during craniotomy; severe dehydration; progressive renal damage or dysfunction after instituting mannitol therapy, including increasing oliguria and azotemia; progressive heart failure or pulmonary congestion after mannitol therapy.

Warnings:

Fluid and electrolyte imbalance: By sustaining diuresis, mannitol may obscure and intensify inadequate hydration or hypovolemia. Excessive loss of water and electrolytes may lead to serious imbalances. Loss of water in excess of electrolytes can cause hypernatremia. Shift of sodium free intracellular fluid into the extracellular compartment following mannitol infusion may lower serum sodium concentration and aggravate preexisting hyponatremia. Also, movement of potassium ions from intracellular to extracellular space may cause hyperkalemia. Electrolyte measurements, including sodium and potassium, are therefore of vital importance in monitoring mannitol infusion.

Renal function impairment: Use a test dose (see Administration and Dosage); try a second test dose if there is an inadequate response, but do not attempt more than 2 test doses.

If urine output continues to decline during infusion, closely review the patient's clinical status and suspend mannitol infusion, if necessary. Accumulation of mannitol may result in overexpansion of the extracellular fluid, which may intensify existing or latent CHF.

Osmotic nephrosis, a reversible vacuolization of the tubules of unknown clinical significance, may proceed to severe irreversible nephrosis; monitor renal function closely.

Pregnancy: Category C. It is not known whether mannitol can cause fetal harm when administered to a pregnant woman or can affect reproduction capacity. Give to a pregnant woman only if clearly needed.

Lactation: It is not known whether this drug is excreted in breast milk; exercise caution when administering to a nursing woman.

Children: Safety and efficacy for patients 12 years of age and younger have not been established.

Precautions:

CHF: Carefully evaluate cardiovascular status before rapid administration of mannitol because sudden expansion of the extracellular fluid may lead to fulminating CHF.

Hypovolemia: By sustaining diuresis, mannitol may obscure and intensify inadequate hydration or hypovolemia.

Pseudoagglutination: Do not give electrolyte free mannitol solutions with blood. If blood is given simultaneously, add at least 20 mEq of sodium chloride to each liter of mannitol solution to avoid pseudoagglutination.

Hemoconcentration: The obligatory diuretic response following rapid infusion of 15%, 20%, or 25% mannitol may further aggravate preexisting hemoconcentration.

Adverse Reactions:

Cardiovascular: Edema; thrombophlebitis; hypotension; hypertension; tachycardia; angina-like chest pains; CHF.

CNS: Headache; blurred vision; convulsions; dizziness.

GI: Nausea; vomiting; diarrhea.

Metabolic: Fluid and electrolyte imbalance; acidosis; electrolyte loss; dehydration.

Renal: Urinary retention; osmotic nephrosis.

Miscellaneous: Pulmonary congestion; dry mouth; thirst; rhinitis; local pain; skin necrosis; chills; urticaria; fever.

Overdosage:

Symptoms: Larger than recommended doses may result in increased electrolyte excretion, particularly sodium, chloride, and potassium. Sodium depletion can result in orthostatic tachycardia or hypotension and decreased central venous pressure. Chloride metabolism closely follows that of sodium. Potassium deficit can impair neuromuscular function and cause intestinal dilation and ileus. If urine flow is inadequate, pulmonary edema or water intoxication may occur. Other symptoms include hypotension, polyuria that rapidly converts to oliguria, stupor, convulsions, hyperosmolality, and hyponatremia.

Treatment: Discontinue infusion immediately. Institute supportive measures to correct fluid and electrolyte imbalances. Hemodialysis is beneficial to clear mannitol and reduce serum osmolality.

Administration and Dosage:

Reduction of IOP: 1.5 to 2 g/kg, as a 20% solution (7.5 to 10 mL/kg) or as a 15% solution (10 to 13 mL/kg) over a period as short as 30 minutes. When used preoperatively, administer 1 to 1.5 hours before surgery to achieve maximal effect.

Preparation of solution: When exposed to low temperatures, mannitol solution may crystallize. Concentrations more than 15% have a greater tendency to crystallize. If crystals are observed, warm the bottle in a hot water bath, a dry heat oven, or autoclave, then cool to at or below body temperature before administering.

When infusing concentrated mannitol, the administration set should include a filter.

Rx	**Osmitrol Viaflex** (Clintec)	**Injection**: 5%	In 1,000 mL.
Rx	**Osmitrol Viaflex** (Clintec)	**Injection**: 10%	In 500 and 1,000 mL.
Rx	**Osmitrol Viaflex** (Clintec)	**Injection**: 15%	In 500 mL.
Rx	**Mannitol** (Various, eg, Astra)	**Injection**: 20%	In 250 and 500 mL.
Rx	**Osmitrol Viaflex** (Clintec)		In 250 and 500 mL.

SODIUM CHLORIDE, HYPERTONIC

Actions:

Pharmacology: A hypertonic (hyperosmolar) solution exerts an osmotic gradient greater than that present in body tissues and fluids, so that water is drawn from body tissues and fluids across semipermeable membranes. Applied topically to the eye, a hypertonicity agent creates an osmotic gradient that draws water out of the cornea.

Indications:

Corneal edema: Temporary relief.

Contraindications:

Hypersensitivity to any component of the product.

Adverse Reactions:

May cause temporary burning and irritation upon instillation.

Patient Information:

To avoid contamination, do not touch tip of container to any surface. Replace cap after using.

Do not use this product except under the advice and supervision of a health care provider. If you experience eye pain, changes in vision, continued redness or irritation of the eye, or if the condition worsens or persists, discontinue use and consult a health care provider.

Product may cause temporary burning and irritation when instilled into the eye.

Do not use if solution changes color or becomes cloudy.

Administration and Dosage:

Solution: Instill 1 or 2 drops in affected eye(s) every 3 or 4 hours, or as directed.

Ointment: Pull down lower eyelid of the affected eye(s) and apply a small amount (approximately 0.25 inch) of ointment to the inside of the affected eye(s) every 3 or 4 hours, or as directed.

Storage/Stability: Store at 8° to 30°C (46° to 86°F). Keep tightly closed. Protect from light.

otc	**Muro 128** (Bausch & Lomb)	**Solution:** 2%	In 15 mL.[1]
otc	**AK-NaCl** (Akorn)	**Solution:** 5%	In 15 mL.[2]
otc	**Muro 128** (Bausch & Lomb)		In 15 and 30 mL.[3]
otc	**Sochlor** (OCuSOFT)		In 15 mL.[2]

otc	**AK-NaCl** (Akorn)	**Ointment:** 5%	Preservative free. In 3.5 g.[4]
otc	**Muro 128** (Bausch & Lomb)		In 3.5 g single and twin packs.[5]
otc	**Sochlor** (OCuSOFT)		In 3.5 g. [4]

[1] With hydroxypropylmethylcellulose 2910, 0.028% methylparaben, 0.012% propylparaben, propylene glycol, boric acid.
[2] With hydroxypropyl methylcellulose 2906, propylene glycol, 0.023% methylparaben, 0.01% propylparaben, boric acid.
[3] Boric acid, hydroxypropyl methylcellulose 2910, propylene glycol, 0.023% methylparaben, 0.01% propylparaben.
[4] With mineral oil, white petrolatum, lanolin oil.
[5] With mineral oil, white petrolatum, lanolin.

Surgical Adjuncts

Irrigating solutions, viscoelastic agents, botulinum toxin type A, absorbable gelatin film, processed pericardium, trypan blue, and proteolytic enzymes are adjuncts to a variety of ophthalmologic procedures and surgeries.

INTRAOCULAR IRRIGATING SOLUTIONS

Irrigating solutions are aqueous solutions used to cleanse and to maintain moisture of ocular tissue. Ideally these solutions are isotonic. The optimum pH is 7.4. A pH less than 7 or more than 8 has caused cellular stress and cellular death when the tissues have been exposed for a prolonged period of time.

The commercially available intraocular irrigating solutions (eg, *BSS, BSS Plus*) are used during ocular surgery to protect the lens, corneal endothelium, and other ocular tissues. Unlike physiological saline and Lactated Ringer's solution, these balanced salt solutions provide the ions magnesium and calcium as cellular nutrients. These nutrients are required for intercellular and intracellular function during prolonged ocular surgery. In addition to magnesium and calcium, bicarbonate, glucose, and glutathione are in these perfusion media (*BSS Plus*). These components help to maintain a deturgesced or thin cornea by avoiding corneal swelling.

For information on extraocular irrigating solutions, see the Miscellaneous Products chapter.

POVIDONE IODINE

An antimicrobial agent effective against a wide range of organisms, povidone iodine has become an important prophylactic adjunct to ophthalmic surgery. This agent is formulated for topical ophthalmic use on the skin of the eyelids and adnexal tissues. The ophthalmic preparation is commonly used to prep the periocular tissues (eyelids, brow, cheek) and to irrigate the ocular surface (cornea, conjunctiva, and fornices).

VISCOELASTIC AGENTS

Viscoelastic agents, sodium hyaluronate, and hydroxypropyl methylcellulose, are used in many ophthalmic surgical procedures, including intraocular lens implantation and keratoplasty. In surgical procedures in the anterior segment of the eye, instillation maintains a deep anterior chamber, allowing for more efficient manipulation with less trauma to the corneal endothelium and surrounding tissues. The viscoelasticity of these agents helps push back the vitreous face and prevent formation of a postoperative flat chamber. The majority of the viscoelastic material is removed from the eye at the end of surgery to diminish the problems of glaucoma.

Viscoelastic agents are tissue-protective substances and do not interfere with normal wound healing. They are nonantigenic and do not contain proteins that may cause inflammation or foreign body reactions.

ABSORBABLE GELATIN FILM

In the dry state, absorbable gelatin film has the appearance and texture of cellophane. When moistened, it assumes a rubbery consistency and can be cut to desired size and shape and fitted to rounded or irregular surfaces.

It is used in many surgical procedures, including glaucoma filtration operations (eg, iridencleisis, trephination), extraocular muscle surgery, and diathermy or scleral "buckling" operations for retinal detachment to aid in preventing formation of adhesions between contiguous ocular structures.

Absence of undue tissue reaction and absorption of gelatin film, with consequent decreased likelihood of developing adhesions, have been found to be of particular value in dural and ocular implants.

NON-PROCESSED AMNIOTIC MEMBRANE

Amniotic membrane is provided as a substrate to facilitate epithelial resurfacing of the cornea and sclera. It is a useful adjunct to limbal stem cell transplantation, chemical injury resurfacing, pterygium removal, corneal ulcers, symblepharon repair, and eyelid reconstruction.

PROCESSED PERICARDIUM

Processed pericardium (*Tutoplast*) is a solvent dehydrated, gamma-irradiated preserved human pericardium. It is indicated for implantation with a specific spectrum of indications. Collagenous connective tissue with multidirectional fibers retains the mechanical strength and elasticity of native pericardium, while providing the basic formative structure to support replacement by new endogenous tissue. This tissue is indicated for use in a variety of surgical applications, including duraplasty (as a substitute for human dura mater), and in abdominal, urological, ophthalmological, and vascular surgery.

INTRAOCULAR ACETYLCHOLINE AND CARBACHOL

Both acetylcholine and carbachol are available for intracameral use to produce complete and rapid miosis following intraocular surgery. Because carbachol is a potent miotic, the intracameral formulation is considerably less concentrated than the solutions prepared for topical use. Intracameral carbachol is available as a 0.01% sterile balanced salt solution with no preservatives and is supplied in a 1.5 mL sterile glass disposable vial. The dose is 0.5 mL applied by gentle irrigation. Acetylcholine is available as a 1:100 solution when reconstituted in a dual chamber vial. The dose is generally 0.5 to 2 mL. Patients treated with intracameral carbachol after phacoemulsification and posterior chamber lens implantation often demonstrate lower IOP during the first postoperative day.

POLYDIMETHYLSILOXANE

Polydimethylsiloxane (silicone oil) is used by retinal surgeons to produce retinal tamponade in selected cases of retinal detachment. This agent is injected directly into the vitreous space in cases of complicated retinal detachment, such as may occur in patients with proliferative vitreoretinopathy, proliferative diabetic retinopathy, cytomegalovirus (CMV) retinitis, giant retinal tears, and following perforating injuries. Silicone oil can also be used as primary therapy in detachments associated with AIDS-related CMV retinitis.

BOTULINUM TOXIN TYPE A

Botulinum toxin is a form of purified botulinum toxin type A produced from a culture of the Hall strain of *Clostridium botulinum*. Botulinum toxin type A blocks neuromuscular conduction by binding to receptor sites on motor nerve terminals, entering the nerve terminals, and inhibiting the release of acetylcholine. When injected IM at therapeutic doses, the drug produces localized chemical denervation muscle paralysis. When the muscle is chemically denervated, it atrophies and may develop extrajunctional acetylcholine receptors. There is evidence that the nerve can sprout and reinnervate the muscle, with reversible weakness. The paralytic effect on muscles injected with botulinum toxin type A is useful in reducing the excessive, abnormal contractions associated with blepharospasm. Induced ptosis to protect the cornea may be provided by *Botox*. Cosmetic use of botulinum increases the spectrum of usefulness. Botulinum toxin type B also exists, but its approved indications are fewer. The potency of A and B are different, and, therefore, a dose of one can not be substituted for the other.

SURGICAL ENZYMES

Two enzymes have been used during ocular surgery: Hyaluronidase and urokinase. Hyaluronidase is added to local anesthetic solutions to increase drug absorption and dispersion. This enzyme hydrolyzes hyaluronic acid in the connective tissue, which increases tissue permeability.

Urokinase has been used to irrigate hyphemas and to treat acute retinal artery and vein occlusions. The conversion of plasminogen to the proteolytic enzyme plasmin by urokinase causes degradation of plasma proteins, fibrinogen, and fibrin clots.

Tissue plasminogen activator (tPA) is an enzyme that has the property of fibrin-enhanced conversion of plasminogen to plasmin. It produces limited conversion of plasminogen in the absence of fibrin. When introduced into the systemic circulation of pharmacologic concentration, it binds to fibrin in a thrombus and converts the entrapped plasminogen to plasmin. This initiates local fibrinolysis with limited systemic proteolysis.

For More Information

Duane TD, ed. *Clinical Ophthalmology*. Philadelphia, PA: Lippincott-Raven; 1987.

Ellis PP. *Ocular Therapeutics and Pharmacology*. 7th ed. St. Louis, MO: C.V. Mosby; 1985.

Goodman & Gilman's. *The Pharmacological Basis of Therapeutics*. 9th ed. New York, NY: McGraw-Hill; 1996.

Havener WH. *Ocular Pharmacology*. 5th ed. St Louis, MO: C.V. Mosby; 1983.

Whikehart DR. Irrigating Solutions. In: Bartlett JD, Jaanus SD, eds. *Clinical Ocular Pharmacology*. 3rd ed. Boston, MA: Butterworth-Heinemann; 1995.

ABSORBABLE GELATIN FILM, STERILE

Actions:

Pharmacology: A sterile, absorbable gelatin film for use in ocular surgery.

In the dry state it has the appearance and texture of cellophane of equivalent thickness; when moistened, it assumes a rubbery consistency and can be cut to desired size and fitted to rounded or irregular surfaces. The rate of absorption after implantation ranges from 1 to 6 months, depending upon the size of the implant and the site of implantation. Pleural and muscle implants are completely absorbed in 8 to 14 days; dural and ocular implants usually require no more than 2 to 5 months for complete absorption. The absence of undue tissue reactions, with the consequent decreased likelihood of developing adhesions, has been of particular value in the case of dural and ocular implants.

Indications:

Ocular surgery: In glaucoma filtration operations (iridencleisis and trephination), extraocular muscle surgery, and diathermy or scleral "buckling" operations for retinal detachment. There is a remarkable lack of cellular reaction to the film implanted subconjunctivally or used as a seton into the anterior chamber. Evidence shows that implants help prevent formation of adhesions between contiguous ocular structures.

Contraindications:

Because the rate of absorption is likely to be increased in the presence of purulent exudation, do not implant in grossly contaminated or infected surgical wounds.

Administration and Dosage:

Preparation: Immerse in sterile saline solution; soak until quite pliable; cut to the desired size and shape; apply as follows:

As a seton in iridencleisis: Place a small piece (approximately 4 mm × 10 mm) over the prolapsed iris pillar parallel to the limbus; Tenon's capsule and the conjunctiva are then closed with continuous absorbable sutures closely spaced to ensure tight wound closure.

Diathermy or scleral "buckling" operations: Place film over the sclera, then suture the muscle and the conjunctiva over the underlying film.

Extraocular muscle surgery: Place film over and beneath the muscle before Tenon's capsule and the conjunctiva are closed in layers.

Storage/Stability: Store at room temperature 15° to 30°C (59° to 86°F). To ensure sterility, use immediately after withdrawal from the envelope.

Rx	**Gelfilm** (Pharmacia)	100 mm × 125 mm	In 1s.
Rx	**Gelfilm Ophthalmic** (Pharmacia)	25 mm × 50 mm	In 6s.

ACETYLCHOLINE CHLORIDE, INTRAOCULAR

Indications:

To produce complete miosis within seconds after delivery of the lens in cataract surgery. In penetrating keratoplasty, iridectomy, and other anterior segment surgery where rapid, complete miosis may be required.

Administration and Dosage:

Solution: Instill the solution into the anterior chamber before or after securing at least 1 suture. The pupil is rapidly constricted and the peripheral iris drawn away from the angle of the anterior chamber if there are no mechanical hindrances. Any anatomical hindrance to miosis may require surgery to permit desired drug effect.

Dose of 0.5 to 2 mL produces satisfactory miosis. Solution need not be flushed from the chamber after miosis occurs. Because acetylcholine has a short duration of action, pilocarpine may be applied topically before dressing to maintain miosis.

Preparation of solution: The aqueous solution of acetylcholine chloride is unstable. Prepare solution immediately before use. Do not use solution that is not clear and colorless. Discard any solution that has not been used. Do not gas sterilize.

Storage/Stability: Store at room temperature 15° to 30°C (59° to 86°F). Do not freeze.

Rx	**Miochol-E** (Novartis)	**Solution**: 1:100 acetylcholine chloride when reconstituted	In 2 mL dual chamber univial (lower chamber 20 mg lyophilized acetylcholine chloride and 56 mg mannitol; upper chamber 2 mL electrolyte diluent[1] and sterile water for injection).

[1] Sodium chloride, potassium chloride, magnesium chloride hexahydrate, calcium chloride dihydrate.

BOTULINUM TOXIN TYPE A

Actions:

Pharmacology: Botulinum toxin is a sterile, lyophilized form of purified botulinum toxin type A, produced from a culture of the Hall strain of *Clostridium botulinum* grown in a medium containing N-Z amine and yeast extract. Botulinum toxin type A blocks neuromuscular conduction by binding to receptor sites on motor nerve terminals, entering the nerve terminals, and inhibiting the release of acetylcholine. When injected IM at therapeutic doses, botulinum toxin type A produces a localized chemical denervation muscle paralysis. When the muscle is chemically denervated, it atrophies and may develop extrajunctional acetylcholine receptors. There is evidence that the nerve can sprout and reinnervate the muscle, reversing the weakness.

The paralytic effect on muscles injected with botulinum toxin type A is useful in reducing the excessive, abnormal contractions associated with blepharospasm.

When used for the treatment of strabismus, the administration of botulinum toxin type A may affect muscle pairs by inducing an atrophic lengthening of the injected muscle and a corresponding shortening of the muscle's antagonist. Following periocular injection of botulinum toxin type A, distant muscles show electrophysiologic changes, but no clinical weakness or other clinical change for a period of several weeks or months, parallel to the duration of local clinical paralysis.

Clinical Trials: In 1 study, botulinum toxin was evaluated in 27 patients with essential blepharospasm; 26 had previously undergone drug treatment utilizing benztropine mesylate, clonazepam, or baclofen without adequate clinical results. Three of these patients then underwent muscle stripping surgery still without an adequate outcome. Upon using botulinum toxin, 25 of the 27 patients reported improvement within 48 hours. One of the other patients was later controlled with a higher dosage. The remaining patient reported only mild improvement but remained functionally impaired.

In another study, 12 patients with blepharospasm were evaluated in a double-blind, placebo-controlled study. All patients receiving botulinum toxin (n = 8) improved compared with no improvements in the placebo group (n = 4). The mean dystonia score improved 72%, the self-assessment score rating improved 61%, and a videotape evaluation rating improved 39%. The effects of the treatment lasted a mean of 12.5 weeks.

Patients with blepharospasm (n = 1,684) evaluated in an open trial showed clinical improvement lasting an average of 12.5 weeks prior to need for retreatment.

Patients with strabismus (n = 677) treated with at least 1 injection of botulinum toxin type A were evaluated in an open trial; 55% were improved to an alignment of 10 prism diopters when evaluated at least 6 months following injection. These results are consistent with results from additional open label trials.

Indications:

Treatment of strabismus and blepharospasm associated with dystonia, including benign essential blepharospasm or VII nerve disorders in patients at least 12 years of age.

Contraindications:

Hypersensitivity to any ingredient in the formulation.

Warnings:

Strabismus: The efficacy of botulinum toxin type A in deviations more than 50 prism diopters, in restrictive strabismus, in Duane syndrome with lateral rectus weakness, and in secondary strabismus caused by prior surgical over-recession of the antagonist is doubtful, or multiple injections over time may be required. Botulinum toxin type A is ineffective in chronic paralytic strabismus except to reduce antagonist contracture in conjunction with surgical repair.

Dosage: Do not exceed the recommended dosages and frequencies of administration. There have been no reported instances of systemic toxicity resulting from accidental injection or oral ingestion of botulinum toxin type A. Should accidental injection or oral ingestion occur, medically supervise the patient for several days on an outpatient basis for signs or symptoms of systemic weakness or muscle paralysis. The entire contents of a vial is below the estimated dose for systemic toxicity in humans weighing at least 6 kg.

Hypersensitivity: As with all biologic products, epinephrine and other precautions should be available should an anaphylactic reaction occur.

Pregnancy: Category C. It is not known whether botulinum toxin type A can cause fetal harm when administered to a pregnant woman or can affect reproduction capacity. Administer to pregnant women only if clearly needed.

Lactation: It is not known whether this drug is excreted in breast milk. Exercise caution when botulinum toxin type A is administered to a breast-feeding woman.

Children: Safety and efficacy in children younger than 12 years of age have not been established.

Precautions:

Safe and effective use: Safe and effective use of botulinum toxin type A depends upon proper storage of the product, selection of the correct dose, and proper reconstitution and administration techniques. Physicians administering botulinum toxin type A must understand the relevant neuromuscular and orbital anatomy and any alterations to the anatomy caused by prior surgical procedures, and standard electromyographic techniques.

Retrobulbar hemorrhages: During the administration of botulinum toxin type A for the treatment of strabismus, retrobulbar hemorrhages sufficient to compromise retinal circulation have occurred from needle penetrations into the orbit. Have appropriate instruments to decompress the orbit accessible. Ocular (globe) penetrations by needles have also occurred. An ophthalmoscope to diagnose this condition should be available.

Reduced blinking: Reduced blinking from botulinum toxin type A injection of the orbicularis muscle can lead to corneal exposure, persistent epithelial defect, and corneal ulceration, especially in patients with VII nerve disorders. One case of corneal perforation in an aphakic eye requiring corneal grafting has occurred because of this effect. Carefully test corneal sensation in eyes previously operated upon, avoid injection into the lower lid area to avoid ectropion, and vigorously treat any epithelial defect. This may require protective drops, ointment, therapeutic soft contact lenses, or closure of the eye by patching or other means.

Antibodies: Presence of antibodies to botulinum toxin type A may reduce the effectiveness of therapy. In clinical studies, reduction in effectiveness because of antibody production has occurred in 1 patient with blepharospasm receiving 3 doses over a 6-week period totaling 92 units and in several patients with torticollis who received multiple doses experimentally, totaling more than 300 units in 1 month. For this reason, keep the dose of botulinum toxin type A for strabismus and blepharospasm as low as possible, in any case less than 200 units in a 1-month period.

Drug Interactions:

Aminoglycosides: The effect of botulinum toxin may be potentiated by aminoglycoside antibiotics or any other drug that interferes with neuromuscular transmission. Exercise caution when botulinum toxin type A is used in patients taking these drugs.

Adverse Reactions:

Ophthalmic:

Strabismus – Inducing paralysis in at least 1 extraocular muscle may produce spatial disorientation, double vision, or past-pointing. Covering the affected eye may alleviate these symptoms. Extraocular muscles adjacent to the injection site are often affected, causing ptosis or vertical deviation, especially with higher doses. Adverse reactions in 2,058 adults who received 3,650 injections for horizontal strabismus included ptosis (15.7%) and vertical deviation (16.9%). The incidence of ptosis was much less after inferior rectus injection (0.9%) and much greater after superior rectus injection (37.7%).

Adverse reactions persisting for longer than 6 months in an enlarged series of 5,587 injections of horizontal muscles in 3,104 patients included ptosis lasting over 180 days (0.3%) and vertical deviation more than 2 prism diopters lasting over 180 days (2.1%).

In these patients, the injection procedure caused 9 scleral perforations. A vitreous hemorrhage occurred and later cleared in 1 case. No retinal detachment or visual loss occurred in any case; 16 retrobulbar hemorrhages occurred. Decompression of the orbit after 5 minutes was done to restore retinal circulation in 1 case. No eye lost vision from retrobulbar hemorrhage. Five eyes had pupillary change consistent with ciliary ganglion damage (Adies pupil).

Blepharospasm – In 1,684 patients who received 4,258 treatments (involving multiple injections) for blepharospasm, incidence of adverse reactions per treated eye was: Ptosis (11%); irritation/tearing, includes dry eye, lagophthalmos, and photophobia (10%); ectropion, keratitis, diplopia, and entropion occurred rarely (less than 1%).

Ecchymosis occurs easily in the soft eyelid tissues. This can be prevented by applying pressure at the injection site immediately after the injection. In 2 cases of VII nerve disorder (1 case of an aphakic eye), reduced blinking from botulinum toxin type A injection of the orbicularis muscle led to serious corneal exposure, persistent epithelial defect, and corneal ulceration. Perforation requiring corneal grafting occurred in 1 case, an aphakic eye (see Precautions).

Two patients previously incapacitated by blepharospasm experienced cardiac collapse attributed to over-exertion within 3 weeks following botulinum toxin type A therapy. Caution sedentary patients to resume activity slowly and carefully following the administration of botulinum toxin type A.

Local: Diffuse skin rash (n = 7) and local swelling of the eyelid skin (n = 2) lasting for several days following eyelid injection have occurred.

Overdosage:

In the event of overdosage or injection into the wrong muscle, additional information may be obtained by contacting Allergan Pharmaceuticals at (800) 347-5063 from 8 am to 4 pm Pacific Time, or at (714) 724-5954 for a recorded message at other times.

Patient Information:

Patients with blepharospasm may have been extremely sedentary for a long time. Caution these patients to resume activity slowly and carefully follow administration.

Administration and Dosage:

Strabismus: Botulinum toxin type A is intended for injection into extraocular muscles utilizing the electrical activity recorded from the tip of the injection needle as a guide to placement within the target muscle. Do not attempt injection without surgical exposure or electromyographic guidance. Physicians should be familiar with electromyographic technique.

Preparation – An injection of botulinum toxin type A is prepared by drawing into a sterile 1 mL tuberculin syringe an amount of the properly diluted toxin (see Dilution Table) slightly greater than the intended dose. Air bubbles in the syringe barrel are expelled and the syringe is attached to the electromyographic injection needle, preferably a 1.5-inch, 27-gauge needle. Injection volume in excess of the intended dose is expelled through the needle into an appropriate waste container to ensure patency of the needle and to confirm that there is no syringe-needle leakage. Use a new, sterile needle and syringe to enter the vial on each occasion for dilution or removal of botulinum toxin type A.

To prepare the eye for botulinum toxin type A injection, give several drops of a local anesthetic and an ocular decongestant several minutes prior to injection.

Note – The volume of botulinum toxin type A injected for treatment of strabismus should be between 0.05 to 0.15 mL per muscle.

The initial listed doses of the diluted botulinum toxin type A (see Dilution table) typically create paralysis of injected muscles beginning 1 to 2 days after injection and increasing in intensity during the first week. The paralysis lasts for 2 to 6 weeks and gradually resolves over a similar time period. Overcorrections lasting longer than 6 months have been rare. Approximately 50% of patients will require subsequent doses because of inadequate paralytic response of the muscle to the initial dose, or because of mechanical factors such as large deviations or restrictions, or because of the lack of binocular motor fusion to stabilize the alignment.

1. Initial doses in units. Use the lower listed doses for treatment of small deviations. Use the larger doses only for large deviations.
   a. For vertical muscles, and for horizontal strabismus of less than 20 prism diopters: 1.25 to 2.5 units in any 1 muscle.
   b. For horizontal strabismus of 20 to 50 prism diopters: 2.5 to 5 units in any 1 muscle.
   c. For persistent VI nerve palsy of at least 1 month duration: 1.25 to 2.5 units in the medial rectus muscle.

2. Subsequent doses for residual or recurrent strabismus.
   a. Re-examine patients 7 to 14 days after each injection to assess the effect of that dose.
   b. Patients experiencing adequate paralysis of the target muscle who require subsequent injections should receive a dose comparable to the initial dose.
   c. Subsequent doses for patients experiencing incomplete paralysis of the target muscle may be increased up to 2-fold the previously administered dose.
   d. Subsequent injections should not be administered until the effects of the previous dose have dissipated as evidenced by substantial function in the injected and adjacent muscles.
   e. Maximum recommended dose as a single injection for any 1 muscle is 25 units.

Blepharospasm: Diluted botulinum toxin type A (see Dilution table) is injected using a sterile, 27- to 30-gauge needle without electromyographic guidance. Initially, 1.25 to 2.5 units (0.05 to 0.1 mL volume at each site) injected into the medial and lateral pre-tarsal orbicularis oculi of the upper lid and into the lateral pre-tarsal orbicularis oculi of the lower lid is the initial recommended dose.

In general, the initial effect of the injections is seen within 3 days and reaches a peak at 1 to 2 weeks post-treatment. Each treatment lasts approximately 3 months, following which the procedure can be repeated indefinitely. At repeat treatment sessions, the dose may be increased up to 2-fold if the response from the initial treatment is considered insufficient (usually defined as an effect that does not last longer than 2 months). However, there appears to be little benefit obtainable from injecting more than 5 units per site. Some tolerance may be found when botulinum toxin type A is used in treating blepharospasm if treatments are given any more frequently than every 3 months; it is rare to have the effect become permanent.

The cumulative dose of botulinum toxin type A in a 30-day period should not exceed 200 units.

Dilution technique: To reconstitute lyophilized botulinum toxin type A, use sterile normal saline without a preservative; 0.9% Sodium Chloride Injection is the recommended diluent. Draw up the proper amount of diluent in the appropriate size syringe. Because botulinum toxin type A is denatured by bubbling or similar violent agitation, inject the diluent into the vial gently. Discard the vial if a vacuum does not pull the diluent into the vial. Record the date and time of reconstitution on the space on the label. Administer within 4 hours after reconstitution.

During this time period, store reconstituted botulinum toxin type A in a refrigerator at 2° to 8°C (36° to 46°F). Reconstituted botulinum toxin type A should be clear, colorless, and free of particulate matter. The use of 1 vial for more than 1 patient is not recommended because the product and diluent do not contain a preservative.

Dilution of Botulinum Toxin Type A	
Diluent added (0.9% Sodium Chloride Injection)	Resulting dose
1 mL	10 units
2 mL	5 units
4 mL	2.5 units
8 mL	1.25 units

These dilutions are calculated for an injection volume of 0.1 mL. A decrease or increase in the botulinum toxin type A dose is also possible by administering a smaller or larger injection volume – from 0.05 mL (50% decrease in dose) to 0.15 mL (50% increase in dose).

Storage/Stability: Store the lyophilized product in a freezer at or below -5°C (23°F). Administer within 4 hours after the vial is removed from the freezer and reconstituted. During these 4 hours, store reconstituted botulinum toxin type A in a refrigerator at 2° to 8°C (36° to 46°F). Reconstituted botulinum toxin type A should be clear, colorless, and free of particulate matter.

Rx	**Botox** (Allergan)	**Powder for Injection (lyophilized)**: 100 units of lyophilized *Clostridium botulinum* toxin type A[1]	Preservative free. 0.05 mg albumin (human), 0.9 mg sodium chloride. In vials.

[1] One unit corresponds to the calculated median lethal intraperitoneal dose (LD_{50}) in mice of the reconstituted drug injected.

CARBACHOL, INTRAOCULAR

For complete prescribing information, refer to the Miotics, Direct-Acting group monograph in the Ocular Hypotensive Agents chapter. The following section is included here for completeness to show all of the clinical uses of this drug class.

Indications:

Miosis: Intraocular use for miosis during surgery.

Administration and Dosage:

For single-dose intraocular use only. Discard unused portion.

Open under aseptic conditions only.

Gently instill no more than 0.5 mL into the anterior chamber before or after securing sutures. Miosis is usually maximal 2 to 5 minutes after application.

Storage/Stability: Store at room temperature 15° to 30°C (59° to 86°F).

Rx	**Miostat** (Alcon)	**Solution:** 0.01%	In 1.5 mL vials.[1]

[1] With 0.64% sodium chloride, 0.075% potassium chloride, 0.048% calcium chloride dihydrate, 0.03% magnesium chloride hexahydrate, 0.39% sodium acetate trihydrate, 0.17% sodium citrate dihydrate, sodium hydroxide, hydrochloric acid.

HYALURONIDASE

Actions:

Pharmacology: Hyaluronidase is a spreading or diffusing substance, which modifies the permeability of connective tissue through the hydrolysis of hyaluronic acid, a polysaccharide found in the intercellular ground substance of connective tissue, and of certain specialized tissues, such as the umbilical cord and vitreous humor.

Indications:

As an adjuvant to increase the absorption and dispersion of other injected drugs.

Contraindications:

Hypersensitivity to hyaluronidase or any other ingredient in the formulation.

Warnings:

Discontinue if sensitization occurs. Do not use to enhance the absorption and dispersion of dopamine and/or alpha agonist drugs. Do not inject into or around an infected or acutely inflamed area because of the danger of spreading a localized infection. Do not apply directly to the cornea. Do not use for intravenous injections because the enzyme is rapidly inactivated.

Pregnancy: Category C. No adequate and well controlled studies have been conducted with *Vitrase* in pregnant women; use during pregnancy only if clearly needed.

Lactation: Exercise caution when administering hyaluronidase to a breast-feeding woman.

Precautions:

Furosemide, benzodiazepines, and phenytoin are incompatible with hyaluronidase.

Drug Interactions:

When hyaluronidase is added to a local anesthetic agent, it hastens the onset of analgesia and tends to reduce the swelling caused by local infiltration, but the wider spread of the local anesthetic solution increases its absorption; this shortens the duration of action and tends to increase the incidence of systemic reaction.

Patients receiving large doses of salicylates, cortisone, ACTH, estrogens, or antihistamines may require larger amounts of hyaluronidase for equivalent dispersing effect, since these drugs apparently render tissues partly resistant to the action of hyaluronidase.

Adverse Reactions:

The most frequently reported adverse experiences have been local injection site reactions. Hyaluronidase has been reported to enhance the adverse reactions associated with coadministered drug products. Allergic reaction (urticaria, angioedema) have been reported in less than 0.1% of patients receiving hyaluronidase. Anaphylactic-like reactions following retrobulbar block or intravenous injections have occurred rarely.

Overdosage:

Symptoms of toxicity consist of local edema or urticaria, erythema, chills, nausea, vomiting, dizziness, tachycardia, and hypotension. Discontinue the enzyme and initiate supportive measures immediately.

Administration and Dosage:

Not recommended for IV use. After reconstitution and further dilution, absorption and dispersion of other injected drugs may be enhanced by adding 50 to 300 units, most typically 150 units, of hyaluronidase into the injection solution. It is recommended that appropriate references be consulted regarding physical or chemical incompatibilities before adding *Vitrase* to a solution containing another drug.

Storage/Stability: Store unopened vial in refrigerator at 2° to 8°C (35° to 46°F). After reconstitution, store at controlled room temperature 20° to 25°C (59° to 77°F), and use within 6 hours. Protect from light.

Rx	**Vitrase** (Ista)	**Injection:** 6,200 units lyophilized ovine hyaluronidase nonpreserved	In single-use 5 mL vial, one 1 mL syringe, one 5 mcm filter needle.

HYDROXYPROPYL METHYLCELLULOSE

Actions:

Pharmacology: Hydroxypropyl methylcellulose is an isotonic, nonpyrogenic viscoelastic solution with a high molecular weight (more than 80,000 daltons). It maintains a deep chamber during anterior segment surgery and allows for more efficient manipulation with less trauma to the corneal endothelium and other ocular tissues. The viscoelasticity helps the vitreous face to be pushed back, preventing formation of a postoperative flat chamber.

Indications:

For professional use in gonioscopic examinations.

Precautions:

Intraocular pressure (IOP): Transient increased IOP may occur following surgery because of pre-existing glaucoma or because of the surgery itself. If the postoperative IOP increases above expected values, administer appropriate therapy.

Adverse Reactions:

Although well tolerated, a transient, postoperative increase in IOP has been reported (see Precautions). Other reactions that have occurred include postoperative inflammatory reactions (iritis, hypopyon), corneal edema, and corneal decompensation.

Administration and Dosage:

Gonioscopic examinations: Fill gonioscopic prism with 2.5% solution, as necessary.

Storage/Stability: If this solution dries on optical surfaces, let them stand in cool water before cleansing. If solution changes color or becomes cloudy, do not use. Not for use with hot laser treatment as solution clouding will occur.

To avoid contamination, do not touch tip of container to any surface. Replace cap after using. Keep container tightly closed. Store at room temperature 15° to 30°C (59° to 86°F). Avoid excessive heat over 60°C (140°F). Protect from light.

otc	**Gonak** (Akorn)	**Solution:** 2.5%	In 15 mL.[1]
otc	**Goniosoft** (OCuSOFT)		In 15 mL.
otc	**Goniosol** (Novartis)		In 15 mL.[2]

[1] With 0.01% benzalkonium chloride, boric acid, KCl, sodium borate, hydrochloric acid or sodium hydroxide, and EDTA.
[2] With 0.01% benzalkonium chloride, boric acid, KCl, EDTA.

INTRAOCULAR IRRIGATING SOLUTIONS

Actions:

Pharmacology: Sterile irrigating solution is a sterile physiological balanced salt solution, each mL containing sodium chloride 0.64%, potassium chloride 0.075%, calcium chloride dihydrate 0.048%, magnesium chloride hexahydrate 0.03%, sodium acetate trihydrate 0.39%, sodium citrate dihydrate 0.17%, sodium hydroxide or hydrochloric acid (to adjust pH), and water. This solution is isotonic to ocular tissue and contains electrolytes required for normal cellular metabolic functions.

Indications:

Irrigation: For irrigation during various ocular surgical procedures. Some products may also be used for ears, nose, and throat (consult specific product labeling).

Warnings:

Route of administration: Not for injection or IV infusion. Use aseptic technique only.

Precautions:

Preservative free solutions: Do not use for more than 1 patient.

Corneal clouding and edema: Corneal clouding and edema have occurred following ocular surgery in which balanced salt solution was used as an irrigating solution. Take appropriate measures to minimize trauma to the cornea and other ocular tissues.

Concomitant medication: Addition of any medication to balanced salt solution may result in damage to intraocular tissue.

Diabetics: Studies suggest that intraocular irrigating solutions which are iso-osmotic with normal aqueous fluids should be used with caution in diabetic patients undergoing vitrectomy as intraoperative lens changes have been observed.

Adverse Reactions:

When corneal endothelium is abnormal, irrigation or any other trauma may result in bullous keratopathy. Postoperative inflammatory reactions and corneal edema and decompensation have occurred. Relationship to balanced salt solution is not established.

Administration and Dosage:

Use balanced salt solution according to the established practices for each surgical procedure. Follow the manufacturer directions for the particular administration set to be used. For products with separate solutions for reconstitution, never use Part I or Part II alone; this could result in damage to the eye.

Storage/Stability: Store at 8° to 30°C (46° to 86°F). Avoid excessive heat. Do not freeze. Discard prepared solution after 6 hours. Do not use if cloudy or if seal or packaging is damaged. Do not use reconstituted solution if it is discolored or contains a precipitate.

Rx	**Balanced Salt Solution** (B. Braun)	**Solution:** 0.64% NaCl, 0.075% KCl, 0.03% magnesium chloride, 0.048% calcium chloride, 0.39% sodium acetate, 0.17% sodium citrate, sodium hydroxide or hydrochloric acid	In 500 mL.
Rx	**BSS** (Alcon)		Preservative free. In 15, 30, 250, and 500 mL.

Rx	**BSS Plus** (Alcon)	**Solution**: Mix aseptically just prior to use. **Part I:** 7.44 mg NaCl, 0.395 mg KCl, 0.433 mg dibasic sodium phosphate, 2.19 mg sodium bicarbonate, hydrochloric acid or sodium hydroxide/mL	Preservative free. In 250 and 500 mL.
		Part II: 3.85 mg calcium chloride dihydrate, 5 mg magnesium chloride hexahydrate, 23 mg dextrose, 4.6 mg glutathione disulfide/mL	Preservative free. In 10 mL.
Rx	**B-Salt Forte** (Akorn)	**Solution**: Mix aseptically just prior to use. **Part I:** 7.14 mg NaCl, 0.38 mg KCl, 0.154 mg calcium chloride dihydrate, 0.2 mg magnesium chloride hexahydrate, 0.92 mg dextrose, hydrochloric acid or sodium hydroxide/mL	Preservative free. In 515 mL.
		Part II: 1081 mg sodium bicarbonate, 216 mg dibasic sodium phosphate (anhydrous), 95 mg glutathione disulfide (oxidized glutathione)/vial	Preservative free. In 60 mL.

MIOTICS, DIRECT-ACTING

For complete prescribing information, see the Miotics, Direct-Acting monograph in the Ocular Hypotensive Agents chapter.

Actions:

Pharmacology: The direct-acting miotics are parasympathomimetic (cholinergic) drugs that duplicate the muscarinic effects of acetylcholine. When applied topically, these drugs produce pupillary constriction, stimulate the ciliary muscles, and increase aqueous humor outflow facility.

Rx	**Carbastat** (Novartis)	**Solution**: 0.01%	In 1.5 mL vials.[1]
Rx	**Miochol-E** (Novartis)	**Solution**: 1:100 acetylcholine chloride when reconstituted	In 2 mL dual chamber univial (lower chamber 20 mg lyophilized acetylcholine chloride and 56 mg mannitol; upper chamber 2 mL electrolyte diluent[2] and sterile water for injection).

[1] With 0.64% sodium chloride, 0.075% potassium chloride, 0.048% calcium chloride dihydrate, 0.03% magnesium chloride hexahydrate, 0.39% sodium acetate trihydrate, 0.17% sodium citrate dihydrate, sodium hydroxide, hydrochloric acid.
[2] Sodium chloride, potassium chloride, magnesium chloride hexahydrate, calcium chloride dihydrate.

POLYDIMETHYLSILOXANE (Silicone Oil)

Actions:

Pharmacology: Polydimethylsiloxane, an oil that is injected into the vitreous space of the eye, is used as a prolonged retinal tamponade in select cases of retinal detachment.

Clinical Trials:

Anatomic reattachment rates – Successful reattachment of the retina occurred in 64% to 75% of the patients who were treated with polydimethylsiloxane. This rate varied depending on the specific etiology of the disease and the severity of the condition. In AIDS CMV retinitis patients receiving silicone oil as a primary means for reattaching the retina, attachment rates were as high as 90% within an average 6-month follow-up period.

Visual acuity outcomes – At 6 months, 45% to 70% of patients showed improvements in visual acuity. In about 15% to 26% of patients, visual acuity did not change and in approximately 15% to 30%, worsening of visual acuity occurred. Deterioration of visual acuity in treated patients appeared to be related to redetachment of the retina, further progression of retinal disease, or to keratopathy and cataract complications. In AIDS CMV retinitis patients, improvement or maintenance of visual acuity was documented in 57% of the patients within an average 6-month follow-up period. In AIDS patients, further decline in visual acuity was seen due to continuing progression of retinal and optic nerve disease and development of oil related cataracts in 33% of patients within 4 to 5 months of oil instillation.

Indications:

Retinal detachments: Prolonged retinal tamponade in selected cases of complicated retinal detachments or early phthisis where other interventions are not appropriate for patient management. Complicated retinal detachments or recurrent retinal detachments occur most commonly in eyes with proliferative vitreoretinopathy (PVR), proliferative diabetic retinopathy (PDR), cytomegalovirus (CMV) retinitis, giant tears, and following perforating injuries.

For primary use in detachments caused by AIDS-related CMV retinitis and other viral infections.

Contraindications:

Pseudophakic patients with silicone intraocular lens (silicone oil can chemically interact and opacify silicone elastomers).

Warnings:

Cataract: Approximately 50% to 70% of phakic patients developed a cataract within 12 months of oil instillation. Approximately 33% of phakic AIDS CMV retinitis patients developed some degree of cataract within an average 4 to 5 month time frame from oil instillation.

Anterior chamber oil migration: In 17% to 20% of patients, oil emulsification or migration into the anterior chamber was observed. Migration into the anterior chamber occurred in both phakic and aphakic patients.

Keratopathy: From 8% to 20% of patients developed keratopathy (0.6%, AIDS patients). This complication occurred most frequently in aphakic patients (18% to 21%) and in the patients in whom oil had migrated into the anterior chamber (30%); the keratopathy in these cases was attributed to prolonged physical contact between the corneal endothelium and the silicone oil.

Glaucoma: Approximately 19% to 20% (0.06%, AIDS patients) of patients developed a persistent elevation in intraocular pressure (more than 23 to 25 mm Hg). The neovascular glaucoma rate was approximately 8%. Moderate temporary postoperative increases occurred within the first 3 weeks of treatment. Thereafter, secondary ocular hypertension occurred by several mechanisms. Glaucoma complications occurred in approximately 30% of patients in which anterior chamber oil is noted. Patients with proliferative diabetic retinopathy were at highest risk for development of glaucoma following silicone oil instillation into the vitreous space.

Precautions:

Long-term use: The safety and efficacy of long-term use have not been established.

Adverse Reactions:

Miscellaneous: The most common adverse reactions include the following: cataract (50% to 70%); anterior chamber oil migration (17% to 20%); keratopathy (8% to 20%); glaucoma (19% to 20%). See Warnings.

Other adverse reactions ranked by frequency of occurrence include the following: Redetachment, optic nerve atrophy, rubeosis iritis, temporary IOP increase, macular pucker, vitreous hemorrhage, phthisis, traction detachment, angle block (more than 2%); subretinal strands, retinal rupture, endophthalmitis, subretinal silicone oil, choroidal detachment, aniridia, PVR reproliferation, cystoid macular edema, enucleation (less than 2%).

Administration and Dosage:

Polydimethylsiloxane can be used in conjunction with or following standard retinal surgical procedures including scleral buckle surgery, vitrectomy, membrane peeling, and retinotomy or relaxing retinectomy.

Avoid introduction of air bubbles into the oil by careful withdrawal or decanting of the oil into the syringe. The oil can be injected into the vitreous from the syringe via a single-use cannulated infusion line or syringe needle. Subretinal fluid can be drained with a flute needle concurrent with polydimethylsiloxane infusion. The vitreous space can be filled with the oil to between 80% and 100% while exchanging for fluid or air, taking necessary precautions to avoid high intraocular pressure from developing during the exchange. Because the polydimethylsiloxane is less dense than the eye aqueous fluid, a basal iridectomy at the 6 o'clock meridian (Ando iridectomy) is recommended to minimize oil-induced pupillary block and early angle-closure glaucoma. Upon choice of the physician, it may be desirable to have the patient assume a face-down posture during the first 24 hours following surgery.

Monitor the patient closely for development of glaucoma, cataract, and keratopathy complications and schedule for follow-up re-examination at regular intervals.

It is recommended that polydimethylsiloxane be removed at an appropriate interval within 1 year following instillation if the retina is stable, attached, and without significant remnants of proliferation. Although there is insufficient clinical evidence to support justification for longer term tamponade, whether or not the oil should be removed in patients at high risk for redetachment or the development of phthisis and shrinkage caused by hypotony must be determined individually by the physician. In order to minimize the number of invasive traumatic experiences for patients with AIDS and CMV retinitis at high risk for redetachment and who have a shortened expected lifespan, avoid silicone oil removal procedures if the patient concurs.

Polydimethylsiloxane can be removed from the posterior chamber by withdrawal with a normal 10 mL syringe and a wide bore 1 mm cannula. By repeated oil-fluid exchange, most of the remaining small silicone oil droplets can subsequently be mobilized and removed from the eye. Alternatively, oil may be passively removed by infusion of an appropriate aqueous solution under the oil bubble, while allowing the oil to effuse out of a sclerotomy incision, or limbal incision in aphakic patients.

As there is a possible correlation between the migration of polydimethylsiloxane into the anterior chamber and the appearance of corneal changes such as edema, hazing or opacification, Descemet folds, or decompensation, perform regular monitoring of the patient's corneal status and take early corrective action if necessary, including extraction of the oil from the anterior chamber. Large bubbles or droplets of oil in the anterior chamber can be removed manually by syringe. Further standard practice for medical treatment of the keratopathy is recommended.

Temporary pressure increases more than 3 weeks after surgery that can normalize spontaneously or be corrected by surgical treatment are those in which the polydimethylsiloxane causes a mechanical blockage of the pupil or inferior iridectomy or causes chamber angle closure by forcing its way anteriorly. In these situations, some of the oil may be withdrawn to relieve the mechanical force of the oil interface. Presence of polydimethylsiloxane droplets in the anterior chamber may also cause a chronic outflow obstruction of the trabecular meshwork. In such situations, elevated intraocular pressure can be managed with antiglaucoma medication in the majority of outflow obstruction patients.

Admixture incompatibility: Do not admix with any other substances prior to injection.

Storage/Stability: Store at room or cool temperature 8° to 24°C (46° to 75°F). Polydimethylsiloxane is supplied in a sterile vial intended for single use only and contains no preservative. Do not resterilize. Discard unused portions. Discard product after expiration date.

Rx	**AdatoSil 5000** (Bausch & Lomb)	**Injection**: Polydimethylsiloxane oil	In single-use 10 and 15 mL vials.

POVIDONE IODINE

Actions:

Pharmacology: Povidone iodine has broad-spectrum antimicrobial action.

Indications:

Ophthalmic preoperative prep: Used prior to eye surgery to prep the periocular region (lids, brow, cheek) and irrigate the ocular surface (cornea, conjunctiva, palpebral fornices).

Contraindications:

Hypersensitivity to iodine.

Warnings:

For external use only: Not for intraocular injection or irrigation.

Pregnancy: Category C. Safety for use during pregnancy has not been established. Use only when clearly needed.

Lactation: Because of the potential for adverse reactions in breast-feeding infants, decide whether to discontinue breast-feeding or discontinue the drug, taking into account the importance of the drug to the mother.

Children: Safety and efficacy have not been established.

Precautions:

Thyroid disorders: Use with caution in patients with thyroid disorders because of the possibility of iodine absorption.

Adverse Reactions:

Local sensitivity has been exhibited by some individuals.

Administration and Dosage:

Do not use in an open globe, as endothelial toxicity may ensue.

Transfer solution to a sterile prep cup. Apply to lashes and lid margins with sterile applicator; repeat once. Apply to lids, brow, and cheek in an ever-expanding circular fashion with sterile applicator; repeat 3 times. While separating the lids, irrigate cornea, conjunctiva, and palpebral fornices with solution and leave in for 2 minutes; flush with sterile saline solution.

Rx	**Betadine 5% Sterile Ophthalmic Prep Solution** (Alcon)	**Solution**: 5% povidone iodine	In 30 mL.[1]

[1] Glycerin, sodium chloride, sodium hydroxide, and sodium phosphate.

SODIUM HYALURONATE

Actions:

Pharmacology: Sodium hyaluronate and sodium chondroitin sulfate are widely distributed in extracellular matrix of connective tissues. They are found in the synovial fluid, skin, umbilical cord, and vitreous and aqueous humor. The cornea is the ocular tissue with the greatest concentration of sodium chondroitin sulfate; the vitreous and aqueous humor contain the greatest concentration of sodium hyaluronate.

This preparation is a specific fraction of sodium hyaluronate developed for use in anterior segment and vitreous procedures as a viscoelastic agent. It has high molecular weight, is nonantigenic, does not cause inflammatory or foreign body reactions, and has a high viscosity. The 1% solution is transparent and remains in the anterior chamber for less than 6 days. It protects corneal endothelial cells and other ocular structures. It does not interfere with epithelialization and normal wound healing.

Indications:

Surgical aid: As a surgical aid in cataract extraction (intra- and extracapsular), intraocular lens implantation (IOL), corneal transplant, glaucoma filtration, retinal attachment surgery, and posterior segment surgery to gently separate, maneuver, and hold tissues.

To maintain a deep anterior chamber in surgical procedures in the anterior segment of the eye, allowing for efficient manipulation with less trauma to the corneal endothelium and other surrounding tissues.

To push back the vitreous face and prevent formation of a postoperative flat chamber.

To create a clear field of vision, facilitating intra- and postoperative inspection of the retina and photocoagulation.

Off-label use(s): Sodium hyaluronate has been used in the treatment of refractory dry eye syndrome.

Warnings:

Hypersensitivity: Because this preparation is extracted from avian tissues and contains minute amounts of protein, risks of hypersensitivity exist.

Precautions:

For intraocular use: Use only if solution is clear. Do not reuse cannulas.

Postoperative intraocular pressure (IOP): Postoperative IOP may be elevated as a result of pre-existing glaucoma, compromised outflow, and by operative procedures and sequelae, including enzymatic zonulysis, absence of an iridectomy, trauma to filtration structures, and by blood and lenticular remnants in the anterior chamber. Because the exact role of these factors is difficult to predict in any individual case, the following precautions are recommended:

> *Do not overfill the anterior chamber* – Do not overfill the anterior chamber (except in glaucoma surgery). (See Administration and Dosage.)
>
> *Monitoring* – Carefully monitor IOP, especially during the immediate postoperative period. Treat significant increases appropriately.
>
> *Posterior segment surgery* – In posterior segment surgery, in aphakic diabetics, exercise special care to avoid using large amounts of the drug. Remove some of the preparation by irrigation or aspiration at the close of surgery (except in glaucoma surgery). (See Administration and Dosage.)
>
> Avoid trapping air bubbles behind the drug.

Cloudiness/Precipitate: Reports indicate that the drug may become cloudy or form a slight precipitate after instillation. The clinical significance is not known because the majority of reports do not indicate any harmful effects on ocular tissues. Be aware of this phenomenon and remove cloudy or precipitated material by irrigation or aspiration. In vitro studies suggest that this phenomenon may be related to interactions with certain concomitantly administered ophthalmic medications.

ProVisc: The device used to obtain *ProVisc* material may cause an allergic reaction in susceptible patients.

Adverse Reactions:

Although well tolerated, a transient postoperative increase of IOP has been reported (see Precautions).

Other reactions that have occurred include postoperative inflammatory reactions (iritis, hypopyon), corneal edema, and corneal decompensation.

Administration and Dosage:

Cataract surgery - IOL implantation: Slowly introduce a sufficient amount (using cannula or needle) into anterior chamber. Inject before or after delivery of lens. Injection before lens delivery protects corneal endothelium from possible damage from removal of the cataractous lens. May use to coat surgical instruments and the IOL prior to insertion. May inject additional amounts during surgery to replace any of the drug lost.

Glaucoma filtration surgery: In conjunction with the performance of the trabeculectomy, inject slowly and carefully through a corneal paracentesis to reconstitute the anterior chamber. Further injection can be continued to allow it to extrude into the subconjunctival filtration site through and around the sutured outer scleral flap.

Corneal transplant surgery: After removal of the corneal button, fill the anterior chamber with the drug. Then, suture the donor graft in place. An additional amount may be injected to replace the lost amount as a result of surgical manipulation.

Sodium hyaluronate has also been used in the anterior chamber of the donor eye prior to trephination to protect the corneal endothelial cells of the graft.

Retinal attachment surgery: Slowly introduce into the vitreous cavity. The injection may be directed to separate membranes from retina for safe excision and release of traction. Also serves to maneuver tissues into desired position (eg, to gently push back a detached retina or unroll a retinal flap); aids in holding retina against the sclera for reattachment.

Storage/Stability:

Amvisc/Amvisc Plus, Coease, Healon/Healon GV – Store at 2° to 8°C (36° to 46°F).

AMO Vitrax – Store at room temperature (15° to 30°C; 59° to 86°F). Do not freeze. Protect from light.

ProVisc – Drug should reach room temperature before use (approximately 20 to 40 minutes, depending on quantity). Store in refrigerator at 2° to 8°C (36° to 46°F).

Rx	**Healon** (AMO)	**Injection:** 10 mg/mL[1]	In 0.4, 0.55, and 0.85 mL disp. syringes.
Rx	**ProVisc** (Alcon)		In 0.4, 0.55, and 0.85 mL disp. glass syringes.
Rx	**Amvisc** (Chiron)	**Injection:** 12 mg/mL[2]	In 0.5 or 0.8 mL disp. syringes.
Rx	**Coease** (Advanced Medical Optics)		In 0.5 or 0.8 mL disp. syringes.
Rx	**Shellgel** (Cytosol Ophthalmics)		In 0.8 mL disp. syringes.
Rx	**Healon GV** (AMO)	**Injection:** 14 mg/mL[1]	In 0.85 mL disp. syringes.
Rx	**Amvisc Plus** (Chiron)	**Injection:** 16 mg/mL[2]	In 0.5 or 8 mL disp. syringes.
Rx	**Healon5** (AMO)	**Injection:** 23 mg/mL[3]	In 0.6 mL disp. syringes.

[1] With 8.5 mg NaCl per mL.
[2] With 9 mg NaCl per mL.
[3] With 8.5 mg NaCl, 0.28 mg disodium hydrogen phosphate dihydrate, 0.04 mg sodium dihydrogen phosphate monohydrate per mL.

SODIUM HYALURONATE AND CHONDROITIN SULFATE

Refer to the Sodium Hyaluronate monograph for more complete information.

Indications:

Surgical aid: A surgical aid in anterior segment procedures, including cataract extraction and intraocular lens implantation.

Off-label use(s): Topical treatment of severe dry eye disorders.

Administration and Dosage:

The higher viscosity materials remain longer in the anterior chamber and will be more difficult to remove from the eye. However, they provide better endothelial protection during phacoemulsification in the presence of Fuch dystrophy.

Carefully introduce (using a 27-gauge cannula) into the anterior chamber. May inject prior to or following delivery of the crystalline lens. Instillation prior to lens delivery provides additional protection to corneal endothelium, protecting it from possible damage arising from surgical instrumentation. May also be used to coat intraocular lens and tips of surgical instruments prior to implantation surgery. Intravitreal injection through the pars plana is helpful in torn capsules to avoid lens sublaxation. May inject additional solution during anterior segment surgery to fully maintain the chamber or to replace solution lost during surgery. At the end of surgery, remove solution by thoroughly irrigating the eye with a balanced salt solution. Alternatively, the solution may be left in the eye when used as directed.

Storage/Stability: Store at 2° to 8°C (36° to 46°F). Do not freeze.

Rx	**Viscoat** (Alcon)	**Solution:** no more than 40 mg sodium chondroitin sulfate, 30 mg sodium hyaluronate per mL	In 0.5 and 0.75 mL disposable syringes.[1]

[1] 0.45 mg sodium dihydrogen phosphate hydrate, 2 mg disodium hydrogen phosphate, 4.3 mg sodium chloride per mL.

TRYPAN BLUE OPHTHALMIC SOLUTION

Refer to the Trypan Blue monograph for more complete information.

Actions:

Pharmacology: Trypan blue selectively stains connective tissue structures in the human eye such as the anterior lens capsule of the human crystalline lens. Trypan blue is intended to be applied directly on the anterior lens capsule, staining any portion of the capsule that comes in contact with the dye. Excess dye is washed out of the anterior chamber. The dye does not penetrate the capsule, permitting visualization of the anterior capsule in contrast to the non-stained cortex and inner lens material.

Indications:

Trypan blue is indicated for the use as an aid in ophthalmic surgery by staining the anterior capsule of the lens.

Contraindications:

Trypan blue is contraindicated when a non-hydrated (dry state), hydrophilic acrylic intraocular lens (IOL) is planned to be inserted into the eye because the dye may be absorbed by the IOL and stain the IOL.

Warnings:

Carcinogenesis: Trypan blue is carcinogenic in rats. Wister/Lewis rats developed lymphomas after receiving subcutaneous injections of 1% trypan blue dosed at 50 mg/kg every other week for 52 weeks (total dose approximately 1,250,000-fold the maximum recommended human dose of 0.06 mg/injection in a 60 kg person, assuming total absorption.)

Mutagenesis: Trypan blue was mutagenic in the Ames test and caused DNA strand breaks in vitro.

Elderly: No overall differences in safety and efficacy have been observed between elderly and younger patients.

Pregnancy: Category C. Trypan blue is teratogenic in rats, mice, rabbits, hamsters, dogs, guinea pigs, pigs, and chickens. The majority of teratogenicity studies performed involve intravenous, intraperitoneal, or subcutaneous administration in the rat. There are no adequate and well-controlled studies in pregnant women. Trypan blue should be given to a pregnant woman only if the potential benefit justifies the potential risk to the fetus.

Lactation: It is not known whether this drug is excreted in human milk. Because many drugs are excreted in human milk, caution should be exercised when trypan blue is administered to a breast-feeding woman.

Children: The safety and efficacy of trypan blue have been established in pediatric patients. Use of trypan blue is supported by evidence from an adequate and well-controlled study in children.

Precautions:

It is recommended that, after injection, all trypan blue be immediately removed from the eye by thorough irrigation of the anterior chamber.

Adverse Reactions:

Adverse reactions reported following use of trypan blue include discoloration of high water content hydrogen intraocular lenses (see Contraindications) and inadvertent staining of the posterior lens capsule and vitreous face. Staining of the posterior lens capsule or staining of the vitreous face is generally self limited, lasting up to 1 week.

Administration and Dosage:

Cataract surgery: Trypan blue is packaged in a 2.25 mL syringe to which a blunt cannula has to be attached. After opening the eye, an air bubble is injected into the anterior chamber of the eye in order to minimize dilution of trypan blue by the aqueous. Trypan blue is carefully applied onto the anterior lens capsule using a blunt cannula. Sufficient staining is achieved as soon as the dye has contacted the capsule. The anterior chamber then is irrigated with balanced salt solution to remove all excess dye. An anterior capsulotomy can then be performed.

Storage/Stability: Trypan blue is stored at 15° to 25°C (59° to 77°F). Protect from direct sunlight.

Rx	**VisionBlue** (Dutch Ophthalmic)	**Solution**: 0.06%	0.5 mL in 2.25 mL single-use *Luer Lok* syringe.

AGENTS FOR RETINAL DISEASE

Historically little attention has been given to the pharmacologic treatment of retinal diseases because most topically applied ophthalmic medications do not penetrate sufficiently to tissues of the retina or posterior pole. In recent years, however, drug delivery systems and appropriate medications have been developed that target several retinal diseases, notably cytomegalovirus (CMV) retinitis and age-related macular disease.

CMV RETINITIS

Before reports of AIDS–related eye disease, CMV retinitis was an obscure condition, occurring in infants born with CMV infection or in patients taking immunosuppressive agents. CMV infects many adults worldwide and is transmitted by close contact with an individual excreting virus in urine, saliva, semen, or other body fluids. Retinitis is the most common form of systemic CMV infection in AIDS. Before the introduction of highly active antiretroviral therapy, CMV retinitis occurred at a frequency of approximately 25% in all patients with AIDS.

CMV retinitis is managed with antiviral medications administered systemically or locally. Current medications include ganciclovir, foscarnet, cidofovir, and fomivirsen. Systemic drug therapy can lead to one or more systemic toxicities, usually hematologic or renal, whereas local delivery is associated with endophthalmitis, retinal detachment, inflammation, or vitreous hemorrhage.

The ophthalmic antiviral preparations appear to interfere with viral reproduction by altering DNA synthesis. Ganciclovir and valganciclovir are indicated for use in immunocompromised patients with CMV retinitis and for prevention of CMV retinitis in transplant patients. Foscarnet and cidofovir are indicated for use in AIDS patients with CMV retinitis.

Antiviral Agents for Ophthalmic Conditions

Generic name	Trade name (manufacturer)	Preparations	Indications
Cidofovir	*Vistide* (Gilead)	Solution for Injection	CMV retinitis
Foscarnet sodium	*Foscavir* (Astra)	Solution for Injection	CMV retinitis
Ganciclovir sodium	*Cytovene* (Syntex)	Reconstituted powder Capsules 250 mg	CMV retinitis
	Vitrasert (Chiron)	Implant	CMV retinitis
Valganciclovir Hydrochloride	*Valcyte* (Roche)	Tablets, film–coated 450 mg	CMV retinitis

AGE-RELATED MACULAR DEGENERATION

Age-related macular degeneration (ARMD) is the leading cause of legal blindness in the United States. It is generally accepted that photooxidative stress underlies the pathogenesis of this disease, with most solar radiation-induced retinal damage resulting from photochemical mechanisms. Choroidal vessels invade Bruch's membrane for unknown reasons, possibly attracted by abnormal excretions from retinal pigment epithelial cells or stimulated by vasoproliferative substances such as vascular endothelial growth factor (VEGF). New blood vessels penetrate the inner collagenase layer of Bruch's membrane, spreading laterally underneath the deposits and within the plane of the drusen. This leads to an increased risk of discrete leakage of blood and serous fluid, detaching both the retinal pigment epithelium and overlying retina.

Historically, management of ARMD due to CNV has depended on laser photocoagulation of the choroidal neovascular membranes. Recently, supplemental antioxidant compounds have been used to protect against oxidative stress, and compounds such as vitamin C, vitamin E, and beta carotene have gained increased acceptance since the 1990s. Photodynamic therapy has also been approved for treatment of exudative ARMD. This approach uses an intravascular compound that causes vascular occlusion after stimulation by a specific wavelength of light at sufficiently low intensity to spare the irradiated tissues from thermal damage. Verteporfin (*Visudyne*) is liposome-encapsulated to enhance delivery to vascular tissue via low-density lipoprotein receptors on proliferating vascular endothelium. Very low laser energy releases the dye from the liposomes and initiates the photodynamic reaction.

Anti-VEGF compounds represent the newest approach to treatment of exudative ARMD, and several such agents are now commercially available. These include pegaptanib sodium (*Macugen*) and ranibizumab (*Lucentis*). These drugs are injected intravitreally at specified intervals.

Bevacizumab (*Avastin*) is a recombinant humanized monoclonal IgG1 antibody that binds to human VEGF and inhibits its biologic activity. The systemic administration is indicated in combination with 5-fluorouracil–based chemotherapy for the first and second-line treatment of metastatic carcinoma of the colon or rectum. It is also indicated in combination with carboplatin and paclitaxel in unresectable, locally advanced, recurrent or metastatic non-squamous, non-small cell lung cancer.

Off-label use of *Avastin* for intravitreal administration in the treatment of chorioretinal diseases was utilized by many retinal specialists until the availability of *Lucentis*. An intravitreal dose of 1.25 mg per 0.05 mL was given although some investigators have used 2.5 mg per 0.1 mL dose. Although results with the intravitreal *Avastin* were very favorable, utilization is cautioned based upon the FDA approval of *Lucentis*.

VERTEPORFIN

CNV associated with age-related macular degeneration is a major cause of visual impairment. This disease is difficult to treat with conventional laser procedures because normal retinal tissues can be destroyed, resulting in central vision loss. Photodynamic therapy offers the opportunity to selectively eradicate neovascular membranes while producing minimal damage to normal retinal and choroidal tissues.

The procedure involves intravenous administration of verteporfin (*Visudyne*) for 10 minutes. Verteporfin is a potent photosensitizing dye. Five minutes after the conclusion of dye administration, during which the drug selectively accumulates in the abnormal, neovascular tissue, nonthermal light at 689 nm is applied to the abnormal tissues for 83 seconds. When activated by light, verteporfin causes the production of singlet oxygen and free radicals that produce cell death and occlusion of abnormal vessels. The use of verteporfin in the photodynamic therapy of neovascular age-related macular degeneration has been shown to be effective in stabilizing the disease in animal models and in human clinical trials.

For More Information

Bashshur ZF, Bazarbachi A, Schakal A, et al. Intravitreal bevacizumab for the management of choroidal neovasularization in age-related macular degeneration. *Am J Ophthalmol.* 2006;142:1-9.

Bright DC. Diseases of the retina. In: Bartlett JD, Jaanus SD, eds. *Clinical Ocular Pharmacology*, 5th ed. St. Louis, MO: Elsevier; 2008.

Eter N, Krohne TU, Holz FG. New pharmacologic approaches to therapy for age-related macular degeneration. *BioDrugs.* 2006;20(3):167-179.

Michels S, Schmidt-Erfurth U, Rosenfeld PJ. Promising new treatments for neovascular age-related macular degeneration. *Expert Opin Investig Drugs.* 2006;15(7):779-793.

Rosenfeld PJ. Intravitreal *Avastin*: The low cost alternative to *Lucentis. Am J Ophthalmol.* 2006:142:141-143.

Steinbrook R. The price of sight — ranibizumab, bevacizumab, and the treatment of macular degeneration. *N Engl J Med.* 2006:355:1409-1412.

CIDOFOVIR

Warning:

Renal impairment is the major toxicity of cidofovir. To minimize possible nephrotoxicity, IV prehydration with Normal Saline and administration of probenecid must be used with each cidofovir infusion. Monitor renal function (serum creatinine and urine protein) within 48 hours prior to each dose of cidofovir and modify the dose for changes in renal function as appropriate.

Granulocytopenia has been observed in association with cidofovir treatment. Monitor neutrophil counts during cidofovir therapy.

Actions:

Pharmacology: Cidofovir is a nucleotide analog. Cidofovir suppresses CMV replication by selective inhibition of viral DNA synthesis. Biochemical data support selective inhibition of CMV DNA polymerase by cidofovir diphosphate, the active intracellular metabolite of cidofovir. Cidofovir diphosphate inhibits herpes virus polymerases at concentrations that are 8- to 600-fold lower than those needed to inhibit human cellular DNA polymerases alpha, beta, and gamma. Incorporation of cidofovir into the growing viral DNA results in reductions in the rate of viral DNA synthesis.

Resistance – CMV isolates with reduced susceptibility to cidofovir have been selected in vitro in the presence of high concentration of cidofovir. IC_{50} values for selected resistant isolates ranged from 7 to 15 mcg.

Cross-resistance – Cidofovir-resistant isolates selected in vitro following exposure to increasing concentrations of cidofovir were assessed for susceptibility to ganciclovir and foscarnet. All were cross-resistant to ganciclovir, but remained susceptible to foscarnet. Ganciclovir or ganciclovir/foscarnet-resistant isolates that are cross-resistant to cidofovir have been obtained from drug-naive patients and from patients following ganciclovir or ganciclovir/foscarnet therapy. To date, the majority of ganciclovir-resistant isolates are UL97 gene product (phosphokinase) mutants and remain susceptible to cidofovir. However, reduced susceptibility to cidofovir has been reported for DNA polymerase mutants of CMV that are resistant to ganciclovir. To date, all clinical isolates that exhibit high level resistance to ganciclovir, because of mutations in the DNA polymerase gene, have been shown to be cross-resistant to cidofovir. Cidofovir is active against some, but not all, CMV isolates that are resistant to foscarnet. The incidence of foscarnet-resistant isolates that are resistant to cidofovir is not known.

A few triple-drug resistant isolates have been described. Genotypic analysis of 2 of these triple-resistant isolates revealed several point mutations in the CMV DNA polymerase gene.

Pharmacokinetics: Cidofovir must be administered with probenecid. Renal tubular secretion contributes to the elimination of cidofovir.

Cidofovir Pharmacokinetic Parameters Following 3 and 5 mg/kg Infusions With and Without Probenecid				
	Cidofovir administered without probenecid		Cidofovir administered with probenecid	
Parameters	3 mg/kg	5 mg/kg	3 mg/kg	5 mg/kg
AUC (mcg•hr/mL)	20	28.3	25.7	40.8
C_{max} (end of infusion) (mcg/mL)	7.3	11.5	9.8	19.6
Vdss (mL/kg)	537		410	
Clearance (mL/min/1.73 m^2)	179		148	
Renal clearance (mL/min/1.73 m^2)	150		98.6	

In vitro, cidofovir was less than 6% bound to plasma or serum proteins over the cidofovir concentration range 0.25 to 25 mcg/mL. CSF concentrations of cidofovir following IV infusion of cidofovir 5 mg/kg with concomitant probenecid and IV hydration were undetectable (less than 0.1 mcg/mL, assay detection threshold) at 15 minutes after the end of a 1 hour infusion in 1 patient whose corresponding serum concentration was 8.7 mcg/mL.

Clinical Trials:

Delayed vs immediate therapy – In an open-label trial, previously untreated patients with peripheral CMV retinitis were randomized to either immediate treatment with cidofovir (5 mg/kg once a week for 2 weeks, then 5 mg/kg every other week), or delayed cidofovir treatment until progression of CMV retinitis occurred. Of 25 and 23 patients in the immediate and delayed groups respectively, 23 and 21 were evaluable for retinitis progression as determined by retinal photography. Based on masked readings of retinal photographs, the median (95% confidence internal [CI]) times to retinitis progression were 120 days (40, 134) and 22 days (10, 27) for the immediate and delayed therapy groups, respectively. This difference was statistically significant. Median (95% CI) times to the alternative endpoint of retinitis progression or study drug discontinuation (including adverse events, withdrawn consent, and systemic CMV disease) were 52 days (37, 85) and 22 days (13, 27) for the immediate and delayed therapy groups, respectively. This difference was statistically significant.

Indications:

CMV retinitis: For the treatment of CMV retinitis in patients with AIDS.

The safety and efficacy of cidofovir have not been established for treatment of other CMV infections (such as pneumonitis or gastroenteritis), congenital or neonatal CMV disease, or CMV disease in non-HIV–infected individuals.

Contraindications:

Hypersensitivity to cidofovir; a history of clinically severe hypersensitivity to probenecid or other sulfa-containing medications; direct intraocular injection. It also is contraindicated in patients receiving other nephrotoxic agents.

Warnings:

Direct intraocular injection: Direct intraocular injection may be associated with significant decreases in intraocular pressure and impairment of vision.

Nephrotoxicity: Dose-dependent nephrotoxicity is the major dose-limiting toxicity related to cidofovir administration. Dose adjustment or discontinuation is required for changes in renal function while on therapy. Proteinuria may be an early indicator of cidofovir-related nephrotoxicity. Continued administration of cidofovir may lead to additional proximal tubular cell injury that may result in glycosuria; decreases in serum phosphate, uric acid, and bicarbonate; and elevations in serum creatinine. Patients with these adverse events occurring concurrently and meeting a criteria of Fanconi's syndrome have been reported. Renal function may not return to baseline after drug discontinuation.

Hematological toxicity: Neutropenia may occur during cidofovir therapy. Monitor neutrophil count while receiving cidofovir therapy.

Metabolic acidosis: Fanconi syndrome and decreases in serum bicarbonate associated with evidence of renal tubular damage have been reported. Serious metabolic acidosis, in association with liver failure, pancreatitis, mucormycosis, aspergillus, disseminated mycobacterial infection, and progression to death occurred in 1 patient.

Ocular hypotony: Among the subset of patients monitored for intraocular pressure changes, ocular hypotony (at least 50% change from baseline) was reported in 5 patients. Hypotony was reported in 1 patient with concomitant diabetes mellitus. Risk of ocular hypotony may be increased in patients with preexisting diabetes.

Renal function impairment: It is recommended that cidofovir not be initiated in patients with baseline serum creatinine more than 1.5 mg/dL or creatinine clearances no more than 55 mL/min. In these patients, use cidofovir when the potential benefits exceed the potential risks.

Carcinogenesis: Mammary adenocarcinomas have occurred in rats and mice, and Zymbal's gland carcinomas have occurred in rats. Studies showed inhibition of spermatogenesis in rats and monkeys. However, no adverse effects on fertility or reproduction were seen following once weekly IV injections of cidofovir in male rats for 13 consecutive weeks.

Elderly: No studies of the safety and efficacy of cidofovir in patients older than 60 years of age have been conducted. Because elderly individuals frequently have reduced glomerular filtration, pay particular attention to assessing renal function before and during cidofovir administration.

Pregnancy: Category C. Cidofovir was embryotoxic (reduced fetal body weights) in rats and in rabbits. An increased incidence of fetal external, soft tissue, and skeletal anomalies (eg, meningocele, short snout, short maxillary bones) occurred in rabbits. There are no adequate and well-controlled studies in pregnant women. Use cidofovir during pregnancy only if potential benefit to the mother justifies the potential risk to the fetus.

Lactation: It is not known whether cidofovir is excreted in breast milk. Because many drugs are excreted in breast milk and because of the potential for adverse reactions as well as the potential for tumorigenicity shown for cidofovir in animal studies, do not administer cidofovir to nursing women. The US Public Health Service Centers for Disease Control and Prevention advises HIV-infected women not to breastfeed and to avoid postnatal transmission of HIV to a child who may not yet be infected.

Children: Safety and effectiveness in children have not been studied. The use of cidofovir in children with AIDS warrants extreme caution because of the risk of long-term carcinogenicity and reproductive toxicity. Administer cidofovir to children only after careful evaluation and only if the potential benefits of treatment outweigh the risks.

Precautions:

Monitoring: Monitor serum creatinine, urine protein and white blood cell counts with differential prior to each dose. In patients with proteinuria, administer IV hydration and repeat the test. Periodically monitor intraocular pressure, visual acuity, and ocular symptoms.

Drug Interactions:

Nephrotoxic agents: Avoid concomitant administration of cidofovir and agents with nephrotoxic potential (eg, amphotericin B, aminoglycosides, foscarnet, IV pentamidine).

Adverse Reactions:

Cardiovascular: Hypotension; postural hypotension; pallor; syncope; tachycardia.

CNS: Asthenia (46%); headache (27%); amnesia; anxiety; confusion; convulsion; depression; dizziness; abnormal gait; hallucinations; insomnia; neuropathy; paresthesia; somnolence; vasodilation.

Dermatologic: Rash (30%); alopecia (25%); acne; skin discoloration; dry skin; herpes simplex; pruritus; rash; sweating; urticaria.

GI: Nausea, vomiting (65%); diarrhea (27%); anorexia (22%); abdominal pain (17%); colitis; constipation; tongue discoloration; dyspepsia; dysphagia; flatulence; gastritis; hepatomegaly; abnormal liver function tests; melena; oral candidiasis; rectal disorder; stomatitis; aphthous stomatitis; mouth ulceration; dry mouth.

GU: Decreased CrCl; glycosuria; hematuria; urinary incontinence; urinary tract infection.

Hematologic/Lymphatic: Thrombocytopenia; neutropenia (less than 750/mm^3; 31%); anemia (20%).

Metabolic/Nutritional: Edema; dehydration; hyperglycemia; hyperlipemia; hypocalcemia; hypokalemia; increased alkaline phosphatase; increased AST; increased ALT; weight loss.

Musculoskeletal: Arthralgia; myasthenia; myalgia.

Renal: Proteinuria (80%); renal toxicity (53%); serum creatinine elevations (29%) (see Warnings).

Respiratory: Asthma; bronchitis; coughing; dyspnea (22%); hiccough; increased sputum; lung disorder; pharyngitis; pneumonia (9%); rhinitis; sinusitis.

Special senses: Amblyopia; conjunctivitis; eye disorder; hypotony (12%) (see Warnings); iritis; retinal detachment; taste perversion; uveitis; abnormal vision.

Miscellaneous: Fever (57%); chills, infections (24%); allergic reaction; face edema; malaise; back, chest, neck pain; sarcoma; sepsis.

Overdosage:

Overdosage with cidofovir has not been reported; however, hemodialysis and hydration may reduce drug plasma concentrations in patients who receive an overdosage of cidofovir. Probenecid may reduce the potential for nephrotoxicity in patients who receive an overdose of cidofovir through reduction of active tubular secretion.

Patient Information:

Advise patients that cidofovir is not a cure for CMV retinitis, and that they may continue to experience progression of retinitis during and following treatment. Advise patients receiving cidofovir to have regular follow-up ophthalmologic examinations. Patients may also experience other manifestations of CMV disease despite cidofovir therapy.

HIV-infected patients may continue taking antiretroviral therapy. However, because probenecid reduces metabolic clearance of zidovudine, advise those taking zidovudine to temporarily discontinue zidovudine administration or decrease their zidovudine dose by 50% on days of cidofovir administration only.

Inform patients of the major toxicity of cidofovir, namely renal impairment, and that dose modification, including reduction, interruption, and possibly discontinuation, may be required. Emphasize close monitoring of renal function (routine urinalysis and serum creatinine) while on therapy.

Emphasize the importance of completing a full course of probenecid with each cidofovir dose. Warn patients of potential adverse events caused by probenecid (eg, headache, nausea, vomiting, hypersensitivity reactions). Hypersensitivity/allergic reactions may include rash, fever, chills, and anaphylaxis. Administration of probenecid after a meal or use of antiemetics may decrease the nausea. Prophylactic or therapeutic antihistamines or acetaminophen may be used to ameliorate hypersensitivity reactions.

Cidofovir caused reduced testes weight and hypospermia in animals. Such changes may occur in humans and cause infertility. Advise women of childbearing potential that cidofovir is embryotoxic in animals and not to use the drug during pregnancy. Women of childbearing potential should use effective contraception during and for 1 month following treatment. Men should practice barrier contraceptive methods during and for 3 months following treatment.

Administration and Dosage:

Do not administer by intraocular injection.

Dosage: The recommended dosage, frequency, or infusion rate must not be exceeded. Cidofovir must be diluted in 0.9% saline solution 100 mL prior to administration. To minimize potential nephrotoxicity, probenecid and IV saline prehydration must be administered with each cidofovir infusion.

Induction treatment: The recommended dose of cidofovir is 5 mg/kg body weight (given as an IV infusion at a constant rate over 1 hour) administered once weekly for 2 consecutive weeks.

Maintenance treatment: The recommended maintenance dose of cidofovir is 5 mg/kg body weight (given as an IV infusion at a constant rate over 1 hour) administered once every 2 weeks.

Probenecid: Probenecid must be administered orally with each cidofovir dose. Two grams must be administered 3 hours prior to the cidofovir dose, and more than 1 g administered at 2 hours and again at 8 hours after completion of the 1 hour cidofovir infusion (for a total of 4 g).

Ingestion of food prior to each dose of probenecid may reduce drug-related nausea and vomiting. Administration of an antiemetic may reduce the potential for nausea associated with probenecid ingestion. In patients who develop allergic or hypersensitivity symptoms to probenecid, consider the use of an appropriate prophylactic or therapeutic antihistamine or acetaminophen.

Hydration: Patients should receive a total of 1 L of 0.9% saline solution IV with each infusion of cidofovir. Infuse the saline solution over a 1- to 2-hour period immediately before the cidofovir infusion. Patients who can tolerate the additional fluid load should receive a second liter. If administered, initiate the second liter of saline at the start of the cidofovir infusion or immediately afterwards, and infuse over a 1- to 3-hour period.

Nephrotoxicity: For increases in serum creatinine (0.3 to 0.4 mg/dL), reduce the cidofovir dose from 5 mg/kg to 3 mg/kg. Discontinue cidofovir therapy for an increase in serum creatinine of at least 0.5 mg/dL or development of at least 3+ proteinuria.

Renal function impairment:

Dosing of Cidofovir with Renal Function Impairment		
CrCl (mL/min)	Induction (once weekly for 2 weeks)	Maintenance (once every 2 weeks)
41 - 55	2 mg/kg	2 mg/kg
30 - 40	1.5 mg/kg	1.5 mg/kg
20-29	1 mg/kg	1 mg/kg
≤ 19	0.5 mg/kg	0.5 mg/kg

Storage/Stability: Store at controlled room temperature 20° to 25°C (68° to 77°F).

Admixtures may be stored under refrigeration (2° to 8°C; 36° to 46°F) for no more than 24 hours. Allow refrigerated admixtures to equilibrate to room temperature prior to use.

Rx	**Vistide** (Gilead Sciences)	**Injection:** 75 mg/mL	In 5 mL amps.

FOSCARNET SODIUM (Phosphonoformic acid)

Warning:

Renal impairment, the major toxicity, occurs to some degree in most patients. Continual assessment of a patient's risk and frequent monitoring of serum creatinine with dose adjustment for changes in renal function are imperative.

Foscarnet causes alterations in plasma minerals and electrolytes that have led to seizures. Monitor patients frequently for such changes and their potential sequelae.

Actions:

Pharmacology: Foscarnet is an organic analog of inorganic pyrophosphate that inhibits replication of all known herpes viruses in vitro including CMV, herpes simplex virus types 1 and 2 (HSV-1, HSV-2), human herpes virus 6 (HHV-6), Epstein-Barr virus (EBV), and varicella-zoster virus (VZV).

Foscarnet exerts its antiviral activity by a selective inhibition at the pyrophosphate binding site on virus-specific DNA polymerases and reverse transcriptases at concentrations that do not affect cellular DNA polymerases. Foscarnet does not require activation (phosphorylation) by thymidine kinase or other kinases, and therefore is active in vitro against HSV mutants deficient in thymidine kinase. CMV strains resistant to ganciclovir may be sensitive to foscarnet.

The quantitative relationship between the in vitro susceptibility of human CMV to foscarnet and clinical response to therapy has not been clearly established and virus sensitivity testing has not been standardized. If no clinical response to foscarnet is observed, test viral isolates for sensitivity to foscarnet; naturally resistant mutants may emerge under selective pressure both in vitro and in vivo. The latent state of any of the human herpes viruses is not known to be sensitive to foscarnet and viral reactivation of CMV occurs after foscarnet therapy is terminated.

Pharmacokinetics: Foscarnet is 14% to 17% bound to plasma protein at plasma drug concentrations of 1 to 1,000 mcM. Plasma foscarnet concentrations in 2 studies are summarized in the following table:

Foscarnet Plasma Concentrations			
Mean dose (infusion time)	Day of sampling	Mean plasma concentration (mcM)	
		C_{max} (range)	C_{min} (range)
57 ± 6 mg/kg every 8 hr (1 hr)	1	573 (213 to 1,305)[1]	78 (< 33 to 139)[3]
47 ± 12 mg/kg every 8 hr (1 hr)	14 or 15	579 (246 to 922)[2]	110 (< 33 to 148)[4]
55 ± 6 mg/kg every 8 hr (hr)	3	445 (306 to 720)[1]	88 (< 33 to 162)[3]
57 ± 7 mg/kg every 8 hr (2 hr)	14 or 15	517 (348 to 789)[2]	105 (43 to 205)[4]

[1] Observed 0.9 to 2.4 hours after start of infusion.
[2] Observed 0.8 to 2.6 hours after start of infusion.
[3] Observed 4 to 8.1 hours after start of infusion.
[4] Observed 6.3 to 8.7 hours after start of infusion.

Mean plasma clearances were 130 ± 44 and 178 ± 48 mL/min/1.73 m^2 in 2 studies in which foscarnet was given by intermittent infusion and 152 ± 59 and 214 ± 25 mL/min/1.73 m^2 in 2 studies using continuous infusion. Approximately 80% to 90% of IV foscarnet is excreted unchanged in the urine of patients with normal renal function. Both tubular secretion and glomerular filtration account for urinary elimination of foscarnet. In one study, plasma clearance was less than creatinine clearance (CrCl), suggesting that foscarnet may also undergo tubular reabsorption. In 3 studies, decreases in plasma clearance of foscarnet were proportional to decreases in CrCl.

Two studies in patients with initially normal renal function who were treated with intermittent infusions showed average drug plasma half-lives of about 3 hours determined on days 1 or 3 of therapy. This may be an underestimate of the effective half-life because of the limited observation period. Plasma half-life increases with the severity of renal impairment. Half-lives of 2 to 8 hours occurred in patients having estimated or measured 24 hour CrCl of 44 to 90 mL/min. Careful monitoring of renal function and dose adjustment is imperative (see Warnings and Administration and Dosage).

Following continuous foscarnet infusion for 72 hours in 6 HIV-positive patients, plasma half-lives of 0.45 ± 0.32 and 3.3 ± 1.3 hours were determined. A terminal half-life of

18 ± 2.8 hours was estimated from foscarnet urinary excretion over 48 hours after stopping infusion. When foscarnet was given as a continuous infusion to 13 patients with HIV infection for 8 to 21 days, plasma half-lives of 1.4 ± 0.6 and 6.8 ± 5 hours were determined. A terminal half-life of 87.5 ± 41.8 hours was estimated from foscarnet urinary excretion over 6 days after the last infusion; however, renal function at the time of discontinuing the infusion was not known.

Measurements of urinary excretion are required to detect the longer terminal half-life assumed to represent release of foscarnet from bone. In animal studies (mice), 40% of an IV dose is deposited in bone in young animals and 7% in adults. Evidence indicates that foscarnet accumulates in human bone; however, the extent to which this occurs has not been determined. Mean volumes of distribution at steady state range from 0.3 to 0.6 L/kg.

Variable penetration into cerebrospinal fluid (CSF) has been observed. Intermittent infusion of 50 mg/kg every 8 hours for 28 days in 9 patients produced CSF levels of 150 to 260 mcM 3 hours after the end of infusion or 39% to 103% of the plasma levels. In another 4 patients, CSF concentrations were 35% to 69% of the plasma drug level after a dose of 230 mg/kg/day by continuous infusion for 2 to 13 days. However, the CSF:plasma ratio was only 13% in one patient receiving a continuous infusion at a rate of 274 mg/kg/day. Disease-related defects in the blood-brain barrier may be responsible for the variations seen.

Clinical Trials: In most clinical studies, treatment for CMV retinitis began with an induction dosage of 60 mg/kg every 8 hours for the first 2 to 3 weeks, followed by a once-daily maintenance at doses ranging from 60 to 120 mg/kg.

A prospective, randomized, masked, controlled clinical trial was conducted in 24 patients with AIDS and CMV retinitis. Patients received induction treatment of 60 mg/kg every 8 hours for 3 weeks, followed by maintenance treatment with 90 mg/kg/day until retinitis progression (appearance of a new lesion or advancement of the border of a posterior lesion more than 750 microns in diameter). The 13 patients randomized to treatment with foscarnet had a significant delay in progression of CMV retinitis compared to untreated controls. Median times to retinitis progression from study entry were 93 days (range, 21 to more than 364) and 22 days (range, 7 to 42), respectively.

In another prospective clinical trial of CMV retinitis in AIDS patients, 33 were treated with 2 to 3 weeks of foscarnet induction (60 mg/kg 3 times a day) and then randomized to 2 maintenance dose groups, 90 and 120 mg/kg/day. Median times from study entry to retinitis progression were 96 days (range, 14 to more than 176) and 140 days (range, 16 to more than 233), respectively. This was not statistically significant.

Indications:

Treatment of CMV retinitis in patients with AIDS.

Contraindications:

Hypersensitivity to foscarnet.

Warnings:

Mineral and electrolyte imbalances: Foscarnet has been associated with changes in serum electrolytes including hypokalemia (16%), hypocalcemia (15%), hypomagnesemia (15%), hypophosphatemia (8%), and hyperphosphatemia (6%). Foscarnet is associated with a transient, dose-related decrease in ionized serum calcium, which may not be reflected in total serum calcium. This effect most likely is related to foscarnet's chelation of divalent metal ions such as calcium. Therefore, advise patients to report symptoms of low ionized calcium such as perioral tingling, numbness in the extremities, and paresthesias. Be prepared to treat these as well as severe manifestations of electrolyte abnormalities, such as tetany and seizures. The rate of infusion may affect the transient decrease in ionized calcium; slowing the rate may decrease or prevent symptoms.

Transient changes in calcium or other electrolytes (including magnesium, potassium, or phosphate) may also contribute to a patient's risk for cardiac disturbances and seizures (see Neurotoxicity and Seizures). Therefore, use particular caution in patients with altered calcium or other electrolyte levels before treatment, especially those with neurologic or cardiac abnormalities and those on other drugs known to influence minerals and electrolytes (see Monitoring and Drug Interactions).

Neurotoxicity and seizures: Foscarnet was associated with seizures in 18/189 (10%) of AIDS patients in 5 controlled studies. Three patients were not taking foscarnet at the time of seizure. In most cases (15/18), the patients had an active CNS condition (eg, toxoplasmosis, HIV encephalopathy) or a history of CNS diseases. The rate of seizures did not increase with duration of treatment. Three cases were associated with overdoses of foscarnet (see Overdosage).

Statistically significant risk factors associated with seizures were low baseline absolute neutrophil count (ANC), impaired baseline renal function, and low total serum calcium. Several cases of seizures were associated with death. However, seizures did not always necessitate drug discontinuation. Ten of 15 patients with seizures while on the drug continued or resumed foscarnet following treatment of their underlying disease, electrolyte disturbances, or dose decreases. If factors predisposing to seizures are present, carefully monitor electrolytes, including calcium and magnesium (see Monitoring).

Other CMV infections: Safety and efficacy have not been established for the treatment of other CMV infections (eg, pneumonitis, gastroenteritis); congenital or neonatal CMV disease; or nonimmunocompromised individuals.

Renal function impairment: The major toxicity of foscarnet is renal impairment, which occurs to some degree in most patients. Approximately 33% of 189 patients with AIDS and CMV retinitis who received IV foscarnet in clinical studies developed significant impairment of renal function, manifested by a rise in serum creatinine concentration to no less than 2 mg/dL. Therefore, use foscarnet with caution in all patients, especially those with a history of renal function impairment. Patients vary in their sensitivity to foscarnet-induced nephrotoxicity, and initial renal function may not be predictive of the potential for drug-induced renal impairment.

Renal impairment is most likely to become clinically evident as assessed by increasing serum creatinine during the second week of induction therapy at 60 mg/kg 3 times a day. However, renal impairment may occur at any time in any patient during treatment; therefore, monitor renal function carefully (see Monitoring).

Elevations in serum creatinine are usually, but not uniformly, reversible following discontinuation or dose adjustment. Recovery of renal function after foscarnet-induced impairment usually occurs within 1 week of drug discontinuation. However, of 35 patients who experienced grade II renal impairment (serum creatinine 2 to 3 times the upper limit of normal), 2 died with renal failure within 4 weeks of stopping foscarnet and 3 others died with renal insufficiency still present less than 4 weeks after drug cessation.

Because of foscarnet's potential to cause renal impairment, dose adjustment for decreased baseline renal function and any change in renal function during treatment is necessary. In addition, it may be beneficial for adequate hydration to be established (eg, by inducing diuresis) prior to and during administration.

Mutagenesis: Foscarnet showed genotoxic effects in an in vitro transformation assay at concentrations greater than 0.5 mcg/mL and an increased frequency of chromosome aberrations in the sister chromatid exchange assay at 1000 mcg/mL. A high dose of foscarnet (350 mg/kg) caused an increase in micronucleated polychromatic erythrocytes in mice at doses that produced exposures comparable to that anticipated clinically.

Elderly: Because these individuals frequently have reduced glomerular filtration, pay particular attention to assessing renal function before and during administration (see Administration and Dosage).

Pregnancy: Category C. Daily subcutaneous doses up to 75 mg/kg administered to female rats prior to and during mating, during gestation, and 21 days postpartum caused a slight increase (less than 5%) in the number of skeletal anomalies compared with the control group. Daily subcutaneous doses up to 75 mg/kg (one-third the maximal daily human exposure) administered to rabbits and 150 mg/kg (one-eighth the maximal daily human exposure) administered to rats during gestation caused an increase in the frequency of skeletal anomalies/variations. These studies are inadequate to define the potential teratogenicity at levels to which women will be exposed. There are no adequate and well-controlled studies in pregnant women. Use during pregnancy only if clearly needed.

Lactation: It is not known whether foscarnet is excreted in breast milk; however, in lactating rats administered 75 mg/kg, foscarnet was excreted in maternal milk at concentrations 3 times higher than peak maternal blood concentrations. Exercise caution if foscarnet is administered to a nursing woman.

Children: The safety and efficacy of foscarnet in children have not been studied. Foscarnet is deposited in teeth and bone, and deposition is greater in young and growing animals. Foscarnet adversely affects development of tooth enamel in mice and rats. The effects of this deposition on skeletal development have not been studied. Because deposition in human bone also occurs, it is likely that it does so to a greater degree in developing bone in children. Administer to children only after careful evaluation and only if the potential benefits for treatment outweigh the risks.

Precautions:

Monitoring: The majority of patients will experience some decrease in renal function because of foscarnet administration. Therefore it is recommended that CrCl, either measured or estimated using the modified Cockcroft and Gault equation based on serum creatinine, be determined at baseline, 2 to 3 times per week during induction therapy and at least once every 1 to 2 weeks during maintenance therapy, with foscarnet dose adjusted accordingly (see Dose Adjustment). More frequent monitoring may be required for some patients. It is also recommended that a 24-hour CrCl be determined at baseline and periodically thereafter to ensure correct dosing. Discontinue foscarnet if CrCl drops to less than 0.4 mL/min/kg.

Because of foscarnet's propensity to chelate divalent metal ions and alter levels of serum electrolytes, closely monitor patients for such changes. It is recommended that a schedule similar to that recommended for serum creatinine (see above) be used to monitor serum calcium, magnesium, potassium, and phosphorus. Particular caution is advised in patients with decreased total serum calcium or other electrolyte levels before treatment, as well as in patients with neurologic or cardiac abnormalities, and in patients receiving other drugs known to influence serum calcium levels.

Correct any clinically significant metabolic changes. Also, patients who experience mild (eg, perioral numbness or paresthesias) or severe symptoms (eg, seizures) of electrolyte abnormalities should have serum electrolyte and mineral levels assessed as close in time to the event as possible.

Careful monitoring and appropriate management of electrolytes, calcium, magnesium, and creatinine are of particular importance in patients with conditions that may predispose them to seizures (see Warnings).

Diagnosis of CMV retinitis: Determine diagnosis by indirect ophthalmoscopy. Other conditions in the differential diagnosis of CMV retinitis include candidiasis, toxoplasmosis, and other diseases producing a similar retinal pattern, any of which may produce a retinal appearance similar to CMV. For this reason it is essential that the diagnosis of CMV retinitis be established by an ophthalmologist familiar with the retinal presentation of these conditions. The diagnosis of CMV retinitis may be supported by culture of CMV from urine, blood, throat, or other sites, but a negative CMV culture does not rule out CMV retinitis.

Toxicity/Local irritation: In controlled clinical studies, the maximum single-dose administered was 120 mg/kg by IV infusion over 2 hours. It is likely that larger doses, or more rapid infusions, would result in increased toxicity. Take care to infuse solutions containing foscarnet only into veins with adequate blood flow to permit rapid dilution and distribution, and avoid local irritation (see Administration and Dosage). Local irritation and ulcerations of penile epithelium have occurred in male patients receiving foscarnet, possibly related to the presence of drug in urine. One case of vulvovaginal ulceration in a female has occurred. Adequate hydration with close attention to personal hygiene may minimize the occurrence of such events.

Anemia: Anemia occurred in 33% of patients. This anemia was usually manageable with transfusions and required discontinuation of foscarnet in less than 1% (1/189) of patients in the studies. Granulocytopenia occurred in 17% of patients; however, only 1% (2/189) were terminated from these studies because of neutropenia.

Drug Interactions:

Nephrotoxic drugs: The elimination of foscarnet may be impaired by drugs that inhibit renal tubular secretion. Because of foscarnet's tendency to cause renal impairment, avoid the use of foscarnet in combination with potentially nephrotoxic drugs such as aminoglycosides, amphotericin B, and IV pentamidine unless the potential benefits outweigh the risks to the patient.

Pentamidine: Concomitant treatment of 4 patients with foscarnet and IV pentamidine may have caused hypocalcemia; 1 patient died with severe hypocalcemia. Toxicity associated with concomitant use of aerosolized pentamidine has not been reported.

Zidovudine: Foscarnet was used concomitantly with zidovudine in approximately one-third of patients in the US studies. Although the combination was generally well tolerated, additive effects on anemia may have occurred. However, no evidence of increased myelosuppression was seen.

Foscarnet decreases serum levels of ionized calcium. Exercise particular caution when other drugs known to influence serum calcium levels are used concurrently.

Adverse Reactions:

The most frequently reported events were the following: fever (65%); nausea (47%); anemia (33%); diarrhea (30%); abnormal renal function including acute renal failure, decreased CrCl, and increased serum creatinine (27%); vomiting, headache (26%); seizure (10%) (see Warnings and Precautions).

Adverse reactions categorized as "severe" were the following: death (14%); abnormal renal function (14%); marrow suppression (10%); anemia (9%); seizures (7%). Although death was specifically attributed to foscarnet in only 1 case, other complications of foscarnet (ie, renal impairment, electrolyte abnormalities, seizures) may have contributed to patient deaths (see Warnings and Precautions).

Cardiovascular: Hypertension, palpitations, ECG abnormalities including sinus tachycardia, first-degree AV block and nonspecific ST-T segment changes, hypotension, flushing, cerebrovascular disorder (see Warnings) (1% to 5%); cardiomyopathy, cardiac failure/arrest, bradycardia, extrasystole, arrhythmias, atrial arrhythmias/fibrillation, phlebitis, superficial thrombophlebitis of arm, mesenteric vein thrombophlebitis (less than 1%).

CNS: Headache, paresthesia, dizziness, involuntary muscle contractions, hypoesthesia, neuropathy, seizures (including grand mal; see Warnings) (at least 5%); tremor, ataxia, dementia, stupor, generalized spasms, sensory disturbances, meningitis, aphasia, abnormal coordination, leg cramps, EEG abnormalities (see Warnings) (1% to 5%); vertigo, coma, encephalopathy, abnormal gait, hyperesthesia, hypertonia, visual field defects, dyskinesia, extrapyramidal disorders, hemiparesis, hyperkinesia, vocal cord paralysis, paralysis, paraplegia, speech disorders, tetany, hyporeflexia, hyperreflexia, neuralgia, neuritis, peripheral neuropathy, cerebral edema, nystagmus (less than 1%).

Dermatologic: Rash, increased sweating (no less than 5%); pruritus, skin ulceration, seborrhea, erythematous rash, maculopapular rash, skin discoloration, facial edema (1% to 5%); acne, alopecia, dermatitis, anal pruritus, genital pruritus, aggravated psoriasis, psoriaform rash, skin disorders, dry skin, urticaria, verruca (less than 1%).

Endocrine: Antidiuretic hormone disorders, decreased gonadotropins, gynecomastia (less than 1%).

GI: Anorexia, nausea, diarrhea, vomiting, abdominal pain (at least 5%); constipation, dysphagia, dyspepsia, rectal hemorrhage, dry mouth, melena, flatulence, ulcerative stomatitis, pancreatitis (1% to 5%); enteritis, enterocolitis, glossitis, proctitis, stomatitis, tenesmus, increased amylase, pseudomembranous colitis, gastroenteritis, oral leukoplakia, oral hemorrhage, rectal disorders, colitis, duodenal ulcer, hematemesis, paralytic ileus, esophageal ulceration, ulcerative proctitis, tongue ulceration (less than 1%).

GU: Alterations in renal function, including serum creatinine, decreased CrCl and abnormal renal function (see Warnings) (at least 5%); albuminuria, dysuria, polyuria, urethral disorder, urinary retention, urinary tract infections, acute renal failure, nocturia (1% to 5%); hematuria, glomerulonephritis, micturition disorders/frequency, toxic nephropathy, nephrosis, urinary incontinence, renal tubular disorders, pyelonephritis, urethral irritation, uremia (less than 1%). Perineal pain in women, penile inflammation (less than 1%).

Hematologic/Lymphatic: Anemia, granulocytopenia, leukopenia (see Precautions) (at least 5%); thrombocytopenia, platelet abnormalities, thrombosis, white blood cell (count) abnormalities, lymphadenopathy (1% to 5%); pulmonary embolism, coagulation disorders, decreased coagulation factors, epistaxis, decreased prothrombin, hypochromic anemia, pancytopenia, hemolysis, leukocytosis, cervical lymphadenopathy, lymphopenia (less than 1%).

Lymphoma-like disorder, sarcoma (1% to 5%); malignant lymphoma, skin hypertrophy (less than 1%).

Hepatic: Abnormal A-G ratio, abnormal hepatic function, increased AST and ALT (1% to 5%); cholecystitis, cholelithiasis, hepatitis, cholestatic hepatitis, hepatosplenomegaly, jaundice (less than 1%).

Local: Injection site pain or inflammation (1% to 5%).

Metabolic/Nutritional: Mineral/electrolyte imbalances (see Warnings), including hypokalemia, hypocalcemia, hypomagnesemia, hypo- or hyperphosphatemia (at least 5%); hyponatremia, decreased weight, increased alkaline phosphatase, LDH and BUN, acidosis, cachexia, thirst, hypercalcemia (1% to 5%); dehydration, glycosuria, increased creatine phosphokinase, diabetes mellitus, abnormal glucose tolerance, hypervolemia, hypochloremia, periorbital edema, hypoproteinemia (less than 1%).

Musculoskeletal: Arthralgia, myalgia (1% to 5%); arthrosis, synovitis, torticollis (less than 1%).

Psychiatric: Depression, confusion, anxiety (no less than 5%); insomnia, somnolence, nervousness, amnesia, agitation, aggressive reaction, hallucination (1% to 5%); impaired concentration, emotional lability, psychosis, suicide attempt, delirium, personality disorders, sleep disorders (less than 1%).

Respiratory: Coughing, dyspnea (at least 5%); pneumonia, sinusitis, pharyngitis, rhinitis, respiratory disorders or insufficiency, pulmonary infiltration, stridor, pneumothorax, hemoptysis, bronchospasm (1% to 5%); bronchitis, laryngitis, respiratory depression, abnormal chest x-ray, pleural effusion, pulmonary hemorrhage, pneumonitis (less than 1%).

Special senses: Vision abnormalities (no less than 5%); taste perversions, eye abnormalities, eye pain, conjunctivitis (1% to 5%); diplopia, blindness, retinal detachment, mydriasis, photophobia, deafness, earache, tinnitus, otitis (less than 1%).

Miscellaneous: Fever, fatigue, rigors, asthenia, malaise, pain, infection, sepsis, death (at least 5%); back/chest pain, edema, influenza-like symptoms, bacterial/fungal infections, moniliasis, abscess (1% to 5%); hypothermia, leg edema, peripheral edema, syncope, ascites, substernal chest pain, abnormal crying, malignant hyperpyrexia, herpes simplex, viral infection, toxoplasmosis (less than 1%).

Overdosage:

Symptoms: In controlled clinical trials, overdosage was reported in 10 patients. All 10 patients experienced adverse reactions and all except 1 made a complete recovery. One patient died after receiving a total daily dose of more than 12.5 for 3 days instead of the intended 10.9 g. The patient suffered a grand mal seizure and became comatose. Three days later the patient died with the cause of death listed as respiratory/cardiac arrest. The other 9 patients received doses ranging from 1.14 times to 8 times their recommended doses with an average of 4 times their recommended doses. Overall, 3 patients had seizures, 3 patients had renal function impairment, 4 patients had paresthesias either in limbs or periorally, and 5 patients had documented electrolyte disturbances primarily involving calcium and phosphate.

Treatment: There is no specific antidote. Hemodialysis and hydration may be of benefit in reducing drug plasma levels in patients who receive an overdosage, but these have not been evaluated in a clinical trial setting. Observe the patient for signs and symptoms of renal impairment and electrolyte imbalance. Institute medical treatment if clinically warranted.

Patient Information:

Foscarnet is not a cure for CMV retinitis; patients may continue to experience progression of retinitis during or following treatment.

Regular ophthalmologic examinations are necessary. The major toxicities of foscarnet are renal impairment, electrolyte disturbances, and seizures; dose modifications and possibly discontinuation may be required.

Close monitoring while on therapy is essential. Advise patients of the importance of perioral tingling, numbness in the extremities, or paresthesias during or after infusion as possible symptoms of electrolyte abnormalities. Should such symptoms occur, stop the infusion, obtain appropriate laboratory samples for assessment of electrolyte concentrations, and consult health care provider before resuming treatment. The rate of infusion must be no more than 1 mg/kg/min.

The potential for renal impairment may be minimized by accompanying administration with hydration adequate to establish and maintain diuresis during dosing.

Administration and Dosage:

Caution: Do not administer by rapid or bolus IV injection. Toxicity may be increased as a result of excessive plasma levels. Take care to avoid unintentional overdose by carefully controlling the rate of infusion. Therefore, an infusion pump must be used. In spite of the use of an infusion pump, overdoses have occurred.

Administer by controlled IV infusion, either by using a central venous line or by using a peripheral vein. The standard 24 mg/mL solution may be used without dilution when using a central venous catheter for infusion. When a peripheral vein catheter is used, dilute the 24 mg/mL solution to 12 mg/mL with 5% dextrose in water or with a normal saline solution prior to administration to avoid local irritation of peripheral veins. Because the dose is calculated on the basis of body weight, it may be desirable to remove and discard any unneeded quantity from the bottle before starting with the infusion to avoid overdosage. Use solutions thus prepared within 24 hours of first entry into a sealed bottle.

Do not exceed the recommended dosage, frequency, or infusion rates. All doses must be individualized for patient's renal function.

Induction treatment: The recommended initial dose for patients with normal renal function is 60 mg/kg, adjusted for individual patient's renal function, given IV at a constant rate over a minimum of 1 hour every 8 hours for 2 to 3 weeks depending on clinical response. An infusion pump must be used to control the rate of infusion. Adequate hydration is recommended to establish diuresis, both prior to and during treatment to minimize renal toxicity (see Warnings), provided there are no clinical contraindications.

Maintenance treatment: 90 to 120 mg/kg/day (individualized for renal function) given as an IV infusion over 2 hours. Because the superiority of the 120 mg/kg/day has not been established in controlled trials, and given the likely relationship of higher plasma foscarnet levels to toxicity, it is recommended that most patients be started on maintenance treatment with a dose of 90 mg/kg/day. Escalation to 120 mg/kg/day may be considered should early reinduction be required because of retinitis progression.

Some patients who show excellent tolerance to foscarnet may benefit from initiation of maintenance treatment at 120 mg/kg/day earlier in their treatment. An infusion pump must be used to control the rate of infusion with all doses. Again, hydration to establish diuresis both prior to and during treatment is recommended to minimize renal toxicity.

Patients who experience progression of retinitis while receiving maintenance therapy may be retreated with the induction and maintenance regimens given above.

Renal function abnormalities: Use with caution in patients with abnormal renal function because reduced plasma clearance of foscarnet will result in elevated plasma levels. In addition, foscarnet has the potential to further impair renal function (see Warnings). Foscarnet has not been specifically studied in patients with CrCl less than 50 mL/min or serum creatinine more than 2.8 mg/dL. Carefully monitor renal function at baseline and during induction and maintenance therapy with appropriate dose adjustments. If CrCl falls below the limits of the dosing nomograms (0.4 mL/min/kg) during therapy, discontinue foscarnet and monitor the patient daily until resolution of renal impairment is ensured.

Dose adjustment in renal impairment: Individualize foscarnet dosing according to the patient's renal function status. Refer to the table below for recommended doses and adjust the dose as indicated.

To use this dosing guide, actual 24 hour CrCl (mL/min) must be divided by body weight (kg) or the estimated CrCl in mL/min/kg can be calculated from serum creatinine (mg/dL) using the following formula (modified Cockcroft and Gault equation).

$$\text{Males: } \frac{\text{Weight (kg)} \times (140 - \text{age})}{72 \times \text{serum creatinine (mg/dL)}} = \text{CrCl}$$

Females: $0.85 \times$ above value

Foscarnet Dosing Guide Based on CrCl	
	Induction
CrCl (mL/min/kg)	Equivalent to 60 mg/kg dose every 8 hours
≥ 1.6	60
1.5	57
1.4	53
1.3	49
1.2	46
1.1	42
1	39
0.9	35
0.8	32
0.7	28
0.6	25
0.5	21
0.4	18

Foscarnet Dosing Guide Based on CrCl		
Maintenance		
CrCl (mL/min/kg)	Equivalent to 90 mg/kg dose every 24 hours	Equivalent to 120 mg/kg dose every 24 hours
≥ 1.4	90	120
1.2-1.4	78	104
1-1.2	75	100
0.8-1	71	94
0.6-0.8	63	84
0.4-0.6	57	76

IV incompatibility: Other drugs and supplements can be administered to a patient receiving foscarnet. However, take care to ensure that foscarnet is only administered with normal saline or dextrose solution 5% and that no other drug or supplement is administered concurrently via the same catheter. Foscarnet is chemically incompatible with dextrose 30%, amphotericin B, and solutions containing calcium such as Ringer's lactate and TPN. Physical incompatibility with other IV drugs includes: Acyclovir sodium, ganciclovir, trimetrexate, pentamidine, vancomycin, trimethoprim/sulfamethoxazole, diazepam, midazolam, digoxin, phenytoin, leucovorin, and prochlorperazine. Because of foscarnet's chelating properties, a precipitate can potentially occur when divalent cations are administered concurrently in the same catheter.

Rx	**Foscavir** (Astra)	**Injection:** 24 mg/mL	In 500 mL bottles.

GANCICLOVIR (DHPG) CAPSULES AND POWDER FOR INJECTION

Warning:

The clinical toxicity of ganciclovir includes granulocytopenia, anemia, and thrombocytopenia. In animal studies, ganciclovir was carcinogenic, teratogenic, and caused aspermatogenesis.

Ganciclovir IV is indicated for use only in the treatment of CMV retinitis in immunocompromised patients and for the prevention of CMV disease in transplant patients at risk for CMV disease.

Because oral ganciclovir is associated with a risk of more rapid rate of CMV retinitis progression, use only in those patients for whom this risk is balanced by the benefit associated with avoiding daily IV infusions.

Actions:

Pharmacology: Ganciclovir, a synthetic guanine derivative active against CMV, is an acyclic nucleoside analog of 2'-deoxyguanosine that inhibits replication of herpes viruses in vitro and in vivo. Sensitive human viruses include CMV, herpes simplex virus-1 and -2, herpes virus type 6, EBV, VZV, and hepatitis B virus.

Ganciclovir must be converted to the corresponding triphosphate in order to exert its antiviral activity. In herpes simplex virus-infected cells, the initial conversion to the monophosphate is catalyzed by a viral thymidine kinase. In contrast, in CMV-infected cells, a protein kinase homologue may be responsible for the initial phosphorylation of ganciclovir. Cellular kinases, in CMV-infected cells, subsequently phosphorylate ganciclovir monophosphate to the diphosphate and active triphosphate moieties. Levels of ganciclovir triphosphate are as much as 100-fold greater in CMV-infected cells than in uninfected cells, indicating a preferential phosphorylation of ganciclovir in virus-infected cells. Ganciclovir triphosphate, once formed, appears quite stable and persists for days in the CMV-infected cell. The antiviral activity of ganciclovir triphosphate is believed to be the result of inhibition of viral DNA synthesis by two known modes: (1) Competitive inhibition of viral DNA polymerases; and (2) direct incorporation into viral DNA, resulting in eventual termination of viral DNA elongation. The cellular DNA polymerase alpha is also inhibited, but at a higher concentration than required for inhibition of viral DNA polymerase.

The median concentration of ganciclovir that effectively inhibits the replication of either laboratory strains or clinical isolates of CMV (ED_{50}) has ranged from 0.02 to 3.48 mcg/mL. The relationship of in vitro sensitivity of CMV to ganciclovir and clinical response has not been established. Ganciclovir inhibits mammalian cell proliferation in vitro at higher concentrations: IC_{50} values range from 30 to 725 mcg/mL, with the exception of bone marrow-derived colony-forming cells that are more sensitive with IC_{50} values ranging from 0.028 to 0.7 mcg/mL.

Pharmacokinetics:

Absorption – The absolute bioavailability of oral ganciclovir under fasting conditions was approximately 5% and following food it was 6% to 9%. When given with a meal containing 602 calories and 46.5% fat, the steady-state area under serum concentration vs time curve (AUC) increased and there was a significant prolongation of time to peak serum concentrations (see Drug Interactions).

At the end of a 1-hour IV infusion of 5 mg/kg, total AUC ranged between 22.1 and 26.8 mcg•hr/mL and C_{max} ranged between 8.27 and 9 mcg/mL.

Distribution – The steady-state volume of distribution after IV administration was 0.74 L/kg. Cerebrospinal fluid concentrations obtained 0.25 and 5.67 hours postdose in 3 patients who received 2.5 mg/kg ganciclovir IV every 8 or 12 hours ranged from 0.31 to 0.68 mcg/mL, representing 24% to 70% of the respective plasma concentrations. Binding to plasma proteins was 1% to 2% over ganciclovir concentrations of 0.5 and 51 mcg/mL.

Metabolism – Following oral administration of a single 1,000 mg dose, 86% of the administered dose was recovered in the feces and 5% was recovered in the urine. No metabolite accounted for 1% to 2% recovered in urine or feces.

Excretion – When administered IV, ganciclovir exhibits linear pharmacokinetics over the range of 1.6 to 5 mg/kg and when administered orally, it exhibits linear kinetics up to a total daily dose of 4 g/day. Renal excretion of unchanged drug by glomerular filtration and active tubular secretion is the major route of elimination. In patients with normal renal function, 91.3% of IV ganciclovir was recovered unmetabolized in the urine. Systemic clearance of IV ganciclovir was 3.52 mL/min/kg while renal clearance was 3.2 mL/min/kg, accounting for 91% of the systemic clearance. After oral administration, steady state is achieved within 24 hours. Renal clearance following oral administration was 3.1 mL/min/kg. Half-life was 3.5 hours following IV administration and 4.8 following oral use.

Renal function impairment – Because the major elimination pathway for ganciclovir is renal, dosage must be reduced according to CrCl (see Administration and Dosage). The pharmacokinetics following IV administration were evaluated in 10 immunocompromised patients with renal impairment who received doses ranging from 1.25 to 5 mg/kg.

IV Ganciclovir Pharmacokinetics in Patients with Renal Impairment			
CrCl (mL/min)	Dose (mg/kg)	Clearance (mL/min)	Half-life (hr)
50-79 (n = 4)	3.2-5	128	4.6
25-49 (n = 3)	3-5	57	4.4
< 25 (n = 3)	1.25-5	30	10.7

The pharmacokinetics following oral administration were evaluated in 8 solid organ transplant recipients; dose was modified according to estimated CrCl.

Oral Ganciclovir in Patients with Renal Impairment			
CrCl (mL/min)	Dose (mg/kg)	AUC_{0-24} (mcg•hr/mL)	Half-life (hr)
50-69 (n = 4)	1,000 mg every 8 hr	49.1 ± 2.2	NC[1]
25-49 (n = 1)	1,000 mg every day	27.4	18.2
10-24 (n = 1)	500 mg every day	10.7	15.7
< 10 (n = 2)	500 mg 3 times weekly[2]	25.6 ± 5.9	NC[1]

[1] NC = Not calculated; half-life exceeded sampling interval.
[2] After hemodialysis.

Hemodialysis reduces plasma concentrations of ganciclovir approximately 50% after IV and oral administration.

Race – The effects of race were studied in subjects receiving a dose regimen of 1,000 mg every 8 hours. Although the numbers of black patients (16%) and Hispanic patients (20%) were small, there appeared to be a trend toward a lower steady-state C_{max} and AUC_{0-8} in these subpopulations as compared with white patients.

Children – At an IV dose of 4 or 6 mg/kg in 27 newborns (2 to 49 days of age), the pharmacokinetic parameters were, respectively, C_{max} of 5.5 and 7 mcg/mL, systemic clearance of 3.14 and 3.56 mL/min/kg, and half-life of 2.4 hours for both.

Clinical Trials:

IV – Immunocompromised patients – Of 314 immunocompromised patients enrolled in an open label study of the treatment of life- or sight-threatening CMV disease, 121 patients had a positive culture for CMV within 7 days prior to treatment.

Virologic Response to IV Ganciclovir Treatment			
Culture source	No. patients cultured	No. (%) patients responding	Median days to response
Urine	107	93 (87%)	8
Blood	41	34 (83%)	8
Throat	21	19 (90%)	7
Semen	6	6 (100%)	15

Transplant recipients – In 149 CMV seropositive heart allograft recipients and 72 CMV culture positive allogeneic bone marrow transplant recipients, ganciclovir prevented recrudescence of CMV shedding in the heart allograft patients and suppressed CMV shedding in the bone marrow allograft patients.

Patients with Positive CMV Cultures Following IV Ganciclovir				
	Heart allograft		Bone marrow allograft	
Time	Ganciclovir	Placebo	Ganciclovir	Placebo
Pretreatment	2%	8%	100%	100%
Week 2	3%	16%	6%	68%
Week 4	5%	43%	0%	80%

Oral – The antiviral activity of ganciclovir capsules was confirmed in 2 randomized, controlled trials comparing IV versus oral ganciclovir for the maintenance treatment of CMV retinitis in patients with AIDS. Only a small proportion of patients remained culture-positive during maintenance therapy with either IV or oral ganciclovir. There were no statistically significant differences in the rates of positive cultures between the treatment groups. The antiviral effect of oral ganciclovir in the patients in the 2 studies is summarized in the following table:

Patients with Positive CMV Following Oral Ganciclovir				
	Patients with newly diagnosed CMV retinitis[1]		Patients with stable, previously treated CMV retinitis[2]	
	IV	Oral	IV	Oral[3]
At start of maintenance	13.5%	24.3%	3%	3.6%
Anytime during maintenance	6.3%	9.1%	2.2%	7.1%

[1] 3 weeks of treatment with IV ganciclovir before start of maintenance.
[2] 4 weeks to 4 months treatment with IV ganciclovir before start of maintenance.
[3] Data from 6 times daily and 3 times daily regimens pooled.

Viral resistance – CMV resistance to ganciclovir in individuals with AIDS and CMV retinitis who have not previously been treated with ganciclovir does occur but appears to be infrequent. Viral resistance has been observed in patients receiving prolonged treatment with ganciclovir IV. However, because of the limited number of viral isolates tested, it is difficult to estimate the overall frequency of reduced sensitivity in patients receiving ganciclovir. Nonetheless, consider the possibility of viral resistance in patients who show poor clinical response or experience persistent viral excretion during therapy. The principal mechanism of resistance to ganciclovir in CMV is the decreased ability to form the active triphosphate moiety. Mutations in the viral DNA polymerase also have been reported to confer viral resistance to ganciclovir. In 2 randomized controlled trials, the incidence of reduced sensitivity appeared to be no more common during treatment with oral ganciclovir than during IV treatment.

Indications:

IV:

CMV retinitis – Treatment of CMV retinitis in immunocompromised patients, including patients with AIDS.

CMV disease – Prevention of CMV disease in transplant recipients at risk for CMV disease.

Oral: Alternative to the IV formulation for maintenance treatment of CMV retinitis in immunocompromised patients, including patients with AIDS, in whom retinitis is stable following appropriate induction therapy and for whom the risk of more rapid progression is balanced by the benefit associated with avoiding daily IV infusions.

Off-label use(s): Ganciclovir also may be beneficial in some immunocompromised patients in the treatment of other CMV infections (eg, pneumonitis, gastroenteritis, hepatitis [see Warnings]).

Contraindications:

Hypersensitivity to ganciclovir or acyclovir.

Warnings:

CMV disease: Safety and efficacy have not been established for congenital or neonatal CMV disease nor for the treatment of established CMV disease other than retinitis nor for use in nonimmunocompromised individuals. The safety and efficacy of oral ganciclovir have not been established for treating any manifestation of CMV disease other than maintenance treatment of CMV retinitis.

Diagnosis of CMV retinitis: Diagnosis is ophthalmologic and should be made by indirect ophthalmoscopy. Other conditions in the differential diagnosis of CMV retinitis include candidiasis, toxoplasmosis, histoplasmosis, retinal scars, and cotton wool spots, any of which may produce a retinal appearance similar to CMV. The diagnosis may be supported by culture of CMV from urine, blood, or throat, but a negative CMV culture does not rule out CMV retinitis.

Retinal detachment: Retinal detachment has been observed in subjects with CMV retinitis both before and after initiation of therapy with ganciclovir. Its relationship to therapy is unknown. Retinal detachment occurred in 11% of patients treated with IV ganciclovir and in 8% of patients treated with oral ganciclovir. Patients with CMV retinitis should have frequent ophthalmologic evaluations to monitor the status of their retinitis and to detect any other retinal pathology.

Hematologic: Do not administer if the absolute neutrophil count is less than 500/mm^3 or the platelet count is less than 25,000/mm^3. Granulocytopenia (neutropenia), anemia, and thrombocytopenia have been observed in patients treated with ganciclovir. The frequency and severity of these events vary widely in different patient populations (see Adverse Reactions). Therefore, use with caution in patients with preexisting cytopenias or with a history of cytopenic reactions to other drugs, chemicals, or irradiation. Granulocytopenia usually occurs during the first or second week of treatment, but may occur at any time during treatment. Cell counts usually begin to recover within 3 to 7 days of discontinuing drug. Colony-stimulating factors have increased neutrophil and WBC counts in patients receiving IV ganciclovir for CMV retinitis.

Renal function impairment: Use ganciclovir with caution because the half-life and plasma/serum concentrations of ganciclovir will be increased because of reduced renal clearance (see Administration and Dosage).

Hemodialysis reduces plasma levels of ganciclovir by about 50%.

Carcinogenesis: In mice, daily oral doses of 1,000 mg/kg may have caused an increased incidence of tumors in the preputial gland of males, nonglandular mucosa of the stomach of males and females, and reproductive tissues (eg, ovaries, uterus, mammary gland, clitoral gland, vagina) and liver in females. A slightly increased incidence of tumors occurred in the preputial gland (males) and nonglandular mucosa (males and females) of the stomach in mice given 20 mg/kg/day. Consider ganciclovir a potential carcinogen in humans.

Mutagenesis: Ganciclovir caused point mutations and chromosomal damage in mammalian cells in vitro and in vivo. Because of the mutagenic and teratogenic potential of ganciclovir, advise women of childbearing potential to use effective contraception during treatment. Similarly, advise men to practice barrier contraception during and for at least 90 days following treatment with ganciclovir.

Fertility impairment: Animal data indicate that ganciclovir causes inhibition of spermatogenesis and subsequent infertility. Ganciclovir caused decreased fertility in male mice and hypospermatogenesis in mice and dogs. These effects were reversible at lower doses and irreversible at higher doses. Although data in humans have not been obtained regarding this effect, ganciclovir, at the recommended doses, may cause temporary or permanent inhibition of spermatogenesis. Animal data also indicate that suppression of fertility in females may occur. Ganciclovir caused decreased mating behavior, decreased fertility, and an increased incidence of embryolethality in female mice following IV doses approximately 1.7 times the mean drug exposure in humans.

Elderly: The pharmacokinetic profile in elderly patients has not been established. Because elderly individuals frequently have a reduced glomerular filtration rate, pay particular attention to assessing renal function before and during administration of ganciclovir (see Administration and Dosage).

Pregnancy: Category C. Ganciclovir is embryotoxic in rabbits and mice following IV administration and teratogenic in rabbits. Fetal resorptions were present in ≥ 85% of rabbits and mice administered 2 times the human exposure. Effects observed in rabbits included the following: Fetal growth retardation, embryolethality, teratogenicity and maternal toxicity. Teratogenic changes included cleft palate, anophthalmia/microphthalmia, aplastic organs (kidney and pancreas), hydrocephaly, and brachygnathia. In mice, effects observed were maternal/fetal toxicity and embryolethality.

Daily IV doses given to female mice prior to mating, during gestation, and during lactation caused hypoplasia of the testes and seminal vesicles in the month-old male offspring, as well as pathologic changes in the nonglandular region of the stomach.

Ganciclovir may be teratogenic or embryotoxic at dose levels recommended for human use. There are no adequate and well-controlled studies in pregnant women. Use during pregnancy only if the potential benefits to the mother justify the potential risk to the fetus.

Lactation: It is not known whether ganciclovir is excreted in breast milk. However, because carcinogenic and teratogenic effects occurred in animals treated with ganciclovir, the possibility of serious adverse reactions from ganciclovir in nursing infants is considered likely. Instruct mothers to discontinue nursing if they are receiving ganciclovir. The minimum interval before nursing can safely be resumed after the last dose of ganciclovir is unknown.

Children: Safety and efficacy in children have not been established. The use of ganciclovir in children warrants extreme caution to the probability of long-term carcinogenicity and reproductive toxicity. Administer to children only after careful evaluation and only if the potential benefits of treatment outweigh the risks. Oral ganciclovir has not been studied in children younger than 13 years of age.

There has been very limited clinical experience using IV ganciclovir for the treatment of CMV retinitis in patients younger than 12 years of age. Two children (9 and 5 years of age) showed improvement or stabilization of retinitis for 23 and 9 months, respectively. These children received induction treatment with 2.5 mg/kg 3 times daily followed by maintenance therapy with 6 to 6.5 mg/kg once a day, 5 to 7 days per week. When retinitis progressed during once-daily maintenance therapy, both children were treated with the 5 mg/kg twice-daily regimen. Two other children (2.5 and 4 years of age) who received similar induction regimens showed only partial or no response to treatment. Another 6-year-old child with T-cell dysfunction showed stabilization of retinitis for 3 months while receiving continuous infusions of IV ganciclovir at doses of 2 to 5 mg/kg/24 hours. Continuous infusion treatment was discontinued because of granulocytopenia.

Eleven of the 72 patients in the placebo-controlled trial in bone marrow transplant recipients were children, ranging from 3 to 10 years of age (5 treated with IV ganciclovir and 6 with placebo). Five of the pediatric patients treated with ganciclovir received 5 mg/kg IV twice daily for up to 7 days; 4 patients went on to receive 5 mg/kg once daily up to day 100 posttransplant. Results were similar to those observed in adult transplant recipients treated with IV ganciclovir. Two of the 6 placebo-treated children developed CMV pneumonia versus none of the 5 treated with ganciclovir. The spectrum of adverse reactions in the children was similar to that observed in the adults.

The spectrum of adverse reactions reported in 120 immunocompromised child clinical trial participants with serious CMV infections receiving IV ganciclovir were similar to those reported in adults. Granulocytopenia (17%) and thrombocytopenia (10%) were the most common adverse reactions reported.

Precautions:

Monitoring: Caused by the frequency of neutropenia, anemia, and thrombocytopenia in patients receiving ganciclovir, it is recommended that complete blood counts and platelet counts be performed frequently, especially in patients in whom ganciclovir or other nucleoside analogs have previously resulted in leukopenia, or in whom neutrophil counts are fewer than 1,000/mm^3 at the beginning of treatment. Because dosing with ganciclovir must be modified in patients with renal impairment, and because of the incidence of increased serum creatinine levels that have been observed in transplant recipients treated with IV ganciclovir, patients should have serum creatinine or creatinine clearance values followed carefully.

Large doses/Rapid infusion: The maximum single dose administered was 6 mg/kg by IV infusion more than 1 hour. Larger doses have resulted in increased toxicity. It is likely that more rapid infusions would also result in increased toxicity (see Overdosage).

Phlebitis/Pain at injection site: Initially, reconstituted solutions of IV ganciclovir have a high pH (pH 11). Despite further dilution in IV fluids, phlebitis or pain may occur at the site of IV infusion. Take care to infuse solutions containing ganciclovir only into veins with adequate blood flow to permit rapid dilution and distribution.

Hydration: Because ganciclovir is excreted by the kidneys and normal clearance depends on adequate renal function, ganciclovir administration should be accompanied by adequate hydration.

Photosensitivity: Photosensitization (photoallergy or phototoxicity) may occur; therefore, caution patients to take protective measures against exposure to ultraviolet or sunlight (ie, sunscreens, protective clothing) until tolerance is determined.

Drug Interactions:

Ganciclovir Drug Interactions

Precipitant drug	Object drug*		Description
Ganciclovir	Cytotoxic drugs	↑	Cytotoxic drugs that inhibit replication of rapidly dividing cell populations such as bone marrow, spermatogonia, and germinal layers of skin and GI mucosa may have additive toxicity when administered concomitantly with ganciclovir. Therefore, consider the concomitant use of drugs such as dapsone, pentamidine, flucytosine, vincristine, vinblastine, adriamycin, amphotericin B, trimethoprim/sulfamethoxazole combinations, or other nucleoside analogs only if potential benefits outweigh the risks.
Imipenem-cilastatin	Ganciclovir	↑	Generalized seizures occurred in patients who received ganciclovir and imipenem-cilastatin. Do not use these drugs concomitantly unless the potential benefits outweigh the risks.
Nephrotoxic drugs	Ganciclovir	↑	Increases in serum creatinine were observed following concurrent use of ganciclovir and either cyclosporine or amphotericin B (see Warnings).
Probenecid	Ganciclovir	↑	Ganciclovir AUC increased 53% (range, -14% to 299%) in the presence of probenecid. Renal clearance of ganciclovir decreased 22% (range, -54% to -4%), which is consistent with an interaction involving competition for renal tubular secretion.
Ganciclovir	Didanosine	↑	Steady-state didanosine AUC increased 111% (range, 10% to 493%) when didanosine was administered either 2 hours prior to or simultaneously with ganciclovir. A decrease in steady-state ganciclovir AUC of 21% (range, -44% to 5%) was observed when didanosine was administered 2 hours prior to administration of ganciclovir, but ganciclovir AUC was not affected by the presence of didanosine when the 2 drugs were administered simultaneously.
Didanosine	Ganciclovir	↓	
Ganciclovir	Zidovudine	↑	Mean steady-state ganciclovir AUC decreased 17% (range, -52% to 23%) in the presence of zidovudine. Steady-state zidovudine AUC increased 19% (range, -11% to 74%) in the presence of ganciclovir. Because both drugs can cause granulocytopenia and anemia, many patients will not tolerate combination therapy at full dosage.
Zidovudine	Ganciclovir	↓	

* ↑ = Object drug increased. ↓ = Object drug decreased.

Drug/Food interactions: When ganciclovir was administered orally with food at a total daily dose of 3 g/day (either 500 mg every 3 hours 6 times daily or 1,000 mg 3 times daily), the steady-state absorption as measured by AUC and C_{max} were similar following both regimens. When ganciclovir capsules were given with a meal containing 602 calories and 46.5% fat at a dose of 1,000 mg every 8 hours to 20 HIV-positive subjects, the steady-state AUC increased 22% (range, 6% to 68%) and there was a significant prolongation of time to peak serum concentrations (T_{max}) from 1.8 to 3 hours and a higher C_{max} (0.85 vs 0.96 mcg/mL).

Adverse Reactions:

Immunologic:

AIDS patients –

Selected Adverse Reactions Reported in 5% of Subjects: Oral vs IV Ganciclovir Maintenance Treatment		
Adverse reaction	Oral (3,000 mg/day) (n = 326)	IV (5 mg/kg/day) (n = 179)
CNS		
Neuropathy	8%	9%
Paresthesia	6%	10%
GI		
Diarrhea	41%	44%
Nausea	26%	25%
Anorexia	15%	14%
Vomiting	13%	13%
Flatulence	6%	3%
Hemic/Lymphatic		
Leukopenia	29%	41%
Anemia	19%	25%
Thrombocytopenia	6%	6%
Miscellaneous		
Fever	38%	48%
Abdominal pain	17%	19%
Rash	15%	10%
Sweating	11%	12%
Infection	9%	13%
Chills	7%	10%
Pneumonia	6%	8%
Pruritus	6%	5%
Vitreous disorder	6%	4%
Sepsis	4%	15%
Catheter-related		
Total catheter events	6%	22%
Catheter infection	4%	9%
Catheter sepsis	1%	8%
Neutropenia (ANC/mm^3)	(n = 320)	(n = 175)
< 500	18	25
500 to < 750	17	14
750 to < 1000	19	26
Total ANC ≤ 1000	54	66
Anemia hemoglobin (g/dL)	(n = 320)	(n = 175)
< 6.5	2	5
6.5 to < 8	10	16
8 to < 9.5	25	26
Total Hb < 9.5	36	46

Overall, subjects treated with IV ganciclovir experienced lower minimum acid-neutralizing capacities (ANCs) and hemoglobin levels, more consistent with neutropenia and anemia, compared with those who received oral ganciclovir.

For the majority of subjects, maximum serum creatinine levels were less than 1.5 mg/dL and no difference was noted between IV and oral ganciclovir for the occurrence of renal impairment. Serum creatinine elevations more than 2.5 mg/dL occurred in less than 2% of all subjects and no significant differences were noted in the time from the start of maintenance to the occurrence of elevations in serum creatinine values.

Transplant recipients –

Granulocytopenia/Thrombocytopenia with IV Ganciclovir				
	Heart allograft[1]		Bone marrow allograft[2]	
Hematologic effect	Ganciclovir (n = 76)	Placebo (n = 73)	Ganciclovir IV (n = 57)	Control (n = 55)
Neutropenia				
Minimum ANC < 500/mm^3	4%	3%	12%	6%
Minimum ANC 500 - 1,000/mm^3	3%	8%	29%	17%
Total ANC ≤ 1,000/mm^3	7%	11%	41%	23%
Thrombocytopenia				
Platelet count < 25,000/mm^3	3%	1%	32%	28%
Platelet count 25,000 - 50,000/mm^3	5%	3%	25%	37%
Total Platelet 50,000/mm^3	8%	4%	57%	65%

[1] Mean duration of treatment = 28 days.
[2] Mean duration of treatment = 45 days.

Elevated Serum Creatinine with IV Ganciclovir						
	Heart allograft		Bone marrow allograft			
Maximum serum creatinine levels	Ganciclovir IV (n = 76)	Placebo (n = 73)	Ganciclovir IV (n = 20)	Control (n = 20)	Ganciclovir IV (n = 37)	Placebo (n = 35)
Serum creatinine ≥ 2.5 mg/dL	18%	4%	20%	0%	0%	0%
Serum creatinine ≥ 1.5 - < 2.5 mg/dL	58%	69%	50%	35%	43%	44%

Cardiovascular: Arrhythmia, deep thrombophlebitis, hypertension, hypotension, vasodilatation (no more than 1%).

CNS: Abnormal dreams, abnormal gait, abnormal thinking, agitation, amnesia, anxiety, ataxia, coma, confusion, depression, dizziness, dry mouth, euphoria, hypertonia, hypesthesia, insomnia, libido decreased, manic reaction, nervousness, psychosis, seizures, somnolence, tremor, trismus (approximately 5%).

Dermatologic: Acne, alopecia, dry skin, fixed eruption, herpes simplex, maculopapular rash, skin discoloration, urticaria, vesiculobullous rash (no more than 1%).

GI: Abnormal liver function test, dyspepsia, nausea, vomiting (2%); constipation, dysphagia, eructation, fecal incontinence, hemorrhage, hepatitis, melena, mouth ulceration, tongue disorder (no more than 1%).

GU: Breast pain, creatinine clearance decreased/increased, hematuria, increased BUN, kidney failure, kidney function abnormal, urinary frequency, urinary tract infection.

Hematologic: Eosinophilia, hypochromic anemia, marrow depression, pancytopenia (no more than 1%).

Metabolic/Nutritional: Increased alkaline phosphatase, creatine phosphokinase, lactic dehydrogenase, AST, ALT (no more than 1%); hypokalemia, pancreatitis, decreased blood sugar (no more than 1%).

Musculoskeletal: Myalgia, myasthenia (no more than 1%).

Respiratory: Cough increased, dyspnea (no more than 1%).

Special senses: Abnormal vision, amblyopia, blindness, conjunctivitis, deafness, eye pain, glaucoma, retinitis, photophobia, taste perversion, tinnitus (no more than 1%).

Miscellaneous: Asthenia (6%); headache (4%); injection site inflammation, pain, phlebitis (2%); enlarged abdomen, abscess, back pain, cellulitis, chest pain, chills, fever, drug level increased (ganciclovir), edema, face edema, injection site abscess/edema/hemorrhage/pain, lab test abnormality, malaise, migraine, photosensitivity reaction, neck pain/rigidity (no more than 1%).

The following adverse reactions may be fatal: pancreatitis, sepsis, and multiple organ failure.

Adverse reactions reported in postmarketing surveillance –

Reported on at least 2 occasions: Acidosis, anaphylactic reaction, cardiac arrest, cataracts, cholestasis, cholangitis, congenital anomaly, encephalopathy, hyponatremia, impotence, infertility, intracranial hypertension, leukemia, lymphoma, myocardial infarction, pericarditis, Stevens-Johnson syndrome, stroke, transverse myelitis, unexplained death.

Reported once: Allograft rejection, arthritis, asthma, bleeding disorder, cachexia, corneal erosion, cyanosis, diplopia, dry eyes, dysesthesia, ear infection, elevated triglyceride levels, endocarditis, exfoliative dermatitis, exacerbation of psoriasis, facial palsy, gangrene, gingival hypertrophy, Guillain-Barre syndrome, hemolytic-uremic syndrome, hypernatremia, hypomagnesemia, icterus, inappropriate serum ADH, increased sweating, irritability, loss of memory, loss of sense of smell, multiple organ failure, myelopathy, myocarditis, nephritis, ophthalmoplegia, parathyroid disorder, Parkinsonism-like reaction, pneumothorax, peripheral ischemia, perforated intestine, pneumonia, proteinuria, pseudotumor cerebri, pulmonary fibrosis, pulmonary embolism, respiratory distress syndrome, rhabdomyolysis, sperm production abnormal, testicular hypotrophy, thyroid disorder, Wolff-Parkinson-White syndrome.

Overdosage:

IV: Overdosage with IV ganciclovir has been reported in 17 patients (13 adults and 4 children younger than 2 years of age). Five patients experienced no adverse reactions following overdosage at the following doses: 7 doses of 11 mg/kg over a 3 day period (adult), single dose of 3,500 mg (adult), single dose of 500 mg (72.5 mg/kg) followed by 48 hours of peritoneal dialysis (4-month-old), single dose of about 60 mg/kg followed by exchange transfusion (18-month-old), 2 doses of 500 mg instead of 31 mg (21-month-old).

Irreversible pancytopenia developed in 1 adult with AIDS and CMV colitis after receiving 3,000 mg IV ganciclovir on each of 2 consecutive days. He experienced worsening GI symptoms and acute renal failure which required short-term dialysis. Pancytopenia developed and persisted until his death from a malignancy several months later. Other adverse reactions reported following overdosage include the following: Persistent bone marrow suppression (1 adult with neutropenia and thrombocytopenia after a single dose of 6,000 mg), reversible neutropenia or granulocytopenia (4 adults, overdoses ranging from 8 mg/kg daily for 4 days to a single dose of 25 mg/kg), hepatitis (1 adult receiving 10 mg/kg daily, and one 2 kg infant after a single 40 mg dose), renal toxicity (1 adult with transient worsening of hematuria after a single 500 mg dose, and 1 adult with elevated creatinine [5.2 mg/dL] after a single 5,000 to 7,000 mg dose) and seizure (1 adult with known seizure disorder after 3 days of 9 mg/kg). In addition, 1 adult received 0.4 mL (instead of 0.1 mL) by intravitreal injection, and experienced temporary loss of vision and central retinal artery occlusion secondary to increased intraocular pressure related to the injected fluid volume.

Oral: There have been no reports of overdosage with oral ganciclovir. Doses no more than 6,000 mg/day did not result in overt toxicity other than transient neutropenia.

Treatment: Dialysis may be useful in reducing serum concentrations. Maintain adequate hydration. Consider the use of hematopoietic growth factors.

Patient Information:

Ganciclovir is not a cure for CMV retinitis, and immunocompromised patients may continue to experience progression of retinitis during or following treatment. Advise patients to have regular ophthalmologic examinations at a minimum of every 6 weeks while being treated.

The major toxicities of ganciclovir are granulocytopenia and thrombocytopenia. Dose modifications may be required, including possible discontinuation. Emphasize the importance of close monitoring of blood counts while on therapy.

Patients with AIDS may be receiving zidovudine. Treatment with zidovudine and ganciclovir will not be tolerated by many patients and may result in severe granulocytopenia.

Advise patients that ganciclovir may cause infertility. Advise women of childbearing potential that ganciclovir should not be used during pregnancy; use effective contraception during ganciclovir treatment. Similarly, advise men to practice barrier contraception during and for at least 90 days following ganciclovir treatment.

Although there is no information, consider ganciclovir a potential carcinogen.

Transplant recipients: Counsel transplant recipients regarding the high frequency of impaired renal function, particularly in patients receiving coadministration of nephrotoxic agents such as cyclosporine and amphotericin B.

Administration and Dosage:

IV: Do not administer by rapid or bolus IV injection. The toxicity may be increased as a result of excessive plasma levels. Do not exceed the recommended infusion rate. IM or subcutaneous injection of reconstituted ganciclovir may result in severe tissue irritation caused by high pH.

CMV retinitis (normal renal function):

Induction – The recommended initial dose is 5 mg/kg (given IV at a constant rate longer than 1 hour) every 12 hours for 14 to 21 days. Do not use oral ganciclovir for induction treatment.

Maintenance –

IV – Following induction treatment, the recommended maintenance dose is 5 mg/kg given as a constant rate IV infusion more than 1 hour once daily 7 days per week, or 6 mg/kg once daily 5 days per week.

Oral – Following induction treatment, the recommended maintenance dose of oral ganciclovir is 1,000 mg 3 times daily with food. Alternatively, the dosing regimen of 500 mg 6 times daily every 3 hours with food, during waking hours, may be used.

For patients who experience progression of CMV retinitis while receiving maintenance treatment with either formulation of ganciclovir, reinduction treatment is recommended.

Prevention of CMV disease in transplant recipients: The recommended initial dose of IV ganciclovir for patients with normal renal function is 5 mg/kg (given IV at a constant rate longer than 1 hour) every 12 hours for 7 to 14 days, followed by 5 mg/kg once daily 7 days per week or 6 mg/kg once daily 5 days per week.

The duration of treatment with IV ganciclovir in transplant recipients is dependent on the duration and degree of immunosuppression. In controlled clinical trials in bone marrow allograft recipients, treatment was continued until day 100 to 120 posttransplantation. CMV disease occurred in several patients who discontinued treatment with ganciclovir prematurely. In heart allograft recipients, the onset of newly diagnosed CMV disease occurred after treatment with ganciclovir was stopped at day 28 posttransplant, suggesting that continued dosing may be necessary to prevent late occurrence of CMV disease in this patient population.

Renal impairment:

IV – Refer to the following table for recommended doses and adjust the dosing interval as indicated.

IV Ganciclovir Dose in Renal Impairment				
CrCl (mL/min)	Ganciclovir induction dose (mg/kg)	Dosing interval (hr)	Ganciclovir maintenance dose (mg/kg)	Dosing interval (hr)
≥ 70	5	12	5	24
50 to 69	2.5	12	2.5	24
25 to 49	2.5	24	1.25	24
10 to 24	1.25	24	0.625	24
< 10	1.25	3 times per week following hemodialysis	0.625	3 times per week following hemodialysis

Hemodialysis: Dosing for patients undergoing hemodialysis should not exceed 1.25 mg/kg 3 times per week, following each hemodialysis session. Give shortly after completion of the hemodialysis session, because hemodialysis reduces plasma levels by approximately 50%.

Oral – In patients with renal impairment, modify the dose of oral ganciclovir as follows:

Oral Ganciclovir Dose in Renal Impairment	
CrCl (mL/min)	Ganciclovir doses
≥ 70	1,000 mg 3 times daily, or 500 mg every 3 hr 6 times daily
50 to 69	1,500 mg 4 times daily, or 500 mg 3 times daily
25 to 49	1,000 mg 4 times daily, or 500 mg twice daily
10 to 24	500 mg 4 times daily
< 10	500 mg 3 times per week, following hemodialysis

CrCl can be related to serum creatinine by the following formula:

$$\text{Males:} \quad \frac{\text{Weight (kg)} \times (140 - \text{age})}{72 \times \text{serum creatinine (mg/dL)}} = \text{CrCl}$$

Females: $0.85 \times$ above value

Patient monitoring: Caused by the frequency of granulocytopenia and thrombocytopenia, it is recommended that neutrophil counts and platelet counts be performed frequently, especially in patients in whom ganciclovir or other nucleoside analogs have previously resulted in leukopenia, or in whom neutrophil counts are less than

1,000/mm^3 at the beginning of treatment. Because dosing with ganciclovir must be modified in patients with renal impairment, and because of the incidence of increased serum creatinine levels that has been observed in transplant recipients treated with IV ganciclovir, patients should have serum creatinine or CrCl values followed carefully.

Reduction of dose: Dose reductions are required for patients with renal impairment and for those with neutropenia or thrombocytopenia. Therefore, perform frequent white blood cell counts. Severe neutropenia (ANC less than 500/mm^3) or severe thrombocytopenia (platelets less than 25,000/mm^3) require a dose interruption until evidence of marrow recovery is observed (ANC more than 750/mm^3).

Preparation of IV solution: Each 10 mL clear glass vial contains ganciclovir sodium equivalent to 500 mg of the free base form of ganciclovir and 46 mg of sodium. Prepare the contents of the vial for administration in the following manner:

Reconstituted solution –

1. Reconstitute lyophilized ganciclovir by injecting 10 mL of sterile water for injection, USP, into the vial. Do not use bacteriostatic water for injection containing parabens; it is incompatible with ganciclovir and may cause precipitation.

2. Shake the vial to dissolve the drug.

3. Visually inspect the reconstituted solution for particulate matter and discoloration prior to proceeding with infusion solution. Discard the vial if particulate matter or discoloration is observed.

4. Reconstituted solution in the vial is stable at room temperature for 12 hours. Do not refrigerate.

Infusion solution – Based on patient weight, remove the appropriate volume of the reconstituted solution (ganciclovir concentration 50 mg/mL) from the vial and add to an acceptable (see below) infusion fluid (typically 100 mL) for delivery over the course of 1 hour. Infusion concentrations greater than 10 mg/mL are not recommended. The following infusion fluids have been determined to be chemically and physically compatible with ganciclovir IV solution: 0.9% sodium chloride, 5% dextrose, Ringer's injection, and lactated Ringer's injection, USP.

Handling and disposal: Exercise caution in the handling and preparation of ganciclovir. Solutions of IV ganciclovir are alkaline (pH 11). Avoid direct contact with the skin or mucous membranes of the powder contained in ganciclovir capsules or of ganciclovir IV solutions. If such contact occurs, wash thoroughly with soap and water; rinse eyes thoroughly with plain water. Do not open or crush ganciclovir capsules.

Because ganciclovir shares some of the properties of antitumor agents (ie, carcinogenicity and mutagenicity), give consideration to handling and disposal according to guidelines issued for antineoplastic drugs.

Storage/Stability: Reconstituted solution in the vial is stable at room temperature for 12 hours. Do not refrigerate. Because nonbacteriostatic infusion fluid must be used with ganciclovir IV solution, the infusion solution must be used within 24 hours of dilution to reduce the risk of bacterial contamination. Refrigerate the infusion solution. Freezing is not recommended.

Rx	**Ganciclovir** (Various, eg, Ranbaxy)	**Capsules:** 250 mg	In 180s.
Rx	**Ganciclovir** (Various, eg, Ranbaxy)	**Capsules:** 500 mg	In 60s, 180s, and 500s.
Rx	**Cytovene** (Roche)	**Powder for injection, lyophilized:** ganciclovir 500 mg/vial (as sodium)	In 10 mL vials.

GANCICLOVIR INTRAVITREAL IMPLANT

Actions:

Pharmacology: Ganciclovir is a synthetic nucleoside analog of 2′-deoxyguanosine that inhibits replication of herpes viruses both in vitro and in vivo. Sensitive human viruses include CMV, herpes simplex virus-1 and -2 (HSV-1, HSV-2), EBV, and VZV.

The median concentration of ganciclovir that effectively inhibits the replication of human CMV (ED_{50}) has ranged from 0.2 to 3 mcg/mL. The relationship of in vitro sensitivity of CMV to ganciclovir and clinical response has not been established. Ganciclovir inhibits mammalian cell proliferation in vitro at higher concentrations: ID_{50} values range from 10 to 60 mcg/mL, with the exception of bone marrow-derived colony-forming cells, which are more sensitive with ID_{50} values more than 10 mcg/mL of the cell types tested.

In vitro sensitivity testing of CMV isolates from patients receiving intravenous ganciclovir has shown emergence of viral resistance. Because the prevalence of resistant isolates is unknown, there is a possibility that some patients may be infected with strains of CMV resistant to ganciclovir. Consequently, consider the possibility of viral resistance in patients showing poor clinical response.

Pharmacokinetics: In one clinical trial, 26 patients (30 eyes treated) received a total of 39 primary implants and 12 exchange implants (performed 32 weeks after the implant was inserted or earlier if progression of CMV retinitis occurred). Precise in vivo release rates of the ganciclovir implant could not be calculated because most of the exchanged implants were empty upon removal. It was unknown at what time the implant ran out of the drug. However, approximate in vivo release rates ranged from 1 mcg/hr to greater than 1.62 mcg/hr for the exchanged implants.

In another study, in 14 implants (3 exchanged, 11 autopsy) in which the in vivo release rate could be accurately calculated, the mean release rate was 1.4 mcg/hr, with a range of 0.5 to 2.88 mcg/hr. The mean vitreous drug levels in 8 eyes (4 collected at time of retinal detachment surgery; 2 collected from autopsy eyes within 6 hours of death and prior to fixation; 2 collected from implant exchange) was 4.1 mcg/mL.

Clinical Trials: Ganciclovir implant (*Vitrasert*) and intravenous (*Cytovene*) were compared in a randomized, controlled parallel group trial conducted between May 1993 and December 1994 in 188 patients with AIDS and newly diagnosed CMV retinitis. Patients in the intravenous treatment group received an induction dose of 5 mg/kg twice daily for 14 days followed by a maintenance dose of 5 mg/kg once daily. The median time to progression was about 210 days for the implant (*Vitrasert*) treatment group, compared with about 120 days for the intravenous (*Cytovene*) ganciclovir treatment group.

Indications:

For the treatment of CMV retinitis in patients with acquired immunodeficiency syndrome (AIDS). The implant is for intravitreal implantation only.

Contraindications:

Hypersensitivity to ganciclovir or acyclovir. Patients contraindicated for intraocular surgery (eg, external infection, severe thrombocytopenia).

Warnings:

Diagnosis of CMV retinitis: Diagnosis is ophthalmologic and should be made by indirect ophthalmoscopy. Other conditions in the differential diagnosis of CMV retinitis include candidiasis, toxoplasmosis, histoplasmosis, retinal scars, and cotton wool spots, any of which may produce a retinal appearance similar to CMV.

CMV retinitis: CMV retinitis may be associated with CMV disease elsewhere in the body. The implant provides localized therapy limited to the implanted eye. The implant does not provide treatment for systemic CMV disease. Monitor patients for extraocular CMV disease.

Surgical procedures: Surgical procedures involve risk. The following complications may occur with intraocular surgery to place the implant into the vitreous cavity: Vitreous loss, vitreous hemorrhage, cataract formation, retinal detachment, uveitis, endophthalmitis, and decrease in visual acuity.

Loss of visual acuity: Loss of visual acuity may occur immediately in the implanted eye of almost all patients postoperatively. This decrease is temporary and lasts for approximately 2 to 4 weeks after implantation. This decrease in visual acuity is probably a result of the surgical implant procedure.

The Vitrasert implant: The *Virasert* implant is sterilized by an ethylene oxide-freon mixture, a substance which harms public health and the environment by destroying ozone in the upper atmosphere.

Carcinogenesis/Mutagenesis/Fertility Impairment: In mice, daily oral doses of 1,000 mg/kg may have caused an increased incidence of tumors in the preputial gland of males, nonglandular mucosa of the stomach of males and females, and reproductive tissues (eg, ovaries, uterus, mammary gland, clitoral gland, vagina) and liver in females. A slightly increased incidence of tumors occurred in the preputial and harderian glands (males), forestomach in males and females, and liver in females in mice given 20 mg/kg/day. Except for histiocytic sarcoma of the liver, ganciclovir-induced tumors were generally of epithelial or vascular origin. Consider ganciclovir a potential carcinogen in humans.

Ganciclovir caused mutations in lymphoma cells in mice and DNA damage in human lymphocytes in vitro at concentrations of 50 to 500 mcg/mL and 250 to 2,000 mcg/mL, respectively. In the mouse micronucleus assay, ganciclovir was clastogenic at doses of 150 and 500 mg/kg (2.8% to 10% human exposure based on AUC), but not

50 mg/kg (exposure approximately comparable to the human, based on AUC). Ganciclovir was not mutagenic in the Ames Salmonella assay at concentrations of 500 to 5,000 mcg/mL.

Ganciclovir caused decreased mating behavior, decreased fertility, and an increased incidence of embryolethality in female mice following intravenous doses of 90 mg/kg/day. Decreased fertility in male mice and hypospermatogenesis in mice and dogs occurred following daily oral or intravenous administration of ganciclovir ranging from 0.2 to 10 mg/kg.

Pregnancy: Category C. Ganciclovir is embryotoxic in rabbits and mice following IV administration and teratogenic in rabbits. Fetal resorptions were present in at least 85% of rabbits and mice administered 60 mg/kg/day and 108 mg/kg/day, respectively. Effects observed in rabbits included the following: Fetal growth retardation, embryolethality, teratogenicity, and maternal toxicity. Teratogenic changes included cleft palate, anophthalmia/microphthalmia, aplastic organs (kidney and pancreas), hydrocephaly, and brachygnathia. In mice, effects observed were maternal/fetal toxicity and embryolethality.

Daily IV doses of 90/mg/kg administered to female mice prior to mating, during gestation and during lactation, caused hypoplasia of the test and seminal vesicles in the month-old male offspring, as well as pathologic changes in the nonglandular region of the stomach.

There are no adequate and well-controlled studies in pregnant women. Use during pregnancy only if the potential benefits to the mother justify the potential risk to the fetus.

Lactation: It is not known whether ganciclovir is excreted in breast milk. However, because carcinogenic and teratogenic effects occurred in animals treated with ganciclovir, the possibility of serious adverse reactions from ganciclovir in nursing infants is considered likely. Instruct mothers to discontinue nursing if they have a ganciclovir implant.

Children: Safety and effectiveness in children younger than 9 years of age have not been established.

Precautions:

As with all intraocular surgery, rigorously maintain sterility of the surgical field and the ganciclovir implant. The implant should be handled only by the suture tab in order to avoid damaging the polymer coatings because this could affect release rate of ganciclovir inside the eye. Do not resterilize the implant by any method.

A high level of surgical skill is required for implantation. A surgeon should have observed or assisted in surgical implantation of the ganciclovir implant prior to attempting the procedure.

Drug Interactions:

No drug interactions have been observed with the ganciclovir implant. There is limited experience with the use of retinal tamponades in conjunction with the ganciclovir implant.

Adverse Reactions:

The most frequent adverse reactions reported involved the eye.

During first 2 months following implantation: Visual acuity loss of at least 3 lines, vitreous hemorrhage, and retinal detachments (about 10% to 20%).

Local: Cataract formation/lens opacities, macular abnormalities, intraocular pressure spikes, optic disk/nerve changes, hyphemas, uveitis (about 1% to 5%). Retinopathy, anterior chamber cell and flare, synechia, hemorrhage (other than vitreous), cotton wool spots, keratophathy, astigmatism, endophthalmitis, microangiopathy, sclerosis, choroiditis, chemosis, phthisis bulbi, angle-closure glaucoma with anterior chamber shallowing, vitreous detachment, vitreous traction, hypotony, severe postoperative inflammation, retinal tear, retinal hole, corneal dellen, choroidal folds, pellet extrusion from scleral wound, gliosis (less than 1%).

Patient Information:

The ganciclovir implant is not a cure for CMV retinitis and immunocompromised patients may continue to experience progression of retinitis with the implant. Advise patients to have regular ophthalmic examinations on both eyes at appropriate intervals following implantation.

As with any surgical procedure, risk is involved. Potential complications accompanying implantation may include intraocular infection or inflammation, retinal detachment, or cataract formation in the natural crystalline lens.

Immediate and temporary decrease in visual acuity in the implanted eye(s) are experienced by almost all patients following implantation. This lasts approximately 2 to 4 weeks postoperatively and is probably a result of the surgical implant procedure.

Administration and Dosage:

Each implant contains a minimum of 4.5 mg of ganciclovir, and is designed to release the drug over a 5- to 8-month period. Following depletion of ganciclovir from the implant, as evidenced by progression of retinitis, the implant may be removed and replaced.

Handling and disposal: Exercise caution in handling the implant in order to avoid damage to the polymer coating on the implant, which may result in an increased rate of drug release from the implant. Handle the implant by the suture tab only. Maintain aseptic technique at all times prior to and during the surgical implantation procedure.

Because the implant contains ganciclovir, which shares some of the properties of antitumor agents (ie, carcinogenicity, mutagenicity), give consideration to handling and disposal of the implant according to guidelines issued for antineoplastic drugs.

Storage/Stability: Store at room temperature 15° to 30°C (59° to 86°F). Do not freeze. Keep away from excessive heat and light.

Rx	**Vitrasert** (Bausch & Lomb Surgical)	**Implant:** Minimum 4.5 mg	In individual unit boxes in a sterile *Tyvek* package.

VALGANCICLOVIR HYDROCHLORIDE

Warning:

The clinical toxicity of valganciclovir, which is metabolized to ganciclovir, includes granulocytopenia, anemia, and thrombocytopenia. In animal studies, ganciclovir was carcinogenic, teratogenic, and caused aspermatogenesis.

Actions:

Pharmacology: Valganciclovir is an L-valyl ester (prodrug) of ganciclovir that exists as a mixture of 2 diastereomers. After oral administration, both diastereomers are rapidly converted to ganciclovir by intestinal and hepatic esterases. Ganciclovir is a synthetic analog of 2′-deoxyguanosine, which inhibits replication of human cytomegalovirus in vitro and in vivo.

In CMV-infected cells ganciclovir is initially phosphorylated to ganciclovir monophosphate by the viral protein kinase pUL97. Further phosphorylation occurs by cellular kinases to produce ganciclovir triphosphate, which is then slowly metabolized intracellularly (half-life, 18 hours). As the phosphorylation is largely dependent on the viral kinase, phosphorylation of ganciclovir occurs preferentially in virus-infected cells. The virustatic activity of ganciclovir is due to inhibition of viral DNA synthesis by ganciclovir triphosphate.

Pharmacokinetics:

Absorption – Valganciclovir is well absorbed from the GI tract and rapidly metabolized in the intestinal wall and liver to ganciclovir. The absolute bioavailability of ganciclovir from valganciclovir tablets following administration with food was approximately 60%. Ganciclovir median T_{max} following administration of 450 mg to 2,625 mg valganciclovir tablets ranged from 1 to 3 hours. Dose proportionality with respect to ganciclovir area under the plasma concentration time curve (AUC) following administration of valganciclovir tablets was demonstrated only under fed conditions. Systemic exposure to the prodrug, valganciclovir, is transient and low, and the AUC_{24} and C_{max} values are approximately 1% and 3% of those of ganciclovir, respectively.

Distribution – Plasma protein binding of ganciclovir is 1% to 2% over concentrations of 0.5 and 51 mcg/mL. When ganciclovir was administered IV, the steady-state volume of distribution of ganciclovir was approximately 0.703 L/kg (n = 69).

Metabolism – Valganciclovir is rapidly hydrolyzed to ganciclovir; no other metabolites have been detected. No metabolite of orally administered radiolabeled ganciclovir (1,000 mg single dose) accounted for more than 1% to 2% of the radioactivity recovered in the feces or urine.

Excretion – The major route of elimination of valganciclovir is by renal excretion as ganciclovir through glomerular filtration and active tubular secretion. Systemic clearance of IV administered ganciclovir was approximately 3.07 mL/min (n = 68) while renal clearance was approximately 2.99 mL/min/kg (n = 16).

The terminal half-life of ganciclovir following oral administration of valganciclovir tablets to either healthy or HIV-positive/CMV-positive subjects was approximately 4.08 hours (n = 73), and that following administration of IV ganciclovir was approximately 3.81 hours (n = 69).

Mean Ganciclovir Pharmacokinetic[1] Measures in Healthy Volunteers and HIV-Positive/CMV-Positive Adults at Maintenance Dosage	
Formulation	Valganciclovir
Dosage	900 mg once daily with food
$AUC_{0\text{-}24\ hr}$ (mcg•hr/mL)	≈ 29.1 (n = 57)
C_{max} (mcg/mL)	≈ 5.61 (n = 58)
Absolute oral bioavailability (%)	≈ 59.4 (n = 32)
Elimination half-life (hr)	≈ 4.08 (n = 73)
Renal clearance (mL/min/kg)	≈ 3.21 (n = 20)

[1] Data were obtained from single and multiple dose studies in healthy volunteers, HIV-positive patients, and HIV-positive/CMV-positive patients with and without retinitis. Patients with CMV retinitis tended to have higher ganciclovir plasma concentrations than patients without CMV retinitis.

Because the major elimination pathway for ganciclovir is renal, dosage reductions according to creatinine clearance are required for valganciclovir tablets. For dosing instructions in patients with renal impairment, refer to Administration and Dosage.

The pharmacokinetics of ganciclovir from a single oral dose of 900 mg valganciclovir tablets were evaluated in 24 otherwise healthy individuals with renal impairment.

Pharmacokinetics of Ganciclovir from a Single Oral Dose of 900 mg Valganciclovir Tablets (n = 6)			
Estimated CrCl (mL/min)	Mean apparent clearance (mL/min)	Mean AUC (mcg•hr/mL)	Mean half-life (hr)
51 to 70	≈ 249	≈ 49.5	≈ 4.85
21 to 50	≈ 136	≈ 91.9	≈ 10.2
11 to 20	≈ 45	≈ 223	≈ 21.8
≤ 10	≈ 12.8	≈ 366	≈ 67.5

Decreased renal function results in decreased clearance of ganciclovir from valganciclovir, and a corresponding increase in terminal half-life. Therefore, dosage adjustment is required for patients with impaired renal function.

Clinical Trials:

Induction therapy of CMV retinitis – In a randomized, open-label controlled study, 160 AIDS patients and newly diagnosed CMV retinitis were randomized to receive treatment with either valganciclovir tablets (900 mg twice daily for 21 days, then 900 mg once daily for 7 days) or with IV ganciclovir solution (5 mg/kg twice daily for 21 days, then 5 mg/kg once daily for 7 days). The median baseline HIV-1 RNA was 4.9 $\log_{10}$, and the median CD4 cell count was 23 cells/mm^3. A determination of CMV retinitis progression by the masked review of retinal photographs taken at baseline and week 4 was the primary outcome measurement of the 3-week induction therapy. The table below provides the outcomes at 4 weeks.

Week 4 Masked Review of Retinal Photographs		
Determination of CMV retinitis progression at Week 4	Ganciclovir (n = 80)	Valganciclovir (n = 80)
Progressor	7	7
Nonprogressor	63	64
Death	2	1
Discontinuations due to adverse reactions	1	2
Failed to return	1	1
CMV not confirmed at baseline or no interpretable baseline photos	6	5

Indications:

CMV retinitis: For the treatment of CMV retinitis in patients with AIDS.

Contraindications:

Hypersensitivity to valganciclovir or ganciclovir.

Warnings:

Toxicity: The clinical toxicity of valganciclovir, which is metabolized to ganciclovir, includes granulocytopenia, anemia, and thrombocytopenia. In animal studies, ganciclovir was carcinogenic, teratogenic, and caused aspermatogenesis.

Hematologic: Valganciclovir tablets should not be administered if the absolute neutrophil count is less than 500 cells/mm^3, the platelet count is less than 25,000/mm^3, or the hemoglobin is less than 8 g/dL.

Severe leukopenia, neutropenia, anemia, thrombocytopenia, pancytopenia, bone marrow depression, and aplastic anemia have been observed in patients treated with valganciclovir tablets (and ganciclovir) (see Precautions and Adverse Reactions).

Therefore, use valganciclovir tablets with caution in patients with pre-existing cytopenias, or in those who have received or are receiving myelosuppressive drugs or irradiation. Cytopenia may occur at any time during treatment and may increase with continued dosing. Cell counts usually begin to recover within 3 to 7 days of discontinuing drug.

Renal function impairment: Because ganciclovir is excreted by the kidneys, normal clearance depends on adequate renal function. If renal function is impaired, dosage adjustments are required for valganciclovir. Such adjustments should be based on measured or estimated CrCl values (see Administration and Dosage). For patients on hemodialysis (CrCl < 10 mL/min) it is recommended that ganciclovir be used (in accordance with the dose-reduction algorithm cited in Administration and Dosage in the ganciclovir package insert) rather than valganciclovir (see Administration and Dosage).

Elderly: The pharmacokinetic characteristics of valganciclovir in elderly patients have not been established. Since elderly individuals frequently have a reduced glomerular filtration rate, particular attention should be paid to assessing renal function before and during administration of valganciclovir.

Lactation: It is not known whether ganciclovir or valganciclovir is excreted in human milk. Because valganciclovir caused granulocytopenia, anemia, and thrombocytopenia in clinical trials and ganciclovir was mutagenic and carcinogenic in animal studies, the possibility of serious adverse reactions from ganciclovir in nursing infants is possible. Because of potential for serious adverse events in nursing infants, mothers should be instructed not to breastfeed if they are receiving valganciclovir tablets. In addition, the Centers for Disease Control and Prevention recommend that HIV-infected mothers not breast-feed their infants to avoid risking postnatal transmission of HIV.

Children: Safety and efficacy of valganciclovir in pediatric patients have not been established.

Precautions:

Monitoring: Because of the frequency of neutropenia, anemia, and thrombocytopenia in patients receiving valganciclovir tablets, it is recommended that complete blood counts and platelet counts be performed frequently, especially in patients in whom ganciclovir or other nucleoside analogs have previously resulted in leukopenia, or in whom neutrophil counts are less than 1,000 cell/mm^3 at the beginning of treatment. Increased monitoring for cytopenias may be warranted if therapy with oral ganciclovir is changed to oral valganciclovir, because of increased plasma concentrations of ganciclovir after valganciclovir administration.

Increased serum creatinine levels have been observed in trials evaluating valganciclovir tablets. Patients should have serum creatinine or CrCl values monitored carefully to allow for dosage adjustments in renally impaired patients. The mechanism of impairment of renal function is not known.

Drug Interactions:

No in vivo drug interaction studies were conducted with valganciclovir. However, because valganciclovir is rapidly and extensively converted to ganciclovir, interactions associated with ganciclovir will be expected for valganciclovir tablets.

Adverse Reactions:

Valganciclovir vs Ganciclovir Selected Adverse Events (%)		
Adverse reaction	Valganciclovir (n = 79)	Ganciclovir IV (n = 79)
Diarrhea	16	10
Neutropenia	11	13
Nausea	8	14
Headache	9	5
Anemia	8	8
Catheter-related infection	3	11

Valganciclovir Adverse Reactions (≥ 5%)	
Adverse reaction	Patients (n = 370)
CNS	
Headache	22
Insomnia	16
Peripheral neuropathy	9
Paresthesia	8
GI	
Diarrhea	41
Nausea	30
Vomiting	21
Abdominal pain	15
Hematologic/Lymphatic	
Neutropenia	27
Anemia	26
Thrombocytopenia	6
Lab test abnormalities	
Neutropenia: ANC/mm^3	
< 500	19
500 to < 750	17
750 to < 1,000	17
Anemia: Hemoglobin g/dL	
< 6.5	7
6.5 to < 8	13
8 to < 9.5	16
Thrombocytopenia: Platelets/mm^3	
< 25,000	4
25,000 to < 50,000	6
50,000 to < 100,000	22
Serum creatinine: mg/dL	
> 2.5	3
> 1.5 to 2.5	12
Miscellaneous	
Pyrexia	31
Retinal detachment	15

Other adverse reactions (less than 5%):

CNS – Convulsion, psychosis, hallucinations, confusion, agitation.

Hematologic/Lymphatic – Pancytopenia, bone marrow depression, aplastic anemia.

Miscellaneous – Decreased CrCl, local and systemic infections and sepsis, potential life-threatening bleeding associated with thrombocytopenia, valganciclovir hypersensitivity.

Refer to the ganciclovir package insert for postmarketing adverse reactions associated with ganciclovir.

Patient Information:

Valganciclovir tablets cannot be substituted for ganciclovir capsules on a one-to-one basis. Inform patients switching from ganciclovir capsules of the risk of overdosage if they take more than the prescribed number of valganciclovir tablets.

Valganciclovir is changed to ganciclovir once it is absorbed into the body. All patients should be informed that the major toxicities of ganciclovir include granulocytopenia (neutropenia), anemia, and thrombocytopenia and that dose modifications may be required, including discontinuation. The importance of close monitoring of blood counts while on therapy should be emphasized. Inform patients that ganciclovir has been associated with elevations in serum creatinine.

Instruct patients to take valganciclovir tablets with food to maximize bioavailability.

Advise patients ganciclovir has caused decreased sperm production in animals and may cause decreased fertility in humans. Advise women of childbearing potential that ganciclovir causes birth defects in animals and should not be used during pregnancy. Because of the potential for serious adverse events in nursing infants, instruct mothers not to breast-feed if they are receiving valganciclovir tablets. Advise women of childbearing potential to use effective contraception during valganciclovir treatment. Similarly, advise men to practice barrier contraception during and for at least 90 days following treatment with valganciclovir tablets.

Although there is no information from human studies, advise patients that ganciclovir should be considered a potential carcinogen.

Convulsions, sedation, dizziness, ataxia, or confusion have been reported with the use of valganciclovir tablets or ganciclovir. If they occur, such effects may affect tasks requiring alertness, including the patient's ability to drive and operate machinery.

Tell patients that ganciclovir is not a cure for CMV retinitis, and that they may continue to experience progression of retinitis during or following treatment. Patients should be advised to have ophthalmologic follow-up examinations at a minimum of every 4 to 6 weeks while being treated with valganciclovir tablets. Some patients will require more frequent follow-up.

Administration and Dosage:

Strict adherence to dosage recommendations is essential to avoid overdose. Valganciclovir tablets cannot be substituted for ganciclovir capsules on a one-to-one basis.

CMV retinitis (normal renal function):

Induction – 900 mg (two 450 mg tablets) twice daily for 21 days with food.

Maintenance – Following induction treatment, or in patients with inactive CMV retinitis, the recommended dosage is 900 mg (two 450 mg tablets) once daily with food.

Renal impairment: Monitor serum creatinine or CrCl levels carefully. Dosage adjustment is required according to CrCl, as shown in the table below. Increased monitoring for cytopenias may be warranted in patients with renal impairment.

Oral Valganciclovir in Renal Impairment

CrCl[1] (mL/min)	Induction dose	Maintenance dose
≥ 60	900 mg twice daily	900 mg once daily
40 to 59	450 mg twice daily	450 mg once daily
25 to 39	450 mg once daily	450 mg every 2 days
10 to 24	450 mg every 2 days	450 mg twice weekly

[1] An estimated CrCl can be related to serum creatinine by the following formulas:

$$\text{Males: } \frac{\text{Weight (kg)} \times (140 - \text{age})}{72 \times \text{serum creatinine (mg/dL)}} = \text{CrCl}$$

$$\text{Females: } 0.85 \times \text{above value}$$

Hemodialysis patients: Do not prescribe valganciclovir to patients receiving hemodialysis.

Handling and disposal: Exercise caution in the handling of valganciclovir tablets. Do not break or crush tablets. Because valganciclovir is considered a potential teratogen and carcinogen in humans, observe caution in handling broken tablets. Avoid direct contact of broken or crushed tablets with skin or mucous membranes. If such contact occurs, wash thoroughly with soap and water, and rinse eyes thoroughly with plain water.

Because ganciclovir shares some of the properties of antitumor agents (ie, carcinogenicity and mutagenicity), consider handling and disposing according to guidelines issued for antineoplastic drugs.

Storage/Stability: Store at 25° to 30°C (59° to 86°F).

Rx	**Valcyte** (Roche)	**Tablets**: 450 mg	In 60s.

VERTEPORFIN

Actions:

Pharmacology: Verteporfin is a light-activated drug used in photodynamic therapy. It consists of a 2-stage process requiring administration of verteporfin for injection and nonthermal red light.

Verteporfin is transported in the plasma primarily by lipoproteins. Once it is activated by light in the presence of oxygen, highly reactive, short-lived singlet oxygen and reactive oxygen radicals are generated.

Light activation of verteporfin results in local damage to neovascular endothelium, resulting in vessel occlusion. Damaged endothelium is known to release procoagulant and vasoactive factors through the lipo-oxygenase (leukotriene) and cyclo-oxygenase (eicosanoids such as thromboxane) pathways, resulting in platelet aggregation, fibrin clot formation, and vasoconstriction. Verteporfin appears to preferentially accumulate in neovasculature, including choroidal neovasculature. However, animal models indicate that the drug is also present in the retina. Therefore, there may be collateral damage to retinal structures following photoactivation including retinal pigmented epithelium and outer nuclear layer of the retina. The temporary occlusion of CNV following verteporfin therapy has been confirmed in humans by fluorescein angiography.

Indications:

Age-related macular degeneration: Treatment of age-related macular degeneration in patients with predominantly classic subfoveal CNV.

During clinical studies, older patients (approximately 75 years of age), patients with dark irides, patients with occult lesions, or patients with less than 50% classic CNV were less likely to benefit from verteporfin therapy.

Contraindications:

Patients with porphyria or a known hypersensitive to any component of this preparation.

Warnings:

Photosensitivity: Following verteporfin injection, avoid exposure of skin or eyes to direct sunlight or bright indoor light for 5 days. If emergency surgery is necessary within 48 hours after treatment, protect as much of the internal tissue as possible from intense light.

Ocular changes: Do not retreat patients who experience severe decrease of vision of at least 4 lines within 1 week after treatment, at least until their vision completely recovers to pretreatment levels and the potential benefits and risks of subsequent treatment are carefully considered by the treating physician.

Lasers: Use of incompatible lasers that do not provide the required characteristics of light for the photoactivation of verteporfin could result in incomplete treatment because of partial photoactivation of verteporfin, overtreatment because of overactivation of verteporfin, or damage to surrounding normal tissue.

Elderly: A reduced treatment effect was seen with increasing age.

Pregnancy: Category C. There are no adequate and well-controlled studies in pregnant women. Use during pregnancy only if the benefit to the mother justifies the potential risk to the fetus.

Lactation: It is not known if verteporfin is excreted in breast milk. Use caution when verteporfin is administered to a woman who is breast-feeding.

Precautions:

Extravasation: Standard precautions to avoid extravasation include the following:

- Establish a free-flowing IV line before starting infusion and carefully monitor the line.
- Because of the possible fragility of vein walls in some elderly patients, use the largest arm vein possible, preferably antecubital.
- Avoid small veins in the back of the hand.

If extravasation does occur, stop the infusion immediately and apply cold compresses. In the event of extravasation during infusion, the extravasation area must be thoroughly protected from direct light until the swelling and discoloration have faded in order to prevent the occurrence of a local burn, which could be severe.

Hepatic Function Impairment: Carefully consider verteporfin therapy in patients with moderate to severe hepatic impairment; there is no clinical experience with verteporfin in these patients.

Adverse Reactions:

The most frequently reported adverse reactions are headaches; injection site reactions (eg, extravasation, rashes); and visual disturbances (eg, blurred vision, decreased visual acuity, visual field defects).

Severe vision decrease, equivalent of at least 4 lines, within 7 days after treatment has been reported. Partial recovery of vision was observed in many patients.

Photosensitivity reactions occurred in the form of skin sunburn following exposure to sunlight.

The higher incidence of back pain in the verteporfin group occurred primarily during infusion.

Overdosage:

Symptoms: Overdose of drug or light in the treated eye may result in nonperfusion of normal retinal vessels with the possibility of severe decrease in vision that could be permanent. An overdose will also result in the prolongation of the period during which the patient remains photosensitive to bright light.

Treatment: Extend photosensitivity precautions for a time proportional to the overdose.

Patient Information:

Advise patients who receive verteporfin that they will become temporarily photosensitive after the infusion. Advise the patient to avoid exposure of unprotected skin, eyes, or other body organs to direct sunlight or bright indoor light for 5 days after treatment. Sources of bright light include, but are not limited to, tanning salons, bright halogen lighting, and high power lighting used in surgical operating rooms and dental offices.

Instruct patients to protect all parts of their skin and their eyes by wearing protective clothing and dark sunglasses if they must go outdoors in daylight during the first 5 days after treatment. UV sunscreens are not effective in protecting against photosensitivity reactions because photoactivation of the residual drug in the skin can be caused by visible light.

Encourage patients not to stay in the dark and to expose their skin to ambient indoor light, as it will help inactivate the drug in the skin through a process called photobleaching.

Administration and Dosage:

A course of verteporfin therapy is a 2-step process: IV infusion of verteporfin and activation of verteporfin with light from a nonthermal diode laser.

Reevaluate patients every 3 months; if choroidal neovascular leakage is detected on fluorescein angiography, repeat therapy.

Verteporfin administration: Reconstitute each vial of verteporfin with 7 mL Sterile Water for Injection to produce 7.5 mL containing 2 mg/mL. Inspect visually for particulate matter and discoloration prior to administration; reconstituted verteporfin is an opaque, dark green solution.

Withdraw the volume of reconstituted verteporfin required to achieve the desired dose of 6 mg/m^2 and dilute with 5% Dextrose for Injection to a total infusion volume of 30 mL. The full infusion volume is administered IV over 10 minutes at a rate of 3 mL/minute, using an appropriate syringe pump and in-line filter.

Take precautions to prevent extravasation at the injection site. If extravasation occurs, protect the site from light.

Light administration: Initiate 689 nm wavelength laser light delivery to the patient 15 minutes after the start of the 10-minute verteporfin infusion.

Photoactivation of verteporfin is controlled by total light dose delivered. In the treatment of choroidal neovascularization (CNV), the recommended light dose is 50 J/cm^2 of neovascular lesion administered at an intensity of 600 mW/cm^2. This dose is administered over 83 seconds.

Light dose, light intensity, ophthalmic lens magnification factor, and zoom-lens setting are important parameters for the appropriate delivery of light to the predetermined treatment spot. Follow the laser system manuals for procedure set up and operation.

The laser system must deliver a stable power output at a wavelength of 689 $\pm$ 3 nm. Light is delivered to the retina as a single circular spot via a fiber optic and a slit lamp, using a suitable ophthalmic magnification lens.

Concurrent bilateral treatment: The controlled trials allowed only the treatment of 1 eye per patient. In patients who present with eligible lesions in both eyes, evaluate the potential benefits and risks of treating both eyes, concurrently. If the patient has already received previous verteporfin therapy in 1 eye with an acceptable safety profile, both eyes can be treated concurrently after a single administration of verteporfin. Treat the more aggressive lesion first at 15 minutes after the start of infusion. Immediately at the end of light application to the first eye, adjust the laser settings to introduce the treatment parameters for the second eye, with the same light dose and intensity as for the first eye, starting at most 20 minutes from the start of infusion.

In patients who present for the first time with eligible lesions in both eyes without prior verteporfin therapy, it is prudent to treat only 1 eye (the most aggressive lesion) at the first course. One week after the first course, if no significant safety issues are identified, the second eye can be treated using the same treatment regimen after a second verteporfin infusion. Approximately 3 months later, both eyes can be evaluated and concurrent treatment following a new verteporfin infusion can be started if both lesions still show evidence of leakage.

Storage/Stability: Use within 4 hours of reconstitution. Store between 20° and 25°C (68° and 77°F). Protect from light.

Rx	**Visudyne** (Novartis)	**Lyophilized cake:** 15 mg (reconstituted to 2 mg/mL)	Egg phosphatidylglycerol. In single-use vials.

PEGAPTANIB SODIUM INJECTION

Refer to the Pegaptanib monograph for more complete information.

Actions:

Pharmacology:

Mechanism of action – Pegaptanib is a selective VEGF antagonist. VEGF is a secreted protein that selectively binds and activates its receptors located primarily on the surface of vascular endothelial cells. VEGF induces angiogenesis, and increases vascular permeability and inflammation, all of which are thought to contribute to the progression of the neovascular (wet) form of age-related macular degeneration (AMD), a leading cause of blindness. VEGF has been implicated in blood retinal barrier breakdown and pathological ocular neovascularization. Pegaptanib is an aptamer, a pegylated modified oligonucleotide, which adopts a 3-dimensional conformation that enables it to bind to extracellular VEGF. Under in vitro testing conditions, pegaptanib binds to the major pathological VEGF isoform, extracellular $VEGF_{165}$, thereby inhibiting $VEGF_{165}$ binding to its VEGF receptors. The inhibition of $VEGF_{164}$, the rodent counterpart of human $VEGF_{165}$, was effective at suppressing pathological neovascularization.

Pharmacokinetics:

Absorption – In animals, pegaptanib is slowly absorbed into the systemic circulation from the eye after intravitreous administration. The rate of absorption from the eye is the rate limiting step in the disposition of pegaptanib in animals and is likely to be the rate limiting step in humans. In humans, a mean maximum plasma concentration of about 80 ng/mL occurs within 1 to 4 days after a 3 mg monocular dose (10 times the recommended dose). The mean area under the plasma concentration-time curve (AUC) is about 25 mcg•hr/mL at this dose.

Distribution – Twenty-four hours after intravitreous administration of a radiolabeled dose of pegaptanib to both eyes of rabbits, radioactivity was mainly distributed in vitreous fluid, retina, and aqueous fluid. After intravitreous and intravenous administrations of radiolabeled pegaptanib to rabbits, the highest concentrations of radioactivity (excluding the eye for the intravitreous dose) were obtained in the kidney.

Metabolism – Based on preclinical data, pegaptanib is metabolized by endo- and exonucleases.

Excretion – In rabbits, the component nucleotide, 2-fluorouridine is found in plasma and urine after single radiolabeled pegaptanib intravenous and intravitreous doses. In rabbits, pegaptanib is eliminated as parent drug and metabolites primarily in the urine.

Special populations – Plasma concentrations do not appear to be affected by age or gender, but have not been studied in patients younger than 50 years of age.

Renal function impairment – Dose adjustment for patients with renal function impairment is not needed when administering the 0.3 mg dose.

Hemodialysis – Pegaptanib has not been studied in patients requiring hemodialysis.

Hepatic function impairment – Pegaptanib has not been studied in patients with hepatic function impairment.

In humans, after a 3 mg monocular dose (10 times the recommended dose), the average ($\pm$ standard deviation) apparent half-life of pegaptanib is 10 ($\pm$ 4) days.

Indications:

Pegaptanib is indicated for the treatment of neovascular (wet) age-related macular degeneration.

Contraindications:

Pegaptanib is contraindicated in patients with ocular or periocular infections.

Warnings:

Intravitreous injections, including those with pegaptanib, have been associated with endophthalmitis. Proper aseptic injection technique should always be utilized when administering pegaptanib. In addition, patients should be monitored during the week following the injection to permit early treatment if an infection occurs (see Dosage and Administration). Increases in intraocular pressure have been seen with 30 minutes of injection of pegaptanib. Therefore, intraocular pressure and the perfusion of the optic nerve head should be monitored and managed appropriately.

Carcinogenesis: Carcinogenicity studies with pegaptanib have not been conducted.

Elderly: Approximately 94% (834 of 892) of patients treated with pegaptanib were at least 65 years of age and approximately 62% (553 of 892) were at least 75 years of age. No difference in treatment effect or systemic exposure was seen with increasing age.

Pregnancy: Category B. There are no studies in pregnant women. The potential risk to humans is unknown. Pegaptanib should be used during pregnancy only if the potential benefit to the mother justifies the potential risk to the fetus.

Lactation: It is not known whether pegaptanib is excreted in human milk. Because many drugs are excreted in human milk, caution should be exercised when pegaptanib is administered to a breast-feeding woman.

Children: Safety and efficacy of pegaptanib in children have not been studied.

Precautions:

For ophthalmic intravitreal injection only.

Drug Interactions:

Drug interaction studies have not been conducted with pegaptanib. Pegaptanib is metabolized by nucleases and is generally not affected by the cytochrome P-450 system. Two early clinical studies conducted in patients who received pegaptanib alone and in combination with PDT revealed no apparent difference in the plasma pharmacokinetics of pegaptanib.

Adverse Reactions:

Serious adverse reactions related to the injection procedure occurring in less than 1% of intravitreous injections included endophthalmitis (see Warnings), retinal detachment, and iatrogenic traumatic cataract.

The most frequently reported adverse reactions in patients treated with pegaptanib 0.3 mg for up to 2 years were anterior chamber inflammation, blurred vision, cataract conjunctival hemorrhage, corneal edema, eye discharge, eye irritation, eye pain, hypertension, increased intraocular pressure (IOP), ocular discomfort, punctate keratitis, reduced visual acuity, visual disturbance, vitreous floaters, and vitreous opacities. These reactions occurred in approximately 10% to 14% of patients.

The following reactions were reported in 6% to 10% of patients receiving pegaptanib 0.3 mg therapy: blepharitis, conjunctivitis, photopsia, vitreous disorder (ocular); bronchitis, diarrhea, dizziness, headache, nausea, urinary tract infection (non-ocular).

The following reactions were reported in 1% to 5% of patients receiving pegaptanib 0.3 mg therapy: allergic conjunctivitis, conjunctival edema, corneal abrasion, corneal deposits, corneal epithelium disorder, endophthalmitis, eye inflammation, eye swelling, eyelid irritation, meibomianitis, mydriasis, periorbital hematoma, retinal edema, vitreous hemorrhage (ocular); arthritis, bone spur, carotid artery occlusion, cerebrovascular accident, chest pain, contact dermatitis, contusion, diabetes mellitus, dyspepsia, hearing loss, pleural effusion, transient ischemic attack, urinary retention, vertigo, vomiting (non-ocular).

Overdosage:

Doses of pegaptanib up to 10 times the recommended dosage of 0.3 mg have been studied. No additional adverse reactions have been noted but there is decreased efficacy with doses higher than 1 mg.

Patient Information:

In the days following pegaptanib administration, patients are at risk for the development of endophthalmitis. If the eye becomes red, sensitive to light, painful, or develops a change in vision, the patient should seek the immediate care of an ophthalmologist.

Administration and Dosage:

Pegaptanib 0.3 mg should be administered once every 6 weeks by intravitreous injection into the eye to be treated.

Pegaptanib should be visually inspected for particulate matter and discoloration prior to administration. Administration of the syringe contents involves attaching the threaded plastic plunger rod to the rubber stopper inside the barrel of the syringe. Do not pull back on the plunger. The syringe needle cap then is removed to allow administration of the product.

The injection procedure should be carried out under controlled aseptic conditions, which includes the use of sterile gloves, a sterile drape, and a sterile eyelid speculum (or equivalent). Adequate anesthesia and a broad-spectrum microbicide should be given prior to the injection.

After the injection, patients should be monitored for elevation in the IOP and for endophthalmitis. Monitoring may consist of a check for perfusion of the optic nerve head immediately after the injection, tonometry within 30 minutes after the injection, and biomicroscopy between 2 and 7 days after the injection. Patients should be instructed to report any symptoms suggestive of endophthalmitis without delay.

No special dosage modification is required for any of the populations that have been studied (eg, gender, elderly).

The safety and efficacy of pegaptanib therapy administered to both eyes concurrently have not been studied.

Storage/Stability: Store in refrigerator at 2° to 8°C (36° to 46°F). Do not freeze or shake vigorously.

Rx	**Macugen** (Eyetech)	**Injection:** 0.3 mg[1]	In 1 mL glass syringe. With 27-gauge needle and shield.

[1] Equivalent to 1.6 mg pegaptanib sodium (pegylated oligonucleotide) or 3.2 mg when expressed as the sodium salt form of the oligonucleotide moiety.

RANIBIZUMAB

Actions:

Pharmacology: Ranibizumab binds to the receptor binding site of active forms of VEGF-A, including the biologically active, cleaved form of this molecule, $VEGF_{110}$. VEGF-A has been shown to cause neovascularization and leakage in models of ocular angiogenesis and is thought to contribute to the progression of the neovascular form of age-related macular degeneration (AMD). The binding of ranibizumab to VEGF-A prevents the interaction of VEGF-A with its receptors (VEGFR1 and VEGFR2) on the surface of endothelial cells, reducing endothelial cell proliferation, vascular leakage, and new blood vessel formation.

Pharmacokinetics: In animal studies, following intravitreal injection, ranibizumab was cleared from the vitreous with a half-life of approximately 3 days. After reaching a maximum at approximately 1 day, the serum concentration of ranibizumab declined in parallel with the vitreous concentration. In these animal studies, systemic exposure of ranibizumab is more than 2,000-fold lower than in the vitreous.

In patients with neovascular AMD, following monthly intravitreal administration, maximum ranibizumab serum concentrations were low (0.3 ng/mL to 2.36 ng/mL). These levels were below the concentration of ranibizumab (11 ng/mL to 27 ng/mL) thought to be necessary to inhibit the biological activity of VEGF-A by 50%, as measured in an in vitro cellular proliferation assay. The maximum observed serum concentration was dose proportional over the dose range of 0.05 to 1 mg/eye. Based on population pharmacokinetic analysis, maximum serum concentrations of 1.5 ng/mL are predicted to be reached at approximately 1 day after monthly intravitreal administration of 0.5 mg/eye. Based on the disappearance of ranibizumab from serum, the estimated average vitreous elimination half-life was approximately 9 days. Steady-state minimum concentration is predicted to be 0.22 ng/mL with a monthly dosing regimen. In humans, serum ranibizumab concentrations are predicted to be approximately 90,000-fold lower than vitreal concentrations.

Indications:

For the treatment of patients with neovascular (wet) age-related macular degeneration.

Contraindications:

Ranibizumab is contraindicated in patients with ocular or periocular infections.

Warnings:

Intravitreous injections, including those with ranibizumab, have been associated with endophthalmitis. Proper aseptic injection technique should always be utilized when administering pegaptanib. In addition, patients should be monitored during the week following the injection to permit early treatment if an infection occurs (see Dosage and Administration). Increases in intraocular pressure have been seen with 60 minutes of injection of pegaptanib. Therefore, intraocular pressure and the perfusion of the optic nerve head should be monitored and managed appropriately. Although there was a low rate (less than 4%) of arterial thromboembolic events observed in clinical trials, there is a theoretical risk of arterial thromboembolic events following intravitreal use of inhibitors of VEGF.

Elderly: In the controlled clinical studies, approximately 94% (822/879) of the patients randomized to treatment with ranibizumab were 65 years of age and older and approximately 68% (601/879) were 75 years and age or older. No notable difference in treatment effect was seen with increasing age in any of the studies. Age did not have a significant effect on systemic exposure in a population pharmacokinetic analysis after correcting for CrCl.

Pregnancy: Category B. There are no studies in pregnant women. The potential risk to humans is unknown. Ranibizumab should be used during pregnancy only if the potential benefit to the mother justifies the potential risk to the fetus.

Lactation: It is not known whether ranibizumab is excreted in human milk. Because many drugs are excreted in human milk, caution should be exercised when ranibizumab is administered to a breast-feeding woman.

Children: Safety and efficacy of ranibizumab in children have not been studied.

Drug Interactions:

Drug interaction studies have not been conducted with ranibizumab. Ranibizumab intravitreal injection has been used adjunctively with verteporfin photodynamic therapy (PDT). Twelve of 105 (11%) patients developed serious intraocular inflammation; in 10 of the 12 patients, this occurred when ranibizumab was administered 7 days (± 2 days) after verteporfin PDT.

Adverse Reactions:

Serious adverse reactions related to the injection procedure occurring in less than 1% of intravitreous injections included endophthalmitis (see Warnings), retinal detachment, and iatrogenic traumatic cataract.

The most frequently reported ocular adverse reactions in 3 separate clinical trails were conjunctival hemorrhage, eye pain, vitreous floaters, retinal hemorrhage, increased intraocular pressure, vitreous detachment, intraocular inflammation, eye irritation, cataract, foreign body sensation, and ocular hyperemia. These reactions were reported in a minimum of 5% of trial patients.

Overdosage:

Planned initial single doses of ranibizumab 1 mg injection were associated with clinically significant intraocular inflammation in 2 of 2 patients injected. With an escalating regimen of doses beginning with initial doses of ranibizumab injection 0.3 mg, doses as high as 2 mg were tolerated in 15 of 20 patients.

Administration and Dosage:

For ophthalmic intravitreal injection only.

0.5 mg (0.05 mL) is recommended to be administered by intravitreal injection once a month. Although less effective, treatment may be reduced to 1 injection every 3 months after the first 4 injections if monthly injections are not feasible. Compared with continued monthly dosing, dosing every 3 months will lead to an approximate 5-letter (1-line) loss of visual acuity benefit, on average, over the following 9 months. Patients should be evaluated regularly.

Using aseptic technique, all (0.2 mL) of the ranibizumab vial contents are withdrawn through a 5-micron 19-gauge filter needle attached to a 1 cc tuberculin syringe. The filter needle should be discarded after withdrawal of the vial contents and should not be used for intravitreal injection. The filter needle should be replaced with a sterile 30-gauge × ½ inch needle for the intravitreal injection. The contents should be expelled until the plunger tip is aligned with the line that marks 0.05 mL on the syringe.

The intravitreal injection procedure should be carried out under controlled aseptic conditions, which include the use of sterile gloves, a sterile drape, and a sterile eyelid speculum (or equivalent). Adequate anesthesia and a broad-spectrum microbicide should be given prior to the injection. Each vial should only be used for the treatment of a single eye. If the contralateral eye requires treatment, a new vial should be used and the sterile field, syringe, gloves, drapes, eyelid speculum, filter, and injection needles should be changed before ranibizumab is administered to the other eye.

Following the intravitreal injection, patients should be monitored for elevation in intraocular pressure and for endophthalmitis. Monitoring may consist of a check for perfusion of the optic nerve head immediately after the injection, tonometry within 30 minutes following the injection, and biomicroscopy between 2 and 7 days following the injection. Patients should be instructed to report any symptoms suggestive of endophthalmitis without delay.

Storage/Stability: Refrigerate at 2° to 8°C (36° to 46°F). Do not freeze. Do not use beyond the date stamped on the label. Protect ranibizumab vials from light. Store in the original carton until time of use.

Rx	**Lucentis** (Genentech)	**Injection**: 10 mg/mL[1]	Preservative-free. In single-use glass vials.

[1] 10% alpha, alpha-trehalose dihydrate, 0.01% polysorbate 20, 10 mM histidine. Designed to deliver 0.05 mL.

Contact Lens Care

More than 36 million Americans wear contact lenses. Contact lenses can offer patients a natural appearance, increased visual performance, and convenience. They can correct most refractive errors such as myopia, hyperopia, and astigmatism. Bifocal contact lenses are available for the presbyopic patient. Tinted contact lenses enhance or completely change the color of a patient's eyes. Research and development by major ophthalmic corporations have produced a variety of new lens materials and designs. With new contact lens products and patient education, contact lens use should continue to grow.

The number of contact lens care products also has increased dramatically. Patients may become confused because there are more than 100 different products sold for contact lens care.

CONTACT LENS MATERIALS AND COMPOSITION

Three types of contact lenses are manufactured: Hard (PMMA), gas permeable (GP), and soft. A recently introduced form of soft lens, the silicone-hydrogel, has exhibited great promise because of unparallel oxygen permeability.

HARD CONTACT LENSES

Hard contact lenses are made from polymethylmethacrylate (PMMA). PMMA does not transmit the oxygen needed for normal corneal integrity. Hard contact lenses have caused chronic corneal edema, corneal distortion, edematous corneal formations, spectacle blur, polymegethism, and corneal abrasions. Because of these ocular complications, hard lenses should not be prescribed for any new contact lens wearer or provided as replacement lenses for existing wearers.

GAS PERMEABLE LENSES

Between 10% and 13% of contact lens patients wear GP lenses. These lenses are oxygen permeable; therefore, the GP patient does not have the moderate physiological complications of the hard lens patient. Several lens polymers with a high degree of oxygen permeability have been FDA-approved for extended wear. GP lenses provide the patient with good vision, durability, and easy care.

The first successful GP lens materials were introduced in 1979 and were of silicone/acrylate (S/A) composition. Also referred to as silicone-based, these copolymers have excellent oxygen permeability characteristics, and actually contain the element silicon as siloxane bonds in side branches of the main carbon-carbon polymer chain. Unlike homogenous PMMA lens materials, S/A materials are polymers with silicone, methacrylate, wetting agents, and cross-linking agents; the latter 2 ingredients are important because of the dryness (hydrophobicity) and flexibility of silicone. Wetting agents, including hydroxyethylmethacrylate (HEMA) and methacrylic acid (the most common), achieve their effect through their strong affinity with water molecules. Cross-linking agents have the ability to strengthen the material; therefore, the flexibility is decreased, machining characteristics are improved, and the material is less sensitive to the effect of solvents.

As it became apparent that higher oxygen permeable (Dk) lens materials would be necessary to meet the cornea's daily wear oxygen requirements and allow for flexible/extended wear schedules, higher Dk lens materials were introduced. However, increasing the siloxane bonding to increase oxygen permeability increased the hydrophobic properties and the flexibility of the lens, resulting in such problems as corneal desiccation, surface deposits, warpage, and flexure with subjective symptoms such as dryness and reduced vision. Increasing the amount of wetting agent to offset these problems typically results in excessive material hydration, causing poor contact lens stability; an excess of cross-linking agents to enhance stability could result in a brittle material. Most of the lenses in use today are fluoro-silicone/acrylate (F-S/A) or modified F-S/A lens materials. They are similar to silicone/acrylates with the notable exception of the addition of fluorine. Fluorine, known for its nonstick properties in Teflon-coated cooking materials, increases the deposit resistance of the lens material by promoting tear film interaction with the lens surface. In addition, low surface tension (energy) is present; in other words, there is a reduced affinity of polarized tear components to become adherent to the contact lens surface. Therefore, the primary problem experienced with S/A lens material—dryness—is often reduced with F-S/A materials. F-S/A lens materials can essentially be divided into three categories based upon their oxygen permeability. Recently introduced F-S/A materials have been copolymerized with less silicone content; in some materials, HEMA has been added. Both of these material composition changes allow for enhanced surface wettability in higher oxygen permeable materials. Low Dk (25 to 50) materials typically provide the greatest stability and surface wettability. They are recommended for myopic daily wear and borderline dry eye patients. High Dk (51 to 100) materials are recommended for hyperopic daily wear and myopic flexible wear and extended wear patients. Hyper Dk (more than 100) materials are recommended for GP extended wear patients. Recently 1 material, Menicon Z by Menicon, has been approved by the Food and Drug Administration (FDA) for 30–day continuous wear.

HYDROGEL (SOFT) CONTACT LENSES

A hydrogel contact lens, sometimes referred to as a soft contact lens, is a flexible lens made of plastic that is able to absorb or bind water. When placed on the eye, it will conform to the shape of the cornea. The water content allows oxygen permeability; the higher the water content, the greater the oxygen permeability. This benefit is often somewhat negated by the greater center thickness often necessary in high water content lens materials reducing the overall oxygen transmission. Introduced in the US in 1971, today soft lenses are manufactured from polymers that contain 38% to 79% water.

Hydrogel lenses are categorized into 4 groups based upon their water content and surface reactivity. Lenses with less than 50% water content are labeled "low water;" lenses with more than 50% water content are labeled "high water." Less reactive surfaces are termed "nonionic" and more reactive materials are labeled "ionic."

HYDROGEL LENS CLASSIFICATION	
Group 1:	Low water (< 50% H_2O) Nonionic polymers
Group 2:	High water (> 50% H_2O) Nonionic polymers
Group 3:	Low water (< 50% H_2O) Ionic polymers
Group 4:	High water (> 50% H_2O) Ionic polymers

Daily wear soft contact lenses are designed to be worn all day (12 to 14 hours), but must be removed nightly to be cleaned and disinfected. Extended wear soft lenses can be worn for more than 24 hours. The FDA and most eye care practitioners recommend a maximum wearing period of 7 days. The lenses must then be removed overnight for cleaning and disinfection. The primary advantage of extended wear lenses is convenience. The popularity of extended wear soft lenses has decreased in recent years because of the reported risk of infection resulting primarily from corneal hypoxia, surface contamination, and limbal compression. The former problem has been minimized by the recent introduction of hyper Dk silicone-hydrogel lens materials. These silicone-hydrogel lenses are Group 3 lenses, which consist of a homogenous combination of the silicone-containing monomer copolymerized with a hydrophilic hydrogel monomer. These are replaced on a monthly basis and FDA-approved for 30-day continuous wear. Disposable toric and multifocal lens designs in this material have recently been introduced, and second and third generation silicone-hydrogel lens materials are currently either being introduced or will soon be brought to market.

Disposable soft contact lenses are designed to eliminate the complications of lens deposits by replacing lenses at frequent intervals. Lens deposits can interfere with vision, cause corneal irritation, and contribute to ocular infection. In addition, disposable lenses offer the patient the convenience of reduced lens care. The introduction of numerous soft toric and bifocal lens designs have allowed more individuals to achieve the benefits of frequent replacement.

Some disposable lenses are approved for daily wear and others for extended wear. It is recommended that conventional soft lenses be discarded after 12 weeks of wear. Replace disposable lenses every 1 to 2 weeks. Planned replacement lenses are replaced every 1, 3, or 6 months. The doctor will prescribe the replacement schedule for each patient. If a disposable lens is not discarded immediately after lens removal, it should be cleaned with a surfactant cleaner and stored in a disinfection solution.

Four companies have introduced a 1-day single-use soft lens, typically available in a 90-pack. This lens is designed to be worn 1 time and then discarded. The patient will apply a fresh, clean, sterile lens each day of lens wear. Contact lens care products (eg, lens case, cleaning solution, disinfection solution) are not needed with these new soft lenses; therefore, compliance is optimized with this modality.

COMPLIANCE

Contact lens success is dependent upon patient compliance in caring for their contact lenses. There are many potential problems with the contact lens cleaning, disinfection, and handling process, including patient noncompliance, solution misuse, concurrent use of incompatible products, preservative sensitivities or allergies, and contamination of solutions. Surveys indicate that 31% to 80% of patients do not care for their lenses in the manner prescribed. Often this pertains to failure to clean or disinfect the lenses as recommended by their practitioner. In some cases, this may be the result of failure to use the quantity of solution as recommended by the manufacturer. It has been found that patients actually spend less than 25% on contact lens solutions as they should be spending if they were following manufacturers' recommendations.

For practitioners today, ensuring compliance with care regimen is one of the major challenges. The risk of corneal infection has been reported to be as much as 80 times that for contact lens wearers versus non-wearers. Failure to adhere to prescribed lens care procedures can lead to a broad range of complications, from mild symptoms of reduced vision and comfort to severe signs of infection and inflammation. It has also been found that improper lens care can result in sight-threatening complications such as corneal ulcer or *Acanthamoeba* keratitis. More recently, it is one of the factors associated with the increased incidence of *Fusarium* keratitis.

The key factor to optimizing patient compliance is thorough education. It is important for practitioners, staff members, and patients to read and adhere to the manufacturers' directions for use of a specific care product. Patients should also understand every component of lens care (ie, wetting, cleaning, disinfection) and why it is important. In addition, they should be able to restate the exact care procedures prior to leaving the office with their contact lenses. When they return for follow-up visits, they should be questioned as to their compliance with lens care (ie, solutions they are using, cleaning upon removal, using fresh solution, cleaning case). In one study, it was found that with patients who did not have their care instructions repeated at follow-up visits, 50% of their solutions, lenses, and cases were contaminated. For those individuals who had these instructions repeated at follow-up visits, only 6% contamination was found. Other preventative measures include instructing patients not to touch the tip of the solution bottle to any surface and to completely close the bottle when not in use. Also, practitioners should routinely remind patients to discard any solution that is beyond the expiration date. Another method to ensure they will comply with using the recommended solutions is to provide a large quantity (a 2- to 3-month supply) initially of solutions and to sell solutions in the office.

It is important to have an effective recall system to ensure that the patient is compliant as well as comfortable with contact lens wear. The recent passing of the Fairness to Contact Lens Consumers Act (FCLCA), which requires that all patients receive a copy of their contact lens prescription once the practitioner has determined that a final prescription has been achieved, could serve as a deterrent for patients to return to their prescribing practitioner unless such a recall system, complemented by a comprehensive patient education program, is in effect.

It is evident that practitioners and their staff members need to be aware of solution costs in their area and the impact they may play on patient compliance. It is important to address patients' temptations to use less expensive saline or homemade saline using salt tablets. Patients must recognize that contamination of these solutions can result in a serious eye infection. Likewise, the use of tap water for any purpose — but especially for wetting, rewetting, or storage — should be avoided because the risk of *Acanthamoeba* keratitis infection. For the same reason, contact lenses should not be used while swimming or when using a hot tub or sauna.

With soft lenses in particular, it is important that the disinfection system is compatible with the type of lens material. Disinfection of low water content FDA Group 1 and Group 3 lenses can usually be performed safely and effectively by thermal, chemical, or hydrogen peroxide systems. High water content Group 2 and Group 4 lenses should not be thermally disinfected, but chemical or hydrogen peroxide systems are usually safe and effective. However, some Group 4 ionic polymers may react negatively with sorbic acid-preserved solutions. Silicone-hydrogel lens materials are compatible with many chemical and oxidative systems, although it is important to utilize the specific care regimen(s) recommended for a given silicone-hydrogel material. It is evident that certain systemic medications can interact negatively with soft contact lenses and result in discoloration and corneal insult. A partial list of these medications and their effect is listed below.

Clinical Effect	Medication
Lens discoloration:	
Green	Topical phenylephrine, epinephrine
Gray-brown	Dopamine, tetracycline, sulfasalazine
Yellow to orange	Phenazopyridine, resorcinol, rifampin, sulfasalazine, tetracycline, systemic beta-blockers
Dryness, increased surface deposits	Antihistamines, anticholinergics, oral contraceptives, beta-blockers, benzodiazepines, phenodiazines, anticholesterol medications
Corneal staining	Beta-blockers, acetylsalicylic acid (aspirin), antihypertensives, tricyclic antidepressants

It is becoming more evident that lens case contamination can result in ocular irritation and infection. Contact lens wearers with eye infections are often found to have lens cases that are contaminated with the same organism as is involved in the eye infection. The most frequently cited source of contamination of the lens case is the patient's own fingers. Therefore, washing hands prior to contact lens application is quite important. Case contamination increases with the number of weeks the patient uses the same case. Therefore, it is important to recommend regular case replacement (preferably monthly but, at minimum, every 3 months) and to provide patients with several cases to encourage disposal. One case (*Proguard*), in combination with

Aquify MPS solution (Ciba Vision), has antimicrobial properties with the lens cap on. Cleaning the lens case regularly prevents a build-up of muco-protein material, which serves as a good culture medium for microbial growth. Once cleaned, sterile saline should be used to rinse the case.

Doctors, pharmacists, and opticians must have a comprehensive understanding of all contact lens materials and systems. With this knowledge, they can educate the patient, increase compliance, and, therefore, decrease lens and solution-related complications. Compliance has been defined by the FDA as the use of an approved contact lens care regimen in agreement with the manufacturer's instructions and consistent with good general hygiene. Compliance must meet the following 4 criteria.

1. The patient should always wash his or her hands before lens manipulation.
2. The patient should use an FDA-approved care system in an appropriate manner.
3. The patient should wear lenses only on a daily wear schedule unless the lenses are approved by the FDA for extended wear.
4. All solutions should be free of bacterial contamination.

There are several consumer education sites provided by manufacturers on the internet. These include the following:

- Patient Education/Contact Lens Care Conditions (Alcon): www.alcon.com/patients-family/contact-lens-wear-conditions.asp
- Refresh Contacts Safety Information (Allergan): www.allergan.com/site/products/consumers/safety.asp?id=refresh_contacts
- Healthy Eye/Eye Insights (American Medical Optics): www.amoeyecare.com/HealthyEyes/HealthyEyes_insights.asp
- Eye Concerns/Infections and Irritations (Bausch & Lomb): www.bausch.com/en_US/consumer/concern/infections_irritations.aspx
- For Your Eyes/Lens Care Guide (Ciba Vision): www.us.cibavision.com/for_your_eyes/lens_care_guide.shtml

CONTACT LENS GUIDELINES

- Proper contact lens care will increase success and decrease complications.
- Cleaning does not disinfect lenses.
- Disinfecting does not clean lenses.
- Enzyme solutions are not a substitute for disinfection.
- Wash and rinse hands thoroughly before handling contact lenses.
- Do not insert contact lenses if eyes are red or irritated. If eyes become painful or vision worsens while wearing lenses, remove lenses and consult eye care practitioner immediately.
- Do not wear contact lenses while sleeping unless they have been prescribed for extended wear.
- For soft lens care, use only products designed for soft lenses.
- For rigid lens care, use only products designed for rigid lenses.
- Do not change or substitute products from a different manufacturer without consulting a doctor.
- Always follow label directions or doctor's recommendations.
- Do not store lenses in tap water.
- Never use saliva to wet contact lenses.
- Keep lens care products out of the reach of children.
- Do not instill topical medications while contact lenses are being worn unless directed by a doctor.
- Do not get cosmetic lotions, creams, or sprays in eyes or on lenses. It is best to put on lenses before putting on makeup and remove them before removing makeup. Water-based cosmetics are less likely to damage lenses than oil-based products.
- Schedule and keep follow-up appointments with an eye-care practitioner (approximately every 6 to 12 months or as recommended).
- Contact lenses wear out with time and should be replaced regularly. Throw away disposable lenses after the recommended wearing period.

CONTACT LENS NONCOMPLIANCE AND MANAGEMENT

Compliance problem	Cause(s)	Management
Discoloration	Inadequate cleaning	Emphasize cleaning upon removal
	Improper solution use	Have patient repeat care instructions
	If oily film, may be lanolin-based	Avoid hand creams/ lanolin-based soaps
Lens parameter change	Group 4 lenses with long H_2O_2 soak cycles	Use non-H_2O_2 or short cycle H_2O_2
	Use of improper H_2O_2 (*AOSept* patient uses another brand)	Patient education on solution compliance
	Soaking lenses in alcohol-based cleaner	Advise patient of consequences
	Patient uses vigorous digital cleaning of GP lenses causing warpage or increase in minus power	Advise patient to clean carefully in palm of hand
Corneal staining	Improper preservative use (*BAK* with soft lenses; purchases improper solutions)	Patient education on proper solution use; provide patient with large initial supply of appropriate solutions; sell solutions in-office
	Patient sensitivity to a specific preservative	Change patient to another preserved system
	Inadequate buffering/ neutralization of H_2O_2	Reeducate patient on proper use and disposal of H_2O_2 solutions
	Use of topical medications that are absorbed by the contact lenses	Discontinue contact lens wear during medication use
	Does not rinse off cleaner adequately or inserts lens with a cleaning/soaking solution (*Claris*/*Optimum*)	Comply with instructions on use of cleaner
Bacterial infection	Case contamination	Clean, rinse with saline every night; dispose of frequently
	Inadequate cleaning	Patient education on proper cleaning upon removal
	Lenses not discarded as often as scheduled	Emphasize proper wear and discard schedule
	Patient "tops off" solution every night	Educate patient to discard old solution and use fresh
	Poor hygiene	Emphasize importance of clean lenses/wash hands prior to lens application
	GP lenses stored dry	Remind patient of need to disinfect GP lenses
	Inadequate disinfection (does not disinfect after cleaning)	Ensure at follow-up visits that patient understands all steps in lens care
	Expired solutions or leaves cap off	Advise patient about the consequences of contamination
Acanthamoeba keratitis	Tap water used for wetting/rewetting/soaking	Tap water use is prohibited
	Patient wears lenses in hot tub or while swimming	Lens wear is not advised for these activities
	Patient makes own saline with salt tablets	Salt tablet use is not recommended
Unilateral redness /reduced wearing time	Left Lens Syndrome	Patient educated to clean left lens as long as right

PRECAUTIONS FOR CONTACT LENS USE

ACANTHAMOEBA KERATITIS

A microorganism of great concern for the contact lens wearer is the protozoan *Acanthamoeba. Acanthamoeba* penetration into the cornea can cause a necrotizing stromal melt and corneal perforations. If not diagnosed in an early state—and it is a difficult condition to detect early—it can result in the need for a corneal transplant. Numerous species of *Acanthamoeba* have been identified; the 2 most common forms associated with contact lens adherence are *castellani* and *polyphagia. Acanthamoeba* can be present in 2 forms: the trophozoite (characteristic ameba presentation) and the rounded cyst form. The latter form is more resistant to disinfection than the trophozoite.

The overall incidence of *Acanthamoeba* infection with contact lens wear is extremely low when compared with the 28 million people in the US who wear contact lenses. However, the incidence is higher in some parts of the world where the domestic tap water is less filtered and exhibits higher contamination. Recently the Centers for Disease Control and Prevention (CDC) reported that the incidence of *Acanthamoeba* keratitis has increased in recent years. This may be, in part, the result of recent changes by the US Environmental Protection Agency (EPA) to reduce the allowable amount of carcinogenic byproducts in the water supply. This change in standards has been hypothesized to be a causative factor in a recent outbreak in the Chicago area, in which an increased risk of *Acanthamoeba* proliferation in the water supply of Lake Michigan was implicated in 40 cases reported over a 30 month period.

It appears that Group 4 (high water ionic) soft lenses are most often associated with *Acanthamoeba* adherence. The least adherent materials are Group 1 (low water non-ionic) soft lenses and GP lens materials. It is most associated with the use of tap water for storing or wetting/rewetting the lenses. Likewise, it often occurs with people who use salt tablets to develop their own saline. There is also a relationship with hot tub water and this infection as well as wearing soft lenses while swimming.

The most effective disinfection method for killing *Acanthamoeba* is heat; however, many lens materials are not compatible with heat disinfection. The use of hydrogen peroxide has a variable effect against *Acanthamoeba.* More than 10 minutes of storage in hydrogen peroxide is necessary for effective killing of the trophozoite form. Hydrogen peroxide does not appear to be effective against the cystic form. Chemical disinfection via nonhydrogen peroxide solutions such as *Opti-Free* and *ReNu* appear to exhibit poor antiacanthamoebal activity. One solution, *Complete Moisture Plus Multi-Purpose Solution* (Advanced Medical Optics) was recalled by the manufacturer in May, 2007 due to its relative ineffectiveness against *Acanthamoeba.* However, when combined with digital cleaning and rinsing, the effect is much greater. The use of *MiraFlow,* with 20% isopropyl alcohol, as a cleaner is highly effective. Even with the recent increase in cases, however, because overall incidence of *Acanthamoeba* keratitis is low, the FDA has not, to date, required efficacy against *Acanthamoeba* for approval of contact lens care systems. Guidelines for minimizing the risk of *Acanthamoeba* infection are listed below.

STEPS TO MINIMIZE RISK OF *ACANTHAMOEBA* KERATITIS ASSOCIATED WITH CONTACT LENS WEAR
Do not wear contact lenses while swimming; if unavoidable, wear airtight goggles over the lenses and dispose of the lenses immediately after swimming
Do not wear contact lenses while in hot tub, spa, while showering, or during exposure to well water
Never use tap water, distilled water, mineral water, or saliva with contact lenses
Use only sterile contact lens solutions; do not top off solutions

STEPS TO MINIMIZE RISK OF *ACANTHAMOEBA* KERATITIS ASSOCIATED WITH CONTACT LENS WEAR
Clean lenses upon removal (at minimum, perform a rub and rinse)
Disinfect lenses after cleaning
Do not use homemade saline (salt tablets)
Wash hands prior to handling lenses
Clean contact lens case daily by rinsing with sterile saline
Replace lens case frequently (at minimum, every 3 months)

HUMAN IMMUNODEFICIENCY VIRUS (HIV)

With as many as 1 in 300 individuals HIV-affected, and the potential impact of the AIDS virus, it is understandable that concern is expressed about contact lens implications. HIV has been isolated in bodily fluids, including tears, and has been located in the conjunctiva, cornea, and on contact lenses. For patients who have the HIV virus, contact lens wear may not be appropriate as the lenses themselves can act as a highly desirable medium for bacteria.

Disinfection of trial lenses and cases used during these fittings is important if, in fact, the lenses are not disposable. Hydrogen peroxide systems approved for contact lenses can be used to disinfect GP and hydrogel lenses. Heat disinfection is recommended for those lenses compatible with this form of disinfection. Chemical disinfection alone appears to have a minimal effect on the AIDS virus. Guidelines for minimizing the risk of *Acanthamoeba* infection are listed below.

IN-OFFICE PRECAUTIONS TO PREVENT THE TRANSMISSION OF THE AIDS VIRUS (Centers for Disease Control and Prevention)
♦ Wash hands with soap and water after procedures involving contact with tears and in between patient visits
♦ Disposable latex gloves may be worn, especially in the presence of cuts or open wounds on the hands
♦ Instruments that come in contact with external surfaces of the eye and can be contaminated by body secretions should be wiped and disinfected; wiping the Goldmann tonometer tip with an isopropyl alcohol swab and then air drying should be sufficient to inactivate the HIV virus
♦ All disposable soft lenses should be discarded after use
♦ Non-disposable and GP lenses can be disinfected with 3% hydrogen peroxide; heat disinfection can also be used with low water content soft lenses

FUSARIUM FUNGAL KERATITIS

The recent dramatic increase in incidence of *Fusarium* fungal-based corneal ulcers associated with contact lens wear has resulted in the importance of educating health care professionals about this sight-threatening complication. The fungus kingdom is large, and contains more than 100,000 species divided into five phyla. The genus *Fusarium* alone currently contains over 20 species, the most common of which is *Fusarium* solani, the organism implicated in the recent outbreak of cases of fungal keratitis. Fusarium is common in warmer climates - such as the southern United States and in South America - and is commonly found in organic matter such as soil and plant material.

In general, fungi survive by producing proteases that specifically digest the tissue in which they grow. In cases of fungal keratitis, these proteases, along with the cornea's own inflammatory response, produce tissue damage, which results in ulceration. *Fusarium* is a filamentary fungi which consists of septate and non-septate organisms which join together to form hyphae. If not treated rapidly, the hyphae possess the ability to penetrate an intact Descemet membrane and are, therefore, capable of spreading into surrounding tissues including the sclera and ciliary body. Permanent vision loss is not uncommon; in 25% to 35% of the cases, a corneal transplant is necessitated. Fungal infection can not be transmitted from person to person.

Natamycin (*Natacyn*) 5% is the drug of choice for filamentous fungal infections and is the sole agent used in 90% of these cases. In non-responsive cases, topical management may need to be supplemented by members of the "azole" class of drugs, including miconazole, ketoconazole, fluconazole and voriconazole. Topical corticosteroids are contraindicated in the treatment of fungal keratitis. Most antifungal agents are fungistatic rather than fungicidal, and the use of corticosteroids will reduce the patient's ability to eliminate the infection and will often worsen the infection.

As of August, 2006, the CDC in Atlanta had confirmed 164 cases of *Fusarium* keratitis in 33 states and one territory, with nearly all of the cases occurring in contact lens wearers. One care system, *ReNu with MoistureLoc* (Bausch and Lomb; Rochester, New York) was found to be associated with a disproportionately high percentage (57%) of cases and has been permanently removed from the world-wide market. It is important to mention that *Fusarium* keratitis has not been commonly associated with any other contact lens care regimen, including the other *ReNu* products. The incidence of this complication can also be minimized when patients adhere to the aforementioned contact lens guidelines, including compliance with the prescribed care regimen, hygiene instructions and wearing and lens replacement schedules. Frequent case replacement — at minimum, every 3 months — is also important as fungal growth has been found in as many as 14% of hydrogel lens cases and 3% of GP lens cases.

IN-OFFICE DISINFECTION

Most trial lenses in use today are used once and then discarded. This is the most acceptable method of diagnostic lens use because there would be no danger of ocular infection spread from one patient to the next because the lenses are packaged in sterile containers. However, there are still some diagnostic lenses that are reused after being disinfected, which does not produce a sterile lens. Large thermal disinfection units are available to disinfect lenses in glass vials, which is an acceptable method of disinfection; however, some lens materials contraindicate thermal disinfection use, primarily those with more than 55% water content. Oxidative disinfection, although an excellent method of disinfection, is difficult to use for diagnostic lenses because of the necessity of disinfecting the lens in a special case and transferring the disinfected lens to a glass vial. The lens may become contaminated in the transfer process or the vial may become contaminated. It is acceptable to store lenses in a glass vial in a chemical disinfecting solution; however, their effects on *Acanthamoeba* and the AIDS virus are questionable. Diagnostic lenses redisinfected with *AOSept* or *ReNu MultiPurpose* solutions (vs thermal disinfection) should be redisinfected at least once a month to prevent contamination.

Arguably, the most effective system is a combination. *Opti-Free Express*, as a result of both the preservative action and the omission of a surfactant, may be used and is approved for use in heat disinfection. The other chemical disinfection systems, conversely, contain a surfactant that, after repeated thermal disinfection cycles, may result in a cloudy lens. The patient should be advised to wash hands prior to handling and, as with any lens worn by the patient, thoroughly clean and rinse the lens prior to disinfection. Lenses of more than 55% water content may be stored in *Opti-Free Express* or other chemical-disinfecting solution without thermal disinfection. The practitioner must keep in mind the limitations of the systems. Any lens used on a known AIDS patient or a patient exposed to *Acanthamoeba* should be disposed of and not reused, even though at the present time it is thought that the risk of transmission via the tears is low. In addition to disinfection of diagnostic lenses after use, diagnostic lenses that are stored in-office and have been opened should be disinfected, at minimum, every 90 days to prevent contamination of the lenses and the vials. In addition, only new, factory-sealed lenses should be dispensed directly to patients.

For More Information

Acanthamoeba: Clinical management, contact lens patient compliance and reporting. *AOA News.* April 16, 2007: 15-18.

Barr JT. Contact lens 2005. *Contact Lens Spectrum.* 2006;21(1):26-34.

Bennett ES. Acanthamoeba keratitis in 2007: stay informed but calm. *Contact Lens Spectrum.* 2007;22(7).

Bennett ES. Lens care and patient education. In: Bennett ES, Henry VA, eds. *Clinical Manual of Contact Lenses*, 2nd ed. Philadelphia, PA: J.B. Lippincott; 2000.

Bennett ES. What we have learned from the fusarium outbreak? *Rev Optom.* 2007;144(4):34-42.

Bennett ES, Schornack MM, Weissman BA. Clinical overview of *Fusarium* keratitis. Submitted to *Optometry: Journal of the American Optometric Association.* Currently under review.

Chun MW, Weissman BA. Compliance in contact lens care. *Am J Optom Physiol Opt.* 1987; 64:274-276.

Collins MJ, Carney LG. Patient compliance and its influence on contact lens wearing problems. *Am J Optom Physiol Opt.* 1986;63:952-956.

De Oliveiva, Temporini-Naster ER, Alves MR, Kara-Jose N. Self evaluation of the contact lens wearing and care by college students and health care workers. *Eye and Contact Lens.* 2003;29:164-167.

Fonn D, Dumbleton K, Jones L, Toit R, Sweeney D. Silicone hydrogel material and surface properties. *Contact Lens Spectrum.* 2002;17:24-29.

Franklin V, Tighe B, Tonge S. Contact lens deposition, discoloration and spoilation mechanisms. *Optician.* 2001;222:16-20.

GP Lens Institute GP Contact Lens Product Guide. http://www.gpli.info. Accessed: July 19, 2007.

Hom MM. *Manual of Contact Lens Prescribing and Fitting with CD-ROM.* 2nd ed. Boston, MA: Butterworth-Heinemann; 2000:235-254.

Kilvingston S, Gray T, Dart J, et al. Acanthamoeba keratitis: the role of domestic tap water contamination in the United Kingdom. *Invest Ophthalmol Vis Sci.* 2004;45:165-169.

Lingel NJ, Casser L. Diseases of the cornea. In: Bartlett JD, Jaanus SD, eds. *Clinical Ocular Pharmacology*, 4th ed. Boston, MA: Butterworth-Heinemann; 2001.

Lowther GE, Shannon BJ, Weisbarth R. *The Pharmacist's Guide to Contact Lenses and Lens Care.* Atlanta, GA: CIBA Vision Corporation; 1988.

Mowrey-McKee M, Sills A, Wright A. Comparative cytotoxicity of soft contact lens care regimens. *CLAO J.* 2002;28:160-164.

Schornack MM. Clinical management of fungal keratitis. *AOA News.* April 24, 2006:17-18.

Seal DV. *Acanthamoeba* keratitis update — incidence, molecular epidemiology and new drugs for treatment. *Eye.* 2003;17:893-905.

Shovlin JP. Acanthanmoeba keratitis in rigid lens wearers: the issue of tap water rinses. *Int Contact Lens Clin.* 1990;17:47.

Shovlin JP. The Contact Lens Prescription Release Bill: our work is not complete. *Rev Contact Lenses.* January 2004:7.

Silbert JA. Medications and contact lens wear. *Contact Lens Spectrum.* 2002;17:26-31.

Teenan DW, Beck L. Contact lens-associated chemical burn. *Contact Lens Ant Eye.* 2001;24:175-176.

Thompson TT. Tyler's quarterly soft contact lens parameter guide. June 2007;24(3):60-64.

Weisbarth R, Henderson B. In: Bennett ES, Weissman BA, eds. *Clinical Contact Lens Practice.* 2nd ed. Philadelphia, PA: Lippincott Williams & Wilkins; 2004:381-419.

Wilson LA, Savant AO, Simmons RB, Ahearn DG. Microbial contamination of contact lens storage cases and solutions. *Am J Ophthalmol.* 1990;109:193.

COMPONENTS IN CONTACT LENS SOLUTIONS

PRESERVATIVES:

Chlorhexidine: Chlorhexidine is bactericidal in action and has been used traditionally in a concentration of 0.005% in hydrogel lens chemical disinfection solutions. However, as gradual binding to hydrogel lenses has been problematic, chlorhexidine is used primarily with GP lenses today. The binding capacity of chlorhexidine to GP lenses appears to be limited because of the wettability of GP lenses and to chlorhexidine's large molecular structure with a weak cationic action. Although chlorhexidine has been reported to have an excellent spectrum of antimicrobial activity, it has limited effectiveness against yeast and fungi; therefore, it often has been combined with ethylenediamine tetra acetate (EDTA) or thimerosal for greater effectiveness. In addition, chlorhexidine has been found to be relatively ineffective against *Serratia marcescens.*

Benzalkonium chloride (BAK): Benzalkonium chloride is a quaternary ammonium compound that is effective against a wide spectrum of bacteria and fungi and normally is used at a concentration of 0.004% in some GP lens solutions. The effectiveness of BAK is enhanced when used in combination with EDTA, allowing a lower concentration than otherwise necessary. It is not used as a preservative with hydrogel lens solutions because the hydrogel plastic will bind the preservative and actually concentrate it, thereby allowing it to potentially reach toxic levels and cause ocular injury.

Thimerosal: Thimerosal is an organic mercurial compound that at one time was a commonly used hydrogel lens solution preservative. However, some patients are sensitive to organic mercurial compounds and experience a burning sensation and associated clinical signs of redness and superficial punctuate keratitis. In addition, it is slow-acting in nature and, in low concentrations, may be ineffective against *Pseudomonas.* Although thimerosal has been found to be compatible with GP lenses, exhibiting only rare sensitivity reactions, for optimal antimicrobial effectiveness it should be used in combination with another preservative such as chlorhexidine.

Ethylenediamine tetra acetate (EDTA): Ethylenediamine tetra acetate is a chelating agent and not a true preservative. However, it is commonly used in combination with BAK and other preservatives in the rigid contact lens solutions because of its synergistic ability to enhance the bacterial action of pure preservatives against *Pseudomonas.*

Benzyl alcohol: Benzyl Alcohol was originally considered for use as a solvent for contact lens materials; however, it also was found to have good disinfection capabilities. Pure benzyl alcohol possesses certain physicochemical characteristics that are regarded as ideal for an ophthalmic preservative, including low molecular weight, bipolarity, and water solubility. It is used in some GP lens combination cleaning/disinfecting solutions. Caution must be used not to wet and insert a lens with a benzyl alcohol-preserved solution because a hypersensitivity reaction may occur.

Polyaminopropyl biguanide (PAPB): Polyaminopropyl biguanide is a high molecular weight preservative that alters the phospholipid groups found in bacterial cell walls. It has been used as a preservative in hydrogel lens disinfection regimens (as DYMED) because of its low sensitivity rate. It has replaced chlorhexidine as a preservative in one of the GP care systems because it exhibits higher antimicrobial effectiveness, notably against *Serratia marcescens.* Some toxic reactions were experienced by patients when it was initially introduced in a GP wetting/soaking solution. However, when reduced in concentration by 66%, it has demonstrated both excellent antimicrobial activity and minimal toxicity when compared with other systems.

Polyquad: Used in both soft and GP lens formulations, polyquad is similar to BAK in composition and action, but appears to minimize the incidence of any adverse reactions. Like PAPB, its high molecular weight prevents it from being absorbed into the contact lens matrix.

Sorbic acid: Typically used in 0.1% concentrations, sorbic acid is a bacteriostatic agent that produces a low incidence of hypersensitive reactions. It is a relatively unstable compound that breaks down into an aldehyde; therefore, through this process it can cause soft lens discoloration when used with hydrogen peroxide.

Actions:

Pharmacology: There are numerous preservatives currently in common use, all differing in their mode of action and efficacy. They are capable of either killing (bactericidal agents) or inhibiting the growth (bacteriostatic agents) of microorganisms. Preservatives are the active ingredients and should perform the following functions:

1. Effectively provide the necessary degree of disinfection in the environment in which it is to be used.
2. Not cause toxic reactions.
3. Be compatible with the lens materials, avoiding adverse effects on surface wettability and lens parameters.
4. Be compatible with the tear film.

Indications:

To be used in contact lens salines, chemical disinfection solutions, and cleaners for the purpose of inhibiting microbial growth in these solutions.

Contraindications:

Hypersensitivity to any specific preservative used in the formulation.

BUFFERS

Actions:

Pharmacology: A weak acid or base and its corresponding salt typically compose the buffer in a contact lens solution. Buffers can be identified by the suffix "-ate" on the label. The borate buffer commonly used in contact lens solutions, which also has some antimicrobial activity, consists of boric acid and sodium borate. Bicarbonate and citrate are other buffers used in these solutions.

Indications:

Buffers are indicated in contact lens solutions to maintain a fairly neutral pH level (6 to 8). Because of their phosphate concentration, the tear layer naturally assists in maintaining a neutral pH.

Contraindications:

None.

WETTING AGENTS

Polyvinyl Alcohol (PVA):

Polyvinyl alcohol has several properties that make it a beneficial additive to GP lens solutions. It is water soluble and is relatively nonviscous and nontoxic to ocular tissues. It has good viscosity-building properties and exhibits good tear spreading on the eye and lens surfaces. It also does not retard regeneration of corneal epithelium.

Methylcellulose:

Methylcellulose derivatives have been used successfully as wetting agents in more viscous GP solutions. They add higher viscosity — and therefore, longer term wettability — than PVA; however, methylcellulose retards epithelial regeneration.

Poloxamer 407:

Poloxamer 407 is used as a viscosity builder and wetting agent in some rewetting drop formulations. It has mucomimetic properties.

Actions:

Pharmacology: GP wetting/rewetting and soft lens rewetting solutions often have wetting agents in the solution itself. These substances typically have good viscosity-building properties and exhibit good spreading and wettability on the eye and lens surfaces.

Indications:

To enhance surface wettability of contact lens materials.

Contraindications:

None.

Wetting/soaking solutions typically contain polyvinyl alcohol or a methylcellulose derivative as a wetting agent.

CONTACT LENS CARE PRODUCTS

Products for use with contact lenses possess the same general characteristics of all ophthalmic products; they are sterile, isotonic, and free of particulate matter. Additionally, product formulations contain various components to achieve specific goals of contact lens care. Although all contact lenses serve similar functions in correcting visual defects, each type of lens material requires a unique lens care program. In selecting appropriate lens care solutions, correctly identifying the type of lens material a patient is wearing is essential.

Individual drug monographs are on the following pages.

GAS PERMEABLE LENSES

Products for use with GP lenses include the following: disinfecting/wetting/soaking, disinfecting/cleaning, surfactant cleaners, enzymatic cleaners, and rewetting drops. All have important functions in maintaining/enhancing the wettability, sterility, and cleanliness of GP lens materials.

DISINFECTING/WETTING/SOAKING SOLUTIONS, GP LENSES

Actions:

Pharmacology: These solutions are formulated for comfort and compatibility with ocular tissues. Therefore, the pH of the solution should be near physiologic pH, or only slightly buffered to allow the pH to rapidly adjust to that of tear film. A wetting agent such as PVA and possibly a viscosity-building agent such as methylcellulose will be used to enhance the tear spreading properties over the surface of the lens. Preservative use is such to disinfect the lens while not being toxic to the eye.

Indications:

These solutions are used for both insertion and soaking/disinfection of GP lenses. They enhance lens surface wettability, maintain lens hydration similar to that achieved during contact lens wear, disinfect the lens, and act as a mechanical buffer between the lens and the cornea.

Warnings:

Almost all of these solutions are not compatible with soft lens material.

otc	**Bausch & Lomb Wetting and Soaking for RGP & Hard Lenses** (Bausch & Lomb)	**Solution:** Buffered, slightly hypertonic, low viscosity. 0.05% EDTA, 0.006% chlorhexidine gluconate. Cationic cellulose derivative polymer.	In 120 mL.
otc	**Bausch & Lomb Boston Conditioning Solution Advance Comfort Formula** (Bausch & Lomb)	**Solution:** Buffered, slightly hypertonic. 0.05% EDTA, 0.003% chlorhexidine gluconate, 0.0005% polyaminopropyl biguanide. Cationic cellulose derivative polymer, PEG, cellulosic viscosifier, polyvinyl alcohol.	In 30, 90, and 120 mL.
otc	**Boston Conditioning Solution** (Bausch & Lomb/ Boston)	**Solution:** Buffered, slightly hypertonic. 0.05% EDTA, 0.006% chlorhexidine gluconate. Cationic cellulose derivative polymer, polyvinyl alcohol, PEG, cellulosic viscosifier.	In 120 mL.
otc	**Boston Simplicity Multi-Action Solution** (Bausch & Lomb/ Boston)	**Solution:** Buffered, slightly hypertonic. 0.05% EDTA, 0.003% chlorhexidine gluconate, 0.0005% polyaminopropyl biguanide. PEO sorbitan monolaurate, betaine surfactant, silicone glycol copolymer, PEG, cellulosic viscosifier.	In 120 mL.
otc	**Boston Simplus** (Bausch & Lomb/ Boston)	**Solution:** Buffered. Chlorhexidine gluconate, polyaminopropyl biguanide. Poloxamine, hydroxyalkylphosphonate, Glucam-20.	In 105 mL.

otc	**Barnes-Hind Comfort-Care GP Wetting & Soaking Solution** (Advanced Medical Optics)	**Solution:** Buffered, isotonic. 0.02% EDTA, 0.005% chlorhexidine gluconate. Oxyethylene, povidone, polyvinyl alcohol, propylene glycol, NaCl, hydroxyethylcellulose, phosphates.	In 240 mL.
otc	**Optimum Cleaning, Disinfecting, and Storage Solution** (Lobob)	**Solution:** 0.3% benzyl alcohol, 0.5% EDTA. Octylphenoxypolyethoxyethanol, lauryl sulfate salt of imidazoline.	In 120 mL.
otc	**Sereine Wetting & Soaking Solution** (Optikem)	**Solution:** Buffered, isotonic, 0.1% EDTA, 0.01% benzalkonium chloride, sodium chloride, polyoxypropylene polyoxyethylene copolymer.	In 120 mL.
otc	**Unique pH Multi-Purpose Solution** (Alcon)	**Solution:** Buffered, 0.0011% polyquad and 0.01% EDTA. Hydroxypropyl guar, polyethylene glycol, *Tetronic*, boric acid, propylene glycol.	In 90 mL.
otc	**Wet-N-Soak Plus Wetting and Soaking Solution** (American Medical Optics)	**Solution:** Buffered, isotonic. 0.003% benzalkonium chloride, polyvinyl alcohol, EDTA.	In 120 mL.

DISINFECTING/CLEANING SOLUTIONS, GP LENSES

Actions:

Pharmacology: These solutions incorporate a mild surfactant cleaner into a preserved-disinfecting solution. With the exception of *Boston Simplicity* (Bausch & Lomb/*Boston*) and *Unique pH* (Alcon), all-in-one products with wetting, cleaning, and disinfecting functions, these solutions are not intended for wetting/rewetting use. Because of the nature and composition of the surfactant cleaning agent(s), these solutions can induce a punctate keratitis if directly instilled into the eye.

Indications:

These solutions are used for disinfecting and cleaning of GP lenses. It may be necessary to add an enzymatic cleaner to the care regimen in some patients.

Warnings:

With the exception of *Boston Simplicity* (Bausch & Lomb/*Boston*) and *Unique pH* (Alcon), which are also wetting solutions, these solutions should not be directly instilled into the eye or a toxic reaction to the surfactant cleaner may result.

otc	**AOSept Clear Care** (Ciba Vision)	**Solution:** Buffered. 3% hydrogen peroxide, 0.79% sodium chloride, phosphonic acid, pluronic 17R4.	In 120, 237, and 355 mL.
otc	**Boston Simplicity Multi-Action Solution** (Bausch & Lomb/ **Boston**)	**Solution:** Buffered, slightly hypertonic. 0.05% EDTA, 0.003% chlorhexidine gluconate, 0.0005% polyaminopropyl biguanide. PEO sorbitan monolaurate, betaine surfactant, silicone glycol copolymer, PEG, cellulosic viscosifier.	In 120 mL.

otc	**Boston Simplus** (Bausch & Lomb/ **Boston**)	**Solution:** Buffered. Chlorhexidine gluconate, polyaminopropyl biguanide. Poloxamine, hydroxyalkylphosphonate, Glucam-20.	In 105 mL.
otc	**Claris Cleaning and Soaking Solution** (Menicon/Allergan)	**Solution:** 0.1% EDTA, 0.1% benzyl alcohol, 0.05% sorbic acid, 0.02% sodium bisulfate, NaCl, potassium chloride, PVA, PVP, hydroxyethylcellulose.	In 120 mL.
otc	**Menicare GP CDS Cleaning, Disinfecting and Storage Solution** (Menicon)	**Solution:** Lauryl salt of imidazoline, octylphenoxypolyethoxyethanol, and preserved with benzyl alcohol 0.3% and disdium edetate 0.5%.	In 118 mL.
otc	**Optimum by Lobob Cleaning, Disinfecting and Storage Solution** (Lobob)	**Solution:** Lauryl salt of imidazoline, octylphenoxypolyethoxyethanol, and preserved with benzyl alcohol 0.3% and disodium edetate 0.5%.	In 118 mL.
otc	**Unique pH Multi-Purpose Solution** (Alcon)	**Solution:** Buffered, 0.0011% polyquad and 0.01% EDTA. Hydroxypropyl guar, polyethylene glycol, *Tetronic*, boric acid, propylene glycol.	Thimerosal free. In 90 mL.

SURFACTANT CLEANING SOLUTIONS, GP LENSES

Actions:

Pharmacology: These solutions use cleaners that typically consist of nonionic surfactant (detergents). Mild abrasive particles are added in some formulations for greater effect against bound muco-protein deposit complexes.

Indications:

All GP wearing patients should use some type of cleaning solution upon lens removal because lipids, mucus, proteins, and other substances such as cosmetics and hand creams can adhere to the lens surface resulting in blurred vision and possibly reduced wearing time. These solutions help maintain a clean, wettable surface and good optics. If an abrasive cleaner is used, do not clean the lens forcefully between the fingers, because increases in minus power and warpage have been reported over time.

Warnings:

Solutions used strictly for cleaning should never be used for wetting/rewetting GP lenses or chemical keratitis may result.

otc	**Bausch & Lomb Concentrated Cleaner for RGP & Hard Lenses** (Bausch & Lomb)	**Solution:** Concentrated homogenous surfactant. Alkyl ether sulfate, ethoxylated alkyl phenol, tri-quaternary cocoa-based phospholipid, silica gel.	In 30 mL.
otc	**Bausch & Lomb Boston Advance Cleaner Solution** (Bausch & Lomb)	**Solution:** Concentrated homogenous surfactant. Alkyl ether sulfate, ethoxylated alkyl phenol, tri-quaternary cocoa-based phospholipid, titanium dioxide, silica gel.	In 30 mL.

otc	**Boston Cleaner Solution** (Polymer Technology)	**Solution**: Concentrated homogenous surfactant. Alkyl ether sulfate, silica gel, titanium dioxide.	In 30 mL.
otc	**Opti-Clean II Daily Cleaner Especially for Sensitive Eyes Solution** (Alcon)	**Solution**: Buffered, isotonic. 0.1% EDTA, 0.001% polyquad. Polysorbate 21, polymeric cleaning agents.	Thimerosal free. In 15 and 30 mL.
otc	**Optimum by Lobob Extra Strength Cleaner** (Lobob)	**Solution**: Slightly alkaline, aqueous solution with cocoamphodiacetate and glycols.	Preservative free. In 60 mL.
otc	**Resolve/GP Daily Cleaner Solution** (Advanced Medical Optics)	**Solution**: Buffered. Cocoamphocarboxyglycinate, sodium lauryl sulfate, hexylene glycol, alkyl ether sulfate, fatty acid amide surfactants.	Preservative free. In 30 mL.
otc	**Sereine Cleaner** (Optikem)	**Solution**: Amphoteric surfactants, edetate disodium 0.1%, benzalkonium chloride 0.01%.	In 60 mL.
otc	**Sereine Soaking & Cleaning Solution** (Optikem)	**Solution**: 0.25% EDTA, 0.01% benzalkonium chloride.	In 120 mL.

ENZYMATIC CLEANERS, GP LENSES

Actions:

Pharmacology: An enzymatic cleaner acts chemically to dissolve adherent mucoprotein complexes on the surface of the lens. Specific enzymes currently in use include papain (from papaya fruit), pancreatin (from hog pancreas), and Subtilisin A and B (produced by microorganisms).

Indications:

Enzyme cleaners are used as an adjunct to surfactant cleaning for the removal of adherent deposits. They are especially beneficial in dry eye patients who are more prone to deposit formation and for individuals who are not compliant with regular surfactant cleaning. Commonly available in tablet form, which dissolves in saline, they are currently available in a liquid form as marketed by 2 companies (*Boston One-Step Liquid Enzyme Cleaner* for weekly use from Bausch & Lomb/Boston; *Opti-Free Supra-Clens Daily Protein Removal* for daily use from Alcon). The liquid enzyme has the benefit of promoting patient compliance via the simplicity of adding a drop of the enzyme solution to the disinfecting solution in each case well for overnight use.

Warnings:

Enzyme solutions are not to be used for wetting or rewetting of GP lenses or chemical keratitis may result.

otc	**Boston One-Step Liquid Enzymatic Cleaner** (Bausch & Lomb/ Boston)	**Solution**: Subtilisin. Glycerol.	Preservative free. In 1 and 2.4 mL.
otc	**Opti-Free Supra Clens Daily Protein Remover** (Alcon)	**Solution**: Propylene glycol, sodium borate, highly purified porcine pancreatin enzymes.	Preservative free. In 3 mL.
otc	**ProFree/GP Weekly Enzymatic Cleaner** (Advanced Medical Optics)	**Tablets**: Papain, NaCl, sodium carbonate, sodium borate, EDTA.	Preservative free. In 16s with vials.
otc	**Ultrazyme Enzymatic Cleaner** (Advanced Medical Optics)	**Tablets**: Subtilisin A. Effervescing, buffering, and tableting agents. To make solution for soaking, dilute in 3% hydrogen peroxide disinfecting solution.	In 5s, 10s, and 20s.

REWETTING SOLUTIONS, GP LENSES

Actions:

Pharmacology: Rewetting drops are usually isotonic or slightly hypertonic. They typically contain a viscosity agent or wetting agent to enhance surface wettability.

Indications:

Rewetting solutions are needed when an GP wearing patient experiences dryness or redness. These solutions rewet the lens surface, rinse away trapped debris, and break up loosely-adherent deposits.

Warnings:

One formulation, *Boston Rewetting Drops*, is not compatible for use with soft lenses.

otc	**Aquify Long Lasting Comfort Drops** (Ciba Vision)	Sodium perborate stabilized with perborate acid.	In 10 mL.
otc	***blink* Contacts Lubricant Eye Drops** (Advanced Medical Optics)	**Solution**: Buffered, isotonic with sodium hyaluronate, sodium chloride, potassium chloride, calcium chloride, magnesium chloride, boric acid, and *OcuPure* (stabilized oxychloro complex) 0.005% as the preservative.	In 10 mL.
otc	**Boston Rewetting Drops** (Bausch & Lomb/ Boston)	**Solution**: Buffered, slightly hypertonic. 0.05% EDTA, 0.006% chlorhexidine gluconate. Cationic cellulose derivative polymer, polyvinyl alcohol, hydroxyethyl cellulose.	In 10 mL.

otc	**Claris Rewetting Drops** (Menicon/Allergan)	**Solution**: Buffered, isotonic, 0.06% polixetonium chloride, hydroxyethylcellulose, borate buffer.	In 15 mL.
otc	**Clerz Plus Lens Drops** (Alcon)	**Solution**: Buffered, isotonic. 0.05% EDTA, 0.001% polyquad. Peg-11 lauryl ether carboxylic acid, *Tetronic* 1304.	In 5, 8, and 15 mL.
otc	**Complete Blink-N-Clean Lens Drops** (Advanced Medical Optics)	**Solution**: Buffered, isotonic. 0.0001% polyhexamethylene biguanide, tromethamine, hydroxypropyl methylcellulose, tyloxapol, EDTA, sodium chloride.	Thimerosal free. In 20 mL.
otc	**Opti-Free RepleniSH Rewetting Drops** (Alcon)	**Solution**: Buffered, Isotonic, aqueous solution with a citrate/borate buffer and sodium chloride, with edetate disodium 0.05% and *Polyquad* (polyquaternium-1) 0.001% as preservatives and RLM-100 (PEG-11 lauryl ether carboxylic acid) and *Tetronic* 1304.	In 10 mL.
otc	**Optimum Wetting and Rewetting Drops** (Lobob)	**Solution**: Sodium and potassium chloride salts, polyvinylpyrrolidone, polyvinyl alcohol, hydroxyethyl cellulose, 0.02% sodium bisulfite. 0.1% benzyl alcohol, 0.5% sorbic acid, 0.1% EDTA.	In 30 mL.
otc	**Sereine Wetting Solution** (Optikem)	**Solution**: Buffered. 0.1% EDTA, 0.01% benzalkonium chloride.	In 60 mL.
otc	**TheraTears Contact Lens Comfort Drops** (Advanced Vision Research)	**Solution**: Sodium carbo methyl cellulose (0.25%), sodium perborate as preservative.	In 15 mL.

HYDROGEL (SOFT) LENSES

Hydrogel contact lens care systems are designed to clean, disinfect, and rewet the lenses. Lenses are cleaned gently in the palm of the hand prior to disinfection. Disinfection of hydrogel lenses is the most important step in the care process. Disinfection is achieved by using a thermal (heat), chemical (non-hydrogen peroxide), or hydrogen peroxide (oxidative) system.

DISINFECTION, CHEMICAL NON-HYDROGEN PEROXIDE, SOFT LENSES

Actions:

Pharmacology: Disinfection is defined as the process whereby vegetative or living microorganisms are completely killed or inactivated. This involves the destruction of microorganisms by attacking the cell wall or membrane, the inhibition of protein synthesis, or both. Current disinfecting products must pass specific FDA and International Organization for Standardization (ISO) microbiological and cleaning efficacy tests in order to gain approval to use particular labeling. Upon passing the appropriate test, a solution may be designated a "multipurpose" solution (MPS), a "multipurpose disinfecting" solution (MPDS), or a "no-rub required" disinfecting solution.

These solutions disinfect via the use of preservatives compatible with hydrogel lens materials. Because many of these solutions combine wetting and, in a few cases, cleaning, they incorporate buffers and a mild surfactant. Typically, a minimum of 4 hours is recommended for disinfection. One faster system, *Quick Care* (Ciba Vision), allows for disinfection and cleaning in a 5-minute period. The starting solution is hypertonic with a surfactant and isopropyl alcohol. Then it is stored for 1 minute in a saline solution with a trace amount of hydrogen peroxide.

Indications:

For disinfection of hydrogel lenses. Other functions—including wetting, rinsing, and cleaning—may be present as well.

Warnings:

Some patients may exhibit a sensitivity to the preservatives in a given system.

otc	**All in One Lite** (Sauflon Pharmaceuticals)	**Solution:** Buffered, isotonic, poloxamer, sodium chloride buffer, sodium chloride and disodium edetate.	9 oz.
otc	**Aquify MPS** (Ciba Vision)	**Solution:** Sterile aqueous solution with sorbitol, tromethamine, pluronic F127, sodium phosphate dihydrogen, Dexpant-5, edetate disodium dehydrate with polyhexanide 0.0001%.	In 118 and 355 mL.
otc	**Complete Moisture Plus Multi-Purpose Solution — No Rub** (Advanced Medical Optics)	**Solution:** Buffered, isotonic. Polyhexamethylene biguanide 0.0001%, edetate disodium, hydroxypropyl methylcellulose, propylene glycol, taurine, phosphate buffers, poloxamer 237, NaCl.	In 118, 355, and 473 mL.
otc	**Opti-Free Express Multi-Purpose Disinfecting No Rub Formula** (Alcon)	**Solution:** Buffered, isotonic. EDTA, 0.001% polyquad, 0.0005% myristamidopropyl dimethylamine. Citrate, NaCl, boric acid, sorbitol, AMP-95, *Tetronic* 1304.	In 118, 355, and 473 mL.
otc	**Opti-Free RepleniSH** (Alcon)	**Solution:** Buffered, isotonic, aqueous solution with sodium citrates, sodium chloride. Sodium borate, propylene glycol, *Tearglyde* (*Tetronic* 1304, nonanoyl ethylenediametriacetic acid) with *Polyquad* (polyquaternium) 0.001% and *Aldox* (myristamidopropyl dimethylamine) 0.0005% as preservatives.	In 118 and 300 mL.
otc	**Opti-Free Rinsing, Disinfecting, and Storage Solution** (Alcon)	**Solution:** Buffered, isotonic. 0.05% EDTA, 0.001% polyquad. Citrates, NaCl.	In 118 and 335 mL.
otc	**Opti-One Multi-Purpose Solution** (Alcon)	**Solution:** Buffered, isotonic. EDTA, polyquad. Borates, citrates, mannitol, NaCl, surfactants, sodium citrate, *Tetronic*, *Pationic*.	In 118 and 355 mL.
otc	**Purilens UV Disinfection System** (Purilens)	**Solution:** Uses cleaning unit with UV-C radiation to disinfect lenses.	
otc	**ReNu MultiPlus Multi-Purpose Solution** (Bausch & Lomb)	**Solution:** Isotonic. 0.0001% polyaminopropyl biguanide (DYMED). Hydroxyalkylphosphonate, boric acid, EDTA, poloxamine, sodium borate, NaCl.	Thimerosal free. In 60, 118, 237, and 355 mL.
otc	**ReNu Multi-Purpose Solution, No Rub Formula** (Bausch & Lomb)	**Solution:** Isotonic, 0.00005% polyaminopropyl biguanide (DYMED). Boric acid, EDTA, sodium borate, NaCl.	In 118 and 355 mL.

DISINFECTION, HYDROGEN PEROXIDE (OXIDATIVE), SOFT LENSES

Actions:

Pharmacology: Oxidative disinfection consists of a 3% hydrogen peroxide solution; neutralizing solution, tablet, or disc; saline; and cleaner. Hydrogen peroxide does not result in clinically significant sensitivity problems when used properly because it breaks down into water and oxygen. Hydrogen peroxide usually is hypotonic and has an approximate pH of 4. It is important that some method of neutralization is present to prevent this acidic solution from direct contact with the eye. Present formulations are stable and newer systems appear to be less complex and more patient-friendly. These chemical properties result in lens expansion and contraction, which is believed to break protein and lipid bonds.

Indications:

For the disinfection of hydrogel lenses. It offers many advantages over other chemical systems. It is safe, very effective, and does not contain sensitizing ingredients. Hydrogen peroxide penetrates into hydrogel lenses and is reported to provide deep-cleaning action by expanding the lens matrix and oxidizing foreign matter.

Warnings:

Punctate keratitis: Hydrogen peroxide will produce a mild to moderate punctate keratitis if not neutralized prior to instillation into the eye. To minimize this problem, many of the hydrogen peroxide solutions are currently packaged in bottles with red tips and warning labels on the bottles that direct the patient not to use the solution directly on the eye.

Discoloration: Use of an *OTC* hydrogen peroxide not formulated for contact lens use may result in discoloration and patient sensitivity because of colorants, incompatible stabilizers, and lack of salts necessary to provide satisfactory saline following neutralization.

otc	**AOSept** (Ciba Vision)	**Disinfecting solution**: Buffered. 3% hydrogen peroxide, 0.85% NaCl, phosphoric acid, phosphates.	Thimerosal free. In 118, 237, 355, and 473 mL.
		AODISC neutralizer: Platinum-coated disc.	Disc good for 100 uses or 3 months of daily use.[1]
otc	**AOSept Clear Care** (Ciba Vision)	**Solution**: Buffered. 3% hydrogen peroxide, 0.79% sodium chloride, phosphonic acid, pluronic 17R4.	In 120, 237, and 355 mL.
otc	**Pure Eyes** (Ciba Vision)	**Disinfectant/Soaking solution**: Buffered. 3% hydrogen peroxide, 0.85% NaCl, phosphonic acid, phosphates.	In 355 mL.
		Cleaner/Rinse solution: Buffered, isotonic. NaCl, boric acid, sodium borate, sodium perborate (generating up to 0.006% hydrogen peroxide stabilized with phosphonic acid), pluronic 407, pluronic 17R4.	Thimerosal free. In 360 mL.

otc	**Sauflon One Step Hydrogen Peroxide Cleaning and Disinfecting System** (Sauflon Pharmaceuticals)	**Solution**: Hydrogen peroxide 3% buffered (with phosphates), stabilized (with phosphonic acid), poloxamer.	In 12 oz.
otc	**UltraCare** (Allergan)	**Disinfecting solution**: Buffered. 3% hydrogen peroxide, sodium stannate, sodium nitrate, phosphates.	In 360 mL.
		Neutralizing tablets: Catalase, hydroxypropyl methylcellulose, cyanocobalamin, buffering and tableting agents.	Beige/pink. In 36s with cup.

[1] For use only with the *AOSept* system.

DISINFECTION, THERMAL (HEAT), SOFT LENSES

Actions:

Pharmacology: Heat disinfection avoids the use of preservatives and their corresponding potential for sensitivity. Heat is the most effective disinfection method, often killing organisms within 15 to 20 minutes compared with several hours with many chemical systems. Most of the units have temperatures reaching a maximum of 80° to 90°C.

Indications:

Heat disinfection is recommended when the other systems are not effective. Lens life is reduced because it heats deposits directly on the lens surface, resulting in discoloration. It is limited to lower water content lens materials.

Warnings:

Heat disinfection should not be used with Group 2 or Group 4 lenses.

PRESERVED SALINE SOLUTIONS, SOFT LENSES

otc	**Sensitive Eyes Plus Saline Solution** (Bausch & Lomb)	**Solution**: Buffered, isotonic. 0.025% EDTA, 0.00003% polyaminopropyl biguanide. Boric acid, sodium borate, potassium chloride, NaCl.	In 118 and 355 mL.
otc	**Sensitive Eyes Saline Solution** (Bausch & Lomb)	**Solution**: Buffered, isotonic. 0.1% sorbic acid, 0.025% EDTA. Boric acid, sodium borate, NaCl.	Thimerosal free. In 118, 237, and 355 mL.
otc	**SoftWear Saline for Sensitive Eyes Solution** (Ciba Vision)	**Solution**: Isotonic. NaCl, boric acid, sodium borate, sodium perborate (generating up to 0.006% hydrogen peroxide stabilized with phosphonic acid).	Thimerosal free. In 118, 237, 355, and 473 mL.

PRESERVATIVE FREE SALINE SOLUTIONS, SOFT LENSES

otc	**Blairex Sterile Saline Solution** (Blairex)	**Solution:** Buffered, isotonic. NaCl, boric acid, sodium borate.	Preservative free. In 90, 240, and 360 mL aerosol.
otc	**Lens Plus Sterile Saline Solution** (Exaeris)	**Solution:** Buffered, isotonic. NaCl, boric acid, nitrogen (as an aerosol propellant).	Preservative free. In 90, 240, 360, and 450 mL aerosol.
otc	**Unisol 4 Solution** (Alcon)	**Solution:** Buffered, isotonic. NaCl, boric acid, sodium borate.	Preservative free. Thimerosal free. In 120 mL.

SURFACTANT CLEANING SOLUTIONS, SOFT LENSES

Actions:

Pharmacology: Similar to GP lens solutions. The purpose of surfactants is to remove loosely adherent deposits and debris, including microorganisms. They act to break up the deposits through the formation of micelles. Most cleaners contain nonionic or ionic detergents, wetting agents, chelating agents, buffers, and preservatives.

Indications:

Similar to GP lens solutions. These solutions help to maintain a clean, wettable surface with good optics. They are typically recommended for use after lens removal.

Warnings:

Same as GP lens solutions.

otc	**Lens Plus Daily Cleaner** (Advanced Medical Optics)	**Solution:** Surface-active, buffered. Cocoamphocarboxyglycinate, sodium lauryl sulfate, hexylene glycol, NaCl, sodium phosphate	Preservative free. In 15 mL.
otc	**MiraFlow Extra-Strength Daily Cleaner** (Ciba Vision)	**Solution:** 15.7% isopropyl alcohol, poloxamer 407, amphoteric 10.	Preservative free. Thimerosal free. In 12 and 20 mL.
otc	**Opti-Clean II Daily Cleaner Especially for Sensitive Eyes** (Alcon)	**Solution:** Buffered, isotonic. 0.1% EDTA, 0.001% polyquad. Polysorbate 21, polymeric cleaning agents.	Thimerosal free. In 20 mL.
otc	**Opti-Free Daily Cleaner** (Alcon)	**Solution:** Buffered, isotonic. 0.1% EDTA, 0.001% polyquad. Polysorbate 21, polymeric cleaning agents.	In 12 and 20 mL.
otc	**Opti-Free Supra Clens Daily Protein Remover** (Alcon)	**Solution:** Propylene glycol, sodium borate, highly purified porcine pancreatin enzymes.	Preservative free. In 3 mL.
otc	**Pliagel Cleaning Solution** (Alcon)	**Solution:** 0.5% EDTA, 0.25% sorbic acid. Poloxamer 407, potassium chloride, NaCl.	Thimerosal free. In 25 mL.
otc	**Sensitive Eyes Daily Cleaner Solution** (Bausch & Lomb)	**Solution:** Buffered, isotonic. 0.5% EDTA, 0.25% sorbic acid. Hydroxypropyl methylcellulose, poloxamine, sodium borate, NaCl.	In 20 mL.

otc	**Sereine Extra-Strength Daily Cleaner** (Optikem, Inc.)	**Solution:** Amphoteric surfactant, poloxamer 407, isopropyl alcohol.	In 1 oz.
otc	**SOF/PRO-CLEAN (Lobob) Sterile Extra Strength Cleaner** (Lobob)	**Solution:** Sorbic acid 0.1%, edetate trisodium 0.25.	In 60 mL.

ENZYMATIC CLEANERS/DAILY PROTEIN REMOVERS, SOFT LENSES

Actions:

Pharmacology: Similar to GP lens solutions. As subtilisin is not deactivated quickly in hydrogen peroxide, it has been incorporated in several systems for use during hydrogen peroxide disinfection, decreasing the number of steps necessary for care and potentially increasing patient compliance. Likewise, commonly used chemical disinfection solutions (eg, *ReNu One-Step*) combine enzymatic cleaning with disinfection. Several daily protein removers are available that use either an enzyme or a surfactant to remove adherent mucoprotein complexes. Several systems have been discontinued in the past year due to the increasing popularity of disposable lenses.

Indications:

Similar to GP lens solutions. It has been estimated that 80% of all clinical complications related to contact lens wear may be attributed to deposits, most often protein deposits. Enzymatic cleaners are most effective against bound tear protein, notably lysozyme. The level of protein deposition on a hydrogel lens surface appears to be directly related to the water content and the ionic nature of the lens.

Warnings:

Same as GP lens solutions.

otc	**Complete MoisturePlus Weekly Enzymatic Cleaner** (American Medical Optics)	**Tablets:** Subtilisin A. Effervescing, buffering, and tableting agents. *To make solution for soaking, dilute in MoisturePlus.*	In 8s.
otc	**Opti-Free Supra Clens Daily Protein Remover** (Alcon)	**Solution:** Propylene glycol, sodium borate, highly purified porcine pancreatin enzymes.	Preservative free. In 5 mL.
otc	**Opti-Free Enzymatic Cleaner** (Alcon)	Highly purified pork pancreatin.	In 18s.
otc	**Opti-Zyme Enzymatic Cleaner Especially for Sensitive Eyes** (Alcon)	**Tablets:** Highly purified pork pancreatin. *To make solution for soaking, dilute in preserved saline or sterile unpreserved saline solution.*	Preservative free. In 24s.
otc	**ReNu 1 Step Daily Liquid Protein Remover** (Bausch & Lomb)	**Liquid:** Proteolytic enzyme (subtilisin) glycerin and borate buffer.	In 7.5 mL.
otc	**Sensitive Eyes Enzymatic Cleaner** (Bausch & Lomb)	**Tablets:** Subtilisin, polyethylene glycol, sodium carbonate, NaCl, tartaric acid. *For use with all disinfection regimens.*	In 8s, 16s, and 40s.

otc	**Ultrazyme Enzymatic Cleaner** (American Medical Optics)	**Tablets:** Subtilisin A. Effervescing, buffering, and tableting agents. *To make solution for soaking, dilute in 3% hydrogen peroxide disinfecting solution.*	In 5s, 10s, and 20s.
otc	**Unizyme Enzymatic Cleaner** (Ciba Vision)	**Tablets:** Subtilisin A. Potassium carbonate, citric acid, polyethylene glycol, sodium benzoate. *For use with all Ciba Vision disinfection systems.*	In 12s.

DISINFECTING/WETTING/SOAKING SOLUTIONS, SOFT LENSES

otc	**ReNu MultiPlus Multi-Purpose Solution** (Bausch & Lomb)	**Solution:** Isotonic. 0.0001% polyaminopropyl biguanide. Hydroxyalkylphosphonate, boric acid, EDTA, poloxamine, sodium borate, NaCl.	Thimerosal free. In 60, 118, 237, and 355 mL.

REWETTING SOLUTIONS, SOFT LENSES

Actions:

Pharmacology: Similar to GP lens solutions. Typically, these products contain a low concentration of a nonionic surfactant to promote cleaning, a polymer to lubricate the lens, buffering agents, and preservatives.

Indications:

Similar to GP lenses with the additional benefit of rehydrating the lens for additional comfort and increased wearing time.

Warnings:

None.

otc	**Aquify Long Lasting Comfort Drops** (Ciba Vision)	**Solution:** Sodium perborate stabilized with perborate acid.	In 10 mL.
otc	**blink Contacts Lubricant Eye Drops** (Advanced Medical Optics)	**Solution:** Buffered, isotonic with sodium hyaluronate, sodium chloride, potassium chloride, calcium chloride, magnesium chloride, boric acid, and *OcuPure* (stabilized oxychloro complex) 0.005% as the preservative.	In 10 mL.
otc	**Clerz Plus Lens Drops** (Alcon)	**Solution:** Buffered, isotonic. With citrate/borate buffer, edetate disodium and polyquad as preservatives, and RLM 10 (PEG-11 laurel ether carboxylic acid) and tectronic 1304.	In 15 mL.
otc	**Complete Blink-N-Clean Lens Drops** (Advanced Medical Optics)	**Solution:** Buffered, isotonic. 0.0001% polyhexamethylene biguanide, tromethamine, hydroxypropyl methylcellulose, tyloxapol, EDTA, sodium chloride.	Thimerosal free. In 20 mL.

otc	**Complete MoisturePlus Lubricating and Rewetting Drops** (Advanced Medical Optics)	**Solution:** Buffered, isotonic. 0.0001% polyhexamethylene biguanide. NaCl, tromethamine, hydroxypropyl methylcellulose, tyloxapol, EDTA.	Thimerosal free. In 15 mL.
otc	**Lens Plus Rewetting Drops** (Advanced Medical Optics)	**Solution:** Buffered, isotonic. NaCl, boric acid.	Preservative free. Thimerosal free. In 0.35 mL (30s).
otc	**Opti-Free Express Rewetting Drops** (Alcon)	**Solution:** Buffered, isotonic. 0.05% EDTA, 0.001% polyquad. Citrate buffer, NaCl.	In 10 and 20 mL.
otc	**Opti-Free RepleniSH Rewetting Drops** (Alcon)	**Solution:** Buffered, isotonic, aqueous solution with a citrate/borate buffer and sodium chloride, with edetate disodium 0.05% and *Polyquad* (polyquaternium-1) 0.001% as preservatives and RLM-100 (PEG-11 lauryl ether carboxylic acid) and *Tetronic* 1304.	In 10 mL.
otc	**Opti-One Rewetting Drops** (Alcon)	**Solution:** Buffered, isotonic aqueous solution with a citrate buffer, NaCl with 0.05% edetate disodium and 0.001% Polyquad (polyquaternium-1) as preservatives.	In 10 mL.
otc	**Refresh Contacts, Contact Lens Comfort Drops** (Allergan)	**Solution:** Buffered, isotonic. 0.005% purite. Carboxymethylcellulose sodium, sodium chloride, boric acid, potassium chloride, calcium chloride, magnesium chloride.	Thimerosal free. In 12 mL.
otc	**Refresh Contacts, Contact Lens Comfort Drops for Sensitive Eyes** (Allergan)	**Solution:** Buffered, isotonic. Carboxymethylcellulose sodium, calcium chloride, magnesium chloride, potassium chloride, sodium chloride, sodium lactate, hydrochloric acid, sodium hydroxide.	Preservative free. In 20 single-use containers.
otc	**ReNu Rewetting Drops** (Bausch & Lomb)	**Solution:** Isotonic. 0.15% sorbic acid, 0.1% EDTA. Boric acid, poloxamine, sodium borate, NaCl.	In 15 mL.
otc	**ReNu MultiPlus Lubricating & Rewetting Drops** (Bausch & Lomb)	**Solution:** Isotonic. 0.1% EDTA, 0.1% sorbic acid. Povidone, boric acid, potassium chloride, sodium borate, NaCl.	In 8 mL.
otc	**Sensitive Eyes Drops** (Bausch & Lomb)	**Solution:** Buffered. 0.1% sorbic acid, 0.025% EDTA. Boric acid, sodium borate, NaCl.	Thimerosal free. In 15 and 30 mL.
otc	**TheraTears Contact Lens Comfort Drops** (Advanced Vision Research)	**Solution:** Sodium carbo methyl cellulose (0.25%), sodium perborate as preservative.	In 15 mL.
otc	**Visine for Contacts** (Pfizer)	**Solution:** Isotonic with a borate buffer system. Hypromellose and glycerin, with potassium sorbate and edetate disodium as preservatives.	In 15 and 30 mL.
otc	**VIVA Comfort Drops** (Vision Pharmaceuticals)	**Solution:** Polysorbate 80 and sodium chloride, citric acid, edetate disodium, purified water, with retinyl palmitate, mannitol, sodium citrate and pyruvate as antioxidants.	Preservative free. In 15 mL.

Miscellaneous Products

Extraocular irrigating solutions, lid scrubs, and vitamins and minerals are adjuncts to a variety of ophthalmic procedures and conditions.

EXTRAOCULAR IRRIGATING SOLUTIONS

Extraocular irrigating solutions are sterile isotonic solutions for general ophthalmic use. Office uses include irrigating procedures following tonometry, gonioscopy, foreign body removal, or use of fluorescein. They are also used to cleanse the eye. Because these solutions have a short contact time with the eye, they do not need to provide nutrients to cells. Unlike intraocular irrigants, irrigants for extraocular use contain preservatives that prevent bacterial contamination. However, the preservatives are exceedingly toxic to the corneal endothelium, and intraocular use of extraocular irrigating fluids is contraindicated.

LID SCRUBS

The mainstay of therapy for blepharitis is careful eyelid hygiene. This is easily accomplished at home by the patient. Although baby shampoo is frequently used for this purpose, commercially available eyelid cleansers are available and are known to be effective with potentially less ocular stinging, burning, and toxicity. Commercial lid scrub products are designed to aid in the removal of oils, debris, or desquamated skin associated with the inflamed eyelid. The lid scrubs can also be used for hygienic eyelid cleansing in contact lens wearers. These products are designed to be used full strength on eyelid tissues but must not be instilled directly into the eyes. Some of the commercial products are packaged with presoaked pads, which provide an abrasive action to augment the cleansing properties of the detergent solution.

VITAMINS AND MINERALS

Deficiencies of vitamin A and zinc have sometimes been associated with certain adverse ocular effects. Beyond replacement of documented deficiencies, however, treatment or prevention of ophthalmic diseases using vitamins and minerals is not clearly established. Various investigators have explored the use of vitamins A, C, and E, as well as zinc or lutein, as preventative measures for degenerative ophthalmic conditions often associated with the aging process. The primary mechanisms of action offered to explain the effectiveness of such therapy include antioxidation and free radical scavenging. Several products are commercially available for the prevention or treatment of nonexudative macular degeneration and ocular surface disorders associated with dry eye, but more data will be required before the efficacy and safety of these products become well established.

For More Information

Age-related Eye Disease Study Research Group. A randomized, placebo-controlled, clinical trial of high-dose supplementation with vitamins C and E, beta carotene, and zinc for age-related macular degeneration and vision loss. *Arch Ophthalmol.* 2001;119:1417-1436.

Allison RW, et al. Reversal of mydriasis by dapiprazole. *Ann Ophthalmol.* 1990;92:131-138.

Arora S, Musadiq M, Mukherji S, et al. Eye nutrient products for age-related macular degeneration: what do they contain? *Eye.* 2004;18:470-473.

Bartlett H, Eperjesi F. Age-related macular degeneration and nutritional supplementation: a review of randomized controlled trials. *Ophthalmic Physiol Opt.* 2003;23:383-399.

Bartlett JD, Classe JG. Dapiprazole: Will it affect the standard of care for pupillary dilation? *Optom Clin.* 1992;2(3):65-75.

Doughty MJ, Lyle WM. A review of the clinical pharmacokinetics of pilocarpine, moxisylyte (thymoxamine), dapiprazole in the reversal of diagnostic pupillary dilation. *Optom Vis Sci.* 1992;69:358-368.

Mares JA, La Rowe TL, Blodi BA. Doctor, what vitamins should I take for my eyes? *Arch Ophthalmol.* 2004;122:628-635.

Polack FM, Goodman DF. Experience with a new detergent lid scrub in the management of chronic blepharitis. *Arch Ophthalmol.* 1988;106:719-720.

Richer S, Stiles W, Statkute L, et al. Double-masked, placebo-controlled, randomized trial of lutein and antioxidant supplementation in the intervention of atrophic age-related macular degeneration: the Veterans LAST study (lutein antioxidant supplementation trial). *Optometry.* 2004;75:216-230.

Semes L, Blaho K. Nutritional agents. In: Bartlett JD, Jaanus SD, eds. *Clinical Ocular Pharmacology.* 5th ed. St. Louis, MO: Elsevier; 2008.

Sperduto RD. Do we have a nutritional treatment for age-related cataract or macular degeneration? *Arch Ophthalmol.* 1990;108:1403-1405.

West AL, Oren GA, Moroi SE. Evidence for the use of nutritional supplements and herbal medicines in common eye diseases. *Am J Ophthalmol.* 2006;141:157-166.

EXTRAOCULAR IRRIGATING SOLUTIONS

Actions:

Pharmacology: These sterile isotonic solutions are for general ophthalmic use. Office uses include irrigating procedures following tonometry, gonioscopy, foreign body removal, or use of fluorescein; they are also used to cleanse the eye. Because these solutions have a short contact time with the eye, they do not need to provide nutrients to cells. Unlike intraocular irrigants, irrigants for extraocular use contain preservatives that prevent bacteriostatic contamination. However, the preservatives are exceedingly toxic to the corneal endothelium and intraocular use of extraocular irrigating fluids is contraindicated.

Indications:

Irrigation: For irrigating the eye to help relieve irritation by removing loose foreign material, air pollutants (eg, smog, pollen), or chlorinated water.

Contraindications:

Hypersensitivity to any component of the formulation; as a saline solution for rinsing and soaking contact lenses; injection or intraocular surgery.

Patient Information:

If you experience eye pain, changes in vision, continued redness or irritation of the eye, or if the condition worsens or persists, consult a doctor.

Obtain immediate medical treatment for all open wounds in or near the eyes.

If solution changes color or becomes cloudy, do not use.

Do not use these products with contact lenses.

To avoid contamination, do not touch tip of the container to any surface. Replace cap after using.

Administration and Dosage:

Solution: Flush the affected eye(s) as needed, controlling the rate of flow of solution by pressure on the bottle.

Eyecup: Fill the sterile eyecup halfway with eye wash. Apply the cup tightly to the affected eye and tilt the head backward. Open eyes wide, rotate eye, and blink several times to ensure that the solution completely floods the eye. Discard the wash. Rinse the cup with clean water and if necessary, repeat the procedure with the other eye.

Rinse the eyecup before and after every use. Avoid contamination of the rim or inside surfaces of the cup.

Storage/Stability: If solution changes color or becomes cloudy, do not use.

otc	**Collyrium for Fresh Eyes Wash** (Bausch & Lomb)	**Solution:** Boric acid, sodium borate, benzalkonium Cl	In 120 mL.
otc	**Eye Stream** (Alcon)	**Solution:** 0.64% NaCl, 0.075% KCl, 0.03% magnesium Cl hexahydrate, 0.048% calcium Cl dihydrate, 0.39% sodium acetate trihydrate, 0.17% sodium citrate dihydrate, 0.013% benzalkonium Cl	In 30 and 120 mL.
otc	**Eye Wash** (Bausch & Lomb)	**Solution:** Boric acid, KCl, EDTA, sodium carbonate, 0.01% benzalkonium Cl	In 118 mL.
otc	**Eye Wash** (Zenith-Goldline)	**Solution:** Boric acid, KCl, EDTA, anhydrous sodium carbonate, 0.01% benzalkonium Cl	In 118 mL.
otc	**Eye Wash** (Altaire)	**Solution:** Edetate disodium, potassium Cl, sodium Cl, sodium phosphate dibasic, sodium phosphate monobasic, benzalkonium Cl	In 118 mL.
otc	**Eye Irrigating Solution** (Rugby)	**Solution:** Sodium borate, NaCl, boric acid, sorbic acid, EDTA	In 118 mL.
otc	**OCuSOFT** (OCuSOFT)	**Solution:** Benzalkonium chloride, edetate disodium, NaCl, sodium phosphate dibasic, sodium phosphate monobasic	In 30 mL.

LID SCRUBS

Indications:

Eyelid cleansing: To aid in the removal of oils, debris, or desquamated skin.

Precautions:

For external use only: Do not instill directly into eye.

Administration and Dosage:

Close eye(s) and gently scrub eyelid(s) and lashes using lateral side-to-side strokes; rinse thoroughly.

otc	**Eye•Scrub** (Novartis)	**Solution:** PEG-200 hydrogenated glyceryl palmate, disodium laureth sulfosuccinate, cocoamidopropylamine oxide, PEG-80 glyceryl cocoate, benzyl alcohol, EDTA	In UD 30s (pads).
otc	**OCuSOFT** (OCuSOFT)	**Solution:** PEG-80, sorbitan laurate, sodium trideceth sulfate, PEG-150 distearate, cocoamidopropyl hydroxysultaine, lauroamphocarboxyglycinate, sodium laureth-13 carboxylate, PEG-15 tallow polyamine, quaternium-15	Alcohol and dye free. In UD 30s (pads) and compliance kit (120 mL and 100 pads).

VITAMINS AND MINERALS

Actions:

Pharmacology: Certain vitamin and mineral deficiencies, most notably vitamin A and zinc, have been associated with adverse ocular effects. Beyond replacement of documented deficiency, treatment or prevention of ophthalmic diseases with vitamins and minerals is not well established.

However, investigators are beginning to explore this area. There is some evidence that vitamins A, C, and E, with zinc or lutein may be preventative for nonexudative age-related macular degeneration. The principal mechanisms of action are offered as antioxidation and free radical scavenging.

Based on the published scientific evidence, more data are required before definitive recommendations can be made. However, products labeled with such claims are available.

Administration and Dosage:

Take with meals.

Adults: 1 to 2 tablets 1 or 2 times daily or as directed by a health care provider.

Storage/Stability: Store at room temperature 15° to 30°C (59° to 86°F) .

otc	**Vitamin A Palmitate** (Freeda)	**Tablets:** 10,000 IU	In 100s and 250s.
		15,000 IU	In 100s and 250s.
otc	**Beta Carotene** (Freeda)	**Tablets:** 10,000 IU	In 100s, 250s, and 500s.
otc	**Palmitate-A** (Akorn)	**Tablets:** 15,000 IU vitamin A palmitate	In 100s.
otc	**Palmitate-A 5000** (Akorn)	**Tablets:** 5,000 IU vitamin A palmitate	In 100s.
otc	**Icaps Plus** (Alcon)	**Tablets:** 6,000 IU vitamin A[1], 200 mg C, 20 mg B_2, 60 IU E, 40 mg Zn[2], 2 mg Cu, 5 mg Mn, 20 mcg Se	In 60s and 120s.
otc	**Icaps Time Release** (Alcon)	**Tablets:** 7,000 IU vitamin A[1], 200 mg C, 20 mg B_2, 100 IU E, 40 mg Zn[2], 2 mg Cu, 20 mcg Se	In 60s and 120s.
otc	**AntiOxidants** (Akorn)	**Caplets:** 5,000 IU vitamin A[1], 400 mg C[3], 200 IU E[4], 40 mg Zn[5], 5 mg L-glutathione, 3 mg sodium pyruvate, 2 mg Cu[6], 40 mcg Se[7]	In 60s.
otc	**Oxi-Freeda** (Freeda)	**Tablets:** 5,000 IU beta carotene, 150 IU E, 20 mg B_1, 20 mg B_2, 20 mg B_6, 10 mcg B_{12}, 15 mg elemental Zn, 50 mcg Se, 20 mg calcium pantothenate, 40 mg glutathione, 40 mg B_3, 100 mg C, 75 mg L-cysteine	In 100s and 250s.
otc	**OCuSoft VMS** (OCu-SOFT)	**Tablets:** 5,000 IU vitamin A, 30 IU E, 60 mg C, 40 mg Zn, 2 mg Cu, 40 mcg Se	Film coated. In 60s.

otc	**Ocuvite** (Bausch & Lomb)	**Tablets:** 40 mg elemental $Zn^{8,}$ 2 mg elemental $Cu^{9,}$ 40 mcg elemental $Se^{10,}$ 5,000 IU vitamin $A^{1,}$ 30 IU $E^{4,}$ 60 mg C^{3}	In 60s and 120s.
otc	**Ocuvite Extra** (Bausch & Lomb)	**Tablets:** 40 mg elemental $Zn^{8,}$ 2 mg elemental $Cu^{9,}$ 200 mg C, 50 IU E, 6,000 IU vitamin $A^{1,}$ 40 mcg elemental Se, 3 mg B_2, 40 mg B_3, 5 mg elemental Mn, 5 mg L-glutathione	In 50s.
otc	**Ocuvite PreserVision** (Bausch & Lomb)	**Tablets:** 7,160 IU vitamin $A^{1,}$ 100 mg E, 113 mg C, 17.4 mg Zn, 0.4 mg Cu, lactose	In 120s.

[1] As beta carotene.
[2] As zinc acetate.
[3] As ascorbic acid.
[4] As dl-alpha tocopheryl acetate.
[5] As zinc ascorbate.
[6] As copper ascorbate.
[7] As L-selenomethionine.
[8] As zinc oxide.
[9] As cupric oxide.
[10] As sodium selenate.

Extemporaneous Preparations

Extemporaneous compounding of ophthalmic solutions may include the preparation of topical, periocular, or intraocular injections. Many topical ophthalmic solutions or suspensions are commercially available. However, certain topical ophthalmic solutions and most periocular and intraocular solutions are neither FDA-approved nor commercially available for ophthalmic administration. When these preparations are required, injectable sources are frequently used. In many cases, this may be limited to dilution of injectable products or the addition of injectable products to commercial ophthalmic preparations to increase their concentration or "fortify" them. These extemporaneously prepared products are considered the community standard based on clinical research and ethical practice, and, as such, may be required to effectively treat a patient with ophthalmic conditions. Considerations for ophthalmic compounding must include topical (usually topical solutions), periocular (subconjunctival or sub-Tenon's; retrobulbar), or intraocular (intravitreal or intracameral) products.

GUIDELINES

Requirements for the preparation of topical ophthalmic preparations are published in the United States Pharmacopoeia (USP). The USP guidelines describe the requirements for the preparation of ophthalmic ointments, solutions, suspensions, and strips. Isotonicity, buffering, sterilization, preservation, and thickening agents are specifically addressed.

Because of concerns for possible eye infections, guidelines for the preparation of all sterile ophthalmic products were published by the American Society of Health-Systems Pharmacists (ASHP). These guidelines state that all extemporaneous ophthalmic products be prepared in an approved and certified laminar airflow or biohazard hood. Proper aseptic technique is essential, as is required for any sterile product. Accuracy is stressed to prevent any miscalculation, which is especially a concern with preparation of intravitreal injections. The use of a 5 micron filter is recommended when a drug is reconstituted or if it is supplied in a glass ampule. When a drug product is not available in a sterile dosage form, use a 0.22 micron filter. The use of a preservative-free product is recommended when feasible. These guidelines are particularly helpful for health care personnel who are not familiar with preparing ophthalmic extemporaneous products. Information on more than 50 ophthalmic medications including topical, subconjunctival, and intraocular formulations, is available in a "cookbook" format by Reynolds. The uses, concentrations, dosing, and references also are included.

References found in the literature for the ocular administration of noncommercial ophthalmic products (eg, acetylcysteine, ceftazidime, disodium EDTA) only provide some assurance that the medication is tolerated in the eye without obvious ocular side effects. Most of these references do not state which vehicles were used, expirations, or other essential information required to properly prepare the product.

STABILITY

Stability data must be based upon concerns for maintaining sterility rather than just the stability of the product itself. Obviously, if sterility cannot be maintained, then stability of the product is secondary. Little published information is available on stability dating of extemporaneously prepared topical ophthalmic solutions. Many institutions have extrapolated from published IV product stability, although this may not always be appropriate. Gentamicin- and tobramycin-fortified ophthalmic solutions are stable at 4° to 8°C for 3 months. The stability of several antibiotics, including vancomycin, gentamicin, bacitracin, and cephalothin, in commercially available 0.5% hydroxypropyl methylcellulose artificial tear solution, demonstrated no significant loss of potency at room temperature for 7 days. However, the use of different vehicles, antibiotic concentrations, storage conditions, and other factors may influence product stability. Frozen and refrigerated stability data may be useful if multiple bottles are prepared. Stability must be established if the product is dispensed for outpatient use or used in a hospital setting. Refrigerate extemporaneously prepared ophthalmic solutions after dispensing to reduce the risk of microbial growth or to ensure minimal loss of potency. A 7-day in-use storage life is acceptable for unpreserved eye drops containing alkaloids or antibiotics if they are stored in the refrigerator after opening.

The stability of periocular or intraocular preparations is usually restricted to 6- to 24-hour expirations because information is limited and these expiration times are commonly used for other extemporaneously prepared injectable products.

Stability and sterility appear to be maintained with some preparations that are aseptically prepared, sealed, and frozen. Frozen stability of products such as periocular mitomycin, intraocular ganciclovir, and topical cefazolin and vancomycin has provided extended dating for these products.

STERILITY

Sterility must be maintained with any extemporaneously prepared ophthalmic product. The USP and ASHP recommend that sterile membrane filtration (0.22 micron filter) be used under aseptic conditions whenever possible. Many institutions prepare extemporaneous ophthalmic products and employ a 0.22 micron filter for the final step to ensure sterilization. Some medications should not be filtered with a 0.22 micron filter. Amphotericin B, a colloidal suspension, should be filtered with nothing smaller than a 5 micron filter to prevent loss of drug. Suspensions and other formulations such as liposomal products should be researched to determine if membrane filtration is acceptable.

PH/BUFFERING

The pH of an extemporaneously prepared topical ophthalmic product is most often considered because of the concern for ocular irritation associated with eyedrops. The eye can tolerate a rather wide range of pH (between 3.5 and 10) for a single drop administration. If the pH is too high or too low, reflex tearing will dilute the drug concentration more quickly than if the pH is in the physiologic range of 7.4 for lacrimal fluid. Some medications require lower pH values to maintain longer shelf lives because they may be chemically unstable at higher pH levels. Buffering systems are not commonly employed in the current practice of preparing extemporaneous ophthalmic preparations. It is important that if a buffer system is used, it is close to pH 7.4, but does not hasten deterioration or precipitation of the drug.

The pH of the eyedrop may influence absorption of a drug into the intraocular fluids and tissues. Generally, the unionized form of a drug will penetrate the lipophilic corneal epithelium, the first significant barrier to intraocular penetration, better than a hydrophilic form will. The cornea contains tight epithelial and endothelial cell junctions that slow or prevent the passage of a drug through the cornea. A drug must penetrate the 3 layers of the cornea, including the epithelium (lipophilic barrier), stroma (water soluble), and endothelium (lipid soluble). Increasing the pH of a solution increases the amount of the unionized form, thereby increasing initial epithelial penetration of the drug.

ISOTONICITY

Isotonicity is not essential even for topical ophthalmic solutions. An acceptable range is from 0.7% to 2% (0.9% sodium chloride is considered isotonic). In fact, some ophthalmic products are produced as hypertonic (sodium chloride 5%) or hypotonic (*Hypotears*) solutions for their desired pharmacologic effects.

VEHICLES

Vehicles used for topical ophthalmic solutions vary and are usually either normal saline, water, various biocompatible polymers used in artificial tears, or, occasionally, balanced salt solution. Artificial tear polymer may provide comfort, prolonged contact time with the eye, the presence of a preservative system, and a neutral pH. However, potential problems include incompatibilities between the active or inactive ingredients and a reduction in preservative effectiveness due to dilution from the active drug. Some artificial tear preparations contain methylcellulose, which is an acceptable thickening agent to increase the viscosity and contact time of the ophthalmic solution. Sterile water or normal saline is often used, but they contain no preservatives. Consider the concern for potential contamination associated with the repeated administration of unpreserved solutions. If the active component has an initial low pH, the lower pH of water and normal saline may further contribute to irritation of the ophthalmic solution. Balanced salt solutions (BSS) contain no preservatives, and consider potential incompatibilities with the various components of the BSS.

Intraocular or periocular preparations most often use sterile water or normal saline as the preferred diluent. Use caution if balanced salt solutions are employed as vehicles because potential incompatibilities, especially with magnesium and calcium salts, may exist with the active ingredient or its inactive components. Do not use balanced salt solution as a diluent for cromolyn sodium or tissue plasminogen activator.

TOPICAL PREPARATIONS

Topical forms of administration include drops, ointments, gels, contact lenses, and collagen shields. The most common extemporaneously prepared product is the topical ophthalmic solution. Topical formulations deliver the drug to the site of action, which reduce the risk of systemic side effects, but do not totally alleviate them.

Extemporaneously prepared topical eye solutions are used most often in the treatment of bacterial keratitis. Until the approval of the fluoroquinolone antibiotics ciprofloxacin and ofloxacin for bacterial keratitis, standard regimens consisted of alternating an aminoglycoside (usually gentamicin- or tobramycin-fortified solutions) with a cephalosporin, most often cefazolin. Some of the most common concentrations of antibiotic drops are gentamicin 13.6 mg/mL, tobramycin 13.6 mg/mL, cefazolin 50 mg/mL, and vancomycin 10 mg/mL.

The aminoglycoside products (usually gentamicin or tobramycin) are fortified to a concentration of 9 to 14 mg/mL from the commercially available strength of 3 mg/mL. An injectable form of the active drug is added under aseptic conditions in a lamellar flow hood to an ophthalmic dropper bottle to "fortify" the commercial strength. Cefazolin ophthalmic solution 25 to 100 mg/mL is made from the injectable product and is reconstituted in water and further diluted in water, normal saline, or artificial tear solution.

Polyhexamethylene biguanide (PHMB 20%) is an environmental biocide for swimming pools. PHMB 0.02% (0.2 mg/mL) is useful in *Acanthamoeba* keratitis as an extemporaneously prepared topical ophthalmic product. Because the initial concentration is 20%, an intermediate dilution is suggested to ensure an accurate final concentration of 0.02% because this is a 1,000-fold difference. Chlorhexidine digluconate is also used in the same concentration of 0.02% as an alternative to PHMB.

Ophthalmic ointments usually consist of a petrolatum and mineral oil base (added to reduce the temperature at which the ointment melts). Some ointments contain lanolin (emulsifier to incorporate water-soluble drugs into the ointment). Allergies to ophthalmic ointments are most often related to the incorporated lanolin. Most drugs are very stable in ointments and do not ionize. Ophthalmic ointments provide longer ocular contact time and comfort. However, contact time may not increase bioavailability because only the drug at the ointment-tear interface will be absorbed. Ointments also are associated with blurred vision and provide poor patient acceptance. Although ointments occasionally are prepared extemporaneously, this is uncommon because of the time required to prepare them, the rare instances of a clinical indication, and the special ophthalmic ointment tubes required.

Antibiotic-soaked collagen shields provide for prolonged topical drug levels. However, potential drug incompatibility problems, loss of the shield from the eye, requirements for rehydration with the antibiotic, and cost have limited their use.

Mitomycin

Mitomycin C is an antitumor antibiotic that is used as an alkylating agent by inhibiting DNA synthesis. Mitomycin C has been used in glaucoma filtering procedures and in the prevention of pterygium recurrence, and some limited use as an adjunctive therapy for the prevention of haze following some refractive surgery procedures. It is believed to act by inhibiting fibroblast activity and thereby prevent the development of fibrosis and slow or prevent wound healing that occurs after glaucoma filtration surgery and after pterygia removal. In contrast to 5-fluorouracil, mitomycin C produces a much more aggressive inhibition of fibroblast activity. Mitomycin C is applied directly to the scleral bed in trabeculectomy and pterygium during the procedures. Doses in the range of 0.2 to 0.4 mg/mL of mitomycin C are applied to the sclera for 2 to 5 minutes and then thoroughly irrigated. A recent study suggested that a subconjunctival dose 1 month prior to pterygium excision reduced fibroblast activity and minimized epithelial toxicity. Topical use of mitomycin C after pterygia removal is not recommended because of the potential for severe ocular complications including corneal edema and perforation, glaucoma, cataract formation, and scleral melts.

PERIOCULAR

Periocular administration includes injections below the conjunctiva or Tenon's capsule. They are given either to prolong administration or to increase penetration of the drug into the eye. Advantages include increased local concentration of the drug, thereby avoiding potential systemic toxicity, and higher intraocular tissue concentrations. Because no FDA-approved formulations are available for periocular administration, injectable preparations are often used. In many cases, the concentration required is drawn directly from a commercial-strength vial. An example of this is gentamicin, which is given in a safe subconjunctival dose of 20 mg/0.5 mL. Direct use from the vial, or sometimes after a single dilution, is often employed with antibiotics, anesthetics, and corticosteroid preparations for use as subconjunctival or sub-Tenon's injections. A common peribulbar or retrobulbar anesthetic combination uses a 50:50 mixture of lidocaine and bupivacaine.

INTRAOCULAR

Intraocular injections are often used in serious eye infections and inflammatory conditions such as endophthalmitis, retinal necrosis, and cytomegalovirus retinitis. Recently, intravitreal steroids such as triamcinolone have been used to treat retinal inflammatory events, including cystoid macular edema and diabetic macular edema, and they have been used in patients with choroidal neovascularization associated with age-related macular degeneration. Intraocular injections provide immediate therapeutic drug levels. It is essential to ensure that the correct dose is prepared to prevent retinal toxicity. The half-life of the drug in the vitreous cavity is a consideration, especially if reinjection may be required. The volume of drug administered is usually in the 0.05 to 0.1 mL range. Proper injection technique is critical to prevent damage to any intraocular structures. Commonly used intraocular medications include vancomycin, ceftazidime, amikacin, ganciclovir, foscarnet, dexamethasone, amphotericin B, and triamcinolone acetonide.

Intraocular doses are often in the microgram to milligram range. The proper dose must be established before the medication is prepared. In some instances, multiple dilutions are required to obtain an accurate concentration for intravitreal injection. Amphotericin B is administered as a 5 mcg injection and must be prepared from a commercial vial of 50 mg. Amikacin is administered in a 400 mcg dose or less and must be diluted from a 500 or 100 mg (pediatric) vial. Vancomycin is injected intravitreally in a dose of 1 mg after being diluted from a vial containing 500 mg. These concentrations may reflect a 10- or even 1,000-fold dilution from the commercial-strength product. Careful calculation and validation from others is appropriate. Syringes must be able to measure low concentrations precisely. An adequate initial volume must be drawn up so that a reasonable volume can be transferred for further dilution. To ensure no loss of drug in the needle hub of a tuberculin syringe, it is more accurate to deliver 0.3 mL from the 0.6 to 0.3 mL gradations on the syringe barrel than from the 0.3 mark to zero. To prevent any miscalculation, no air bubbles should be left in the syringe or needle when preparing the injection. It is prudent to add both drug and diluent to a single sterile vial to prevent any miscalculation in volume. A larger volume of the final concentration of drug should be dispensed (eg, draw up 0.4 mL of a 1 mg/0.1 mL vancomycin) and labeled appropriately. The larger volume will allow for easy transfer of the final concentration of drug to another syringe, should this be required. Please refer to the compounding guidelines issued by the United States Pharmacopoeia in 2004.

OCULAR DOSAGE FORM *Drug Class*	Commercial Strength	Ophthalmic Strength	Dilution Directions	Special Instructions	Comments
TOPICAL					
Antibiotics					
Gentamicin (or Tobramycin)	40 mg/mL (injection) and 3 mg/mL (ophth soln)	9 to 14 mg/mL	Add 2 mL of injectable to 5 mL bottle (7 mL or 13.6 mg/mL)		Use same bottle eyedrops came in
Cefazolin	1 gram (vial-recon)	25 to 100 mg/mL as eye drop	Recon vial with 3 mL water, qs to 10 mL with water - transfer to ophthalmic bottle	Artificial tear used to qs	Frozen stability appears to be good for ≥ 28 days - concerns are to ensure sterility when frozen
Vancomycin	500 mg (vial-recon)	25 mg/mL	Recon with 10 mL sterile water (50 mg/mL), transfer to ophthalmic bottle and shake. Transfer 5 mL to an ophthalmic dropper bottle and add 5 mL of sterile water		Frozen stability good for 28 days Must ensure sterility when frozen Unbuffered pH is in 4 to 4.5 range
Antifungals					
Amphotericin B	50 mg/mL (injection)	1 to 5 mg/mL	Add 10 mL of sterile water to 50 mg bottle (further dilute with sterile water for lower concentration)	Do not dilute with saline or BSS. Must use sterile water or dextrose. Product is colloidal dispersion. Do not filter with less than 5 micron filter	Refrigeration required. Refrigerated stability for 7 days, but no preservative; may require 24 hour expiration
Other					
PHMB	20% solution	0.02% (some have used 0.04% or 0.06% also)	Dilution with sterile water is best	First dilute an intermediate solution of *0.5% PHMB*, then further dilute to 0.02% with sterile water	Stability is very good (30 days) Intermediate dilution is more accurate
Chlorhexidine	20% solution	0.02%	Dilution with sterile water is best	First dilute with an intermediate solution of 0.5%, then further dilute to 0.02%	Stability is very good (30 days) Intermediate dilution is more accurate with sterile water
PERIOCULAR					
Antibiotics					
Gentamicin	40 mg/mL vial	20 mg per 0.5 mL	No dilution required		
Cefazolin	1 g vial (recon)	100 mg per 0.5 mL	Recon with sterile water		
Corticosteroids					
Dexamethasone	4 mg/mL or 10 mg/mL	2 mg per 0.5 mL 5 mg per 0.5 mL	No dilution required	Given sub-conjunctivally	Short half life - 24 to 48 hours

OCULAR DOSAGE FORM *Drug Class*	Commercial Strength	Ophthalmic Strength	Dilution Directions	Special Instructions	Comments
Triamcinolone acetonide	40 mg/mL	20 mg per 0.5 mL	No dilution required	Given sub-Tenon's	Long half life - may last weeks to months
Antimetabolites					
Mitomycin	5 mg vial (recon)	0.2-0.4 mg/mL	Dilute with sterile water	Solution soaked into sponge	Frozen stability in 0.2 to 0.4 mg range is good for 60 days[9]
INTRAOCULAR					
Antibiotics					
Vancomycin	500 mg (recon)	1 mg per 0.05 to 0.1 mL	Recon with 10 mL normal saline	Take 2 mL of reconstituted solution add sterile vial; add 8 mL of sterile water (final conc. = 1 mg/0.1 mL)	Double check dilution; filter
Amikacin	100 mg/2 mL vial	400 mcg per 0.05 to 0.1 mL	Dilute with sterile normal saline (NS)	Take 1 mL of amikacin, add 11.5 mL saline in vial (final conc. = 400 mcg/0.1 mL)	Double check dilution
Cefazolin	500 mg vial	1 to 2.5 mg per 0.1 mL	Dilute 500 mg with 2 mL of sterile water. Concentration is 225 mg/mL. Must be further diluted.	Take 1 mL of solution and dilute with 9 cc of sterile saline to approximately 2.5 mg/0.1 mL.	For intracameral use
Ceftazidime	1 > vial (recon)	2 mg per 0.05 to 0.1 mL	Dilute with sterile water	Add 9.4 mL of water to > 1 ceftazidime vial. Transfer 2 mL of solution to vial, add 8 mL of NS (final conc. = 2 mg/0.1 mL)	Double check dilution
Cefuroxime sodium	750 mg or 1.5 g vial	1 mg per 0.1 mL	Dilute with sterile water 8 mL or 16 mL, respectively	Add 3.3 mL of sterile normal saline to 0.5 mL	For intracameral use
Antivirals					
Ganciclovir	500 mg vial (recon)	200 to 2,000 mcg per 0.05 to 0.1 mL	Dilute with sterile water	Recon with 2.5 mL NS; transfer 0.1 mL to sterile vial, add 9.9 mL NS *(final conc. = 200 mcg/0.1 mL)* or transfer 1 mL and add 9 mL NS *(final conc. = 2,000 mcg/0.1 mL)*	Refrigerate for storage
Foscarnet	Solution 24 mg/mL	1,200 to 2,400 mcg per 0.05 to 0.1 mL	Use directly from vial		
Others					
Bevacizumab (*Avastin*)	100 or 400 mg preservative free 4 and 16 mL vials (25 mg/mL)	1.25 mg per 0.05 mL	Use directly from vial		Refrigerated stability for at least 14 days

OCULAR DOSAGE FORM *Drug Class*	Commercial Strength	Ophthalmic Strength	Dilution Directions	Special Instructions	Comments
Tissue plasminogen activator (tPA) (alteplase)	20 mg vial	6.25 to 25 mcg per 0.1 mL	Dilute 20 mg vial with 20 mL sterile water as per directions; further dilute 1 mL of above with 3 mL of NS (250 mcg/mL)		Frozen stability good for ≥ 1 year
Voriconazole (*Vfend*)	200 mg vial preservative free	100 mcg per 0.1mL	Dilute vial with 19 mL of water for injection (10 mg/mL). Take 1 mL and add 9 mL of saline so final concentration (100 mcg/0.1 mL)		Single use non-preserved vial

For More Information

Bakri SJ, Snyder MR, Pulido JS, et al. Six-month stability of bevacizumab (*Avastin*) binding to vascular endothelial growth factor after withdrawal into a syringe and refrigeration or freezing. *Retina.* 2006;26:519-522.

Chen CW, Huang HT, Bair JS, Lee CC. Trabeculectomy with simultaneous topical application of mitomycin-C in refractory glaucoma. *J Ocul Pharmacol.* 1990;6:175-182.

Donnenfeld ED, Perry HD, Fromer S, et al. Subconjunctival mitomycin C as adjunctive therapy before pterygium excision. *Ophthalmology.* 2003;110:1012-1016.

Fiscella RG, Proffitt DF, Weisbecker CA. Stability of mitomycin for ophthalmic use. *Am J Hosp Pharm.* 1992;49:2440.

Fiscella RG, Aramwit P. Ganciclovir for intravitreal injection. *Am J Health-Syst Pharm.* 1995;52:422.

Frucht-Pery J, Ilsar M. The use of low-dose mitomycin C for prevention of recurrent pterygium. *Ophthalmology.* 1994;101:759-762.

Glasser DB, Baum J. In: *Antibacterial Agents in Infections of the Eye.* 2nd ed. Tabbara KF, Hyndiuk RA, eds. Boston MA: Little, Brown and Company; 1996:207-31.

Kramer M, Kramer MR, Blau H, et al. Intravitreal voriconazole for the treatment of endogenous *Aspergillus* endophthalmitis. *Ophthalmology.* 2006;113:1184-1186.

Liesegang TJ. Bacterial keratitis. *Infec Dis Clin NA.* 1992;6:815-830.

Mathers W. *Archives of Ophthalmol.* 2006;124:923.

McBride HA, Martinez DR, Trang JM, Lander RD, Helms HA. Stability of gentamicin sulfate and tobramycin sulfate in extemporaneously prepared ophthalmic solutions at 8 degrees C. *Am J Hosp Pharm.* 1991;48:507-509.

Muller LT, Candal EM, Epstein RJ, et al. Transepithelial phototherapeutic keratectomy/photorefractive keratectomy with adjunctive mitomycin-C for complicated LASIK flaps. *J Cataract Refract Surg.* 2005;31:291-296.

O'Brien TP, Maguire MG, Fink NE, Alfonso E, McDonnell P. Efficacy of ofloxacin vs cefazolin and tobramycin in the therapy for bacterial keratitis. Report from the Bacterial Keratitis Study Research Group.*Arch Ophthalmol.* 1995;113:1257-1265.

Oldham GB, Andrews V. The control of microbial contamination in unpreserved eye drops. *Br J Ophthalmol.* 1996;80:583-584.

Osborn E, Baum JL, Ernst C, Koch P. The stability of ten antibiotics in artificial tear solutions. *Am J Ophthalmol.* 1976;82:775-780.

Parks DJ, Abrams DA, Sarfarazi FA, Katz HR. Comparison of topical ciprofloxacin to conventional antibiotic therapy in the treatment of ulcerative keratitis. *Am J Ophthalmol.* 1993;115:471-477.

Reynolds LA. Guidelines for the preparation of sterile ophthalmic products. *Am J Hosp Pharm.* 1991;48:2438-2439.

Reynolds LA, Closson RG, eds. *Extemporaneous Ophthalmic Preparations.* Vancouver, Canada: Applied Therapeutics, Inc.; 1993.

Rubinfeld RS, Pfister R, Stein RM, et al. Serious complications of topical mitomycin-C after pterygium surgery. *Ophthalmology.* 1992;99:1647-1654.

Trissel LA. *Handbook on Injectable Drugs,* 8th ed. Bethesda, MD: American Society of Hospital Pharmacists; 1994.

The United States Pharmacopoeia 27 — National Formulary 22 (USP-NF). Chapter 797: Pharmaceutical Compounding. 2004.

Ward C, Weck S. Dilution and storage of recombinant tissue plasminogen activator (*Activase*) in balanced salt solutions. *Am J Ophthalmol.* 1990;109:98-99.

Yee E, Fiscella R, Winarko TK. Topical polyhexamethylene biguanide (pool cleaner) for treatment of *Ananthamoeba* keratitis. *Am J Hosp Pharm.* 1993;50:2522-2523.

Systemic Drugs Affecting the Eye

The eye is highly susceptible to toxic substances because of its rich blood supply, multiple tissue types, and relatively small size. Many systemically administered drugs have the potential to cause adverse ocular effects, and nearly all ocular structures are vulnerable. This section considers the most common drugs that are documented to cause ocular toxicities and summarizes the salient features of those effects.

DRUGS AFFECTING THE CORNEA AND LENS

Antimalarial Drugs

Quinacrine and hydroxychloroquine can cause changes in the cornea. In the early stages, diffuse punctate deposits appear in the corneal epithelium; later, the deposits aggregate into curved lines that converge and coalesce just below the central cornea. These opacities take on a whorl-like configuration. Less than half of patients affected by corneal changes have visual symptoms consisting of halos around lights, glare, and photophobia. Visual acuity usually remains unchanged. Once drug therapy is discontinued, both subjective symptoms and objective corneal signs disappear.

Chlorpromazine

Chlorpromazine is the only phenothiazine that causes changes in the cornea and lens. Lenticular pigmentation can vary from fine, dot-like opacities on the anterior lens surface to a central, lightly pigmented, pearl-like, opaque mass surrounded by smaller clumps of pigment. Corneal pigmentary changes almost invariably occur only in patients who have concomitant lens opacities. Corneal pigmentation occurs at the level of the endothelium and Descemet's membrane, primarily in the interpalpebral fissure area. These ocular changes rarely reduce visual acuity, but patients may occasionally report glare, halos around lights, or hazy vision. The pigmentary deposits are generally irreversible even when drug therapy is reduced or discontinued.

Systemic Drugs Affecting The Eye

Systemic drug	Examples	Structure/Function affected
Alcohol	alcohol	Extraocular muscles
Amiodarone	*Cordarone*	Cornea and lens
Antianxiety agents	chlordiazepoxide (eg, *Librium*)	Extraocular muscles Causes cycloplegia
Anticholinergics	atropine, scopolamine	Tear secretion Pupil (mydriasis) Causes cycloplegia
Antidepressants	amitriptyline (eg, *Elavil*)	Extraocular muscles Causes cycloplegia
Antihistamines	chlorpheniramine (eg, *Chlor-Trimeton*) diphenhydramine (eg, *Benadryl*)	Tear secretion Extraocular muscles Pupil (mydriasis) Causes cycloplegia
Antimalarials	hydroxychloroquine (eg, *Plaquenil Sulfate*) quinacrine (eg, *Atabrine HCl*)	Cornea, lids, retina
Barbiturates	phenobarbital	Extraocular muscles
Beta-blockers	atenolol (eg, *Tenormin*)	Tear secretion Reduces intraocular pressure
Carbonic anhydrase inhibitors	acetazolamide (eg, *Diamox*)	Causes myopia

Systemic Drugs Affecting The Eye		
Systemic drug	**Examples**	**Structure/Function affected**
CNS stimulants	amphetamines (eg, *Dexedrine*), cocaine, methylphenidate (eg, *Ritalin*)	Pupil (mydriasis) Lowers intraocular pressure
Chloramphenicol	*Chloromycetin*	Optic nerve
Chlorpromazine	*Thorazine*	Cornea and lens, lids Extraocular muscles
Cocaine	crack cocaine	Cornea and conjunctiva
Corticosteroids	prednisone cortisol	Lens Elevates intraocular pressure
Digitalis glycosides	digoxin (eg, *Lanoxin*)	Retina
Diuretics	hydrochlorothiazide (eg, *HydroDIURIL*)	Causes myopia
Ethambutol	*Myambutol*	Optic nerve
Gold salts	auranofin (*Ridaura*) gold sodium thiomalate (*Aurolate*)	Cornea and lens Conjunctiva and lids Extraocular muscles
Indomethacin	*Indocin*	Cornea, retina
Isotretinoin	*Accutane*	Conjunctiva and lids Tear secretion Retina
Minocycline	*Dynacin, Minocin*	Sclera, blue-gray or brownish Papilledema
Opiates	morphine, codeine, heroin	Pupil (miosis)
Phenytoin	*Dilantin*	Extraocular muscles
Psoralens	methoxsalen (*Oxsoralen*)	Cornea and lens
Quinine	*Quinamm*	Retina
Salicylates	aspirin (eg, *Bayer*)	Extraocular muscles
Sildenafil	*Viagra*	Retina, vision color disturbances
Sulfonamides	sulfisoxazole (*Gantrisin*)	Causes myopia
Tamoxifen	*Nolvadex*	Retina
Tamsulosin	*Flomax*	Intraoperative floppy iris syndrome (IFIS)
Tetracycline	*Sumycin*	Conjunctiva and lens
Thioridazine	*Mellaril*	Retina
Topiramate	*Topamax*	Causes myopia and angle-closure glaucoma
Vigabatrin	*Sabril*	Symptomatic or asymptomatic field loss

Indomethacin

The incidence of corneal toxicity associated with indomethacin therapy is 11% to 16%. The corneal lesions appear as either fine stromal, speckled opacities or have a whorl-like distribution resembling that of chloroquine keratopathy. These changes diminish or disappear within 6 months after discontinuing indomethacin. No definite relationship has been established between dosage of drug and corneal changes.

Photosensitizing Drugs

Photosensitizing drugs are compounds that absorb optical radiation and undergo a photochemical reaction, resulting in chemical modifications of tissue. The psoralen compounds are classic examples of photosensitizing drugs and are widely used by dermatologists to treat psoriasis and vitiligo. This treatment, commonly referred to as PUVA therapy, involves administering methoxsalen (*Oxsoralen*) or related compounds, followed by exposure to UV radiation. Cataract formation is well documented in patients undergoing PUVA therapy.

Gold Salts

Following prolonged administration, gold salts can be deposited in various tissues of the body, a condition known as chrysiasis. Ocular chrysiasis can involve the conjunctiva, cornea, and lens. Corneal chrysiasis consists of numerous gold deposits that appear as yellowish-brown, violet, or red particles distributed irregularly in the stroma. The deposition of gold usually spares the peripheral 1 to 3 mm and superior 25% to 50% of the cornea, and the deposits tend to localize to the posterior stroma. Lenticular chrysiasis appears as fine dust-like, yellowish, glistening deposits in the anterior capsule or anterior subcapsular region.

Corticosteroids

Systemic steroids can produce posterior subcapsular (PSC) cataracts that are clinically indistinguishable from complicated cataracts and cataracts caused by exposure to ionizing radiation. They often cannot be distinguished from age-related PSC cataracts. Even if the steroid dosage is reduced or discontinued, the cataract usually remains unchanged. Visual impairment is rare in patients with steroid-induced PSC cataracts. Most patients retain visual acuity of 20/40 or better, but patients may report light sensitivity, photophobia, reading difficulty, or glare. Inhaled steroids may be associated with increased risk of cataract.

Amiodarone

Cases of optic neuropathy or optic neuritis, usually resulting in visual impairment, have occurred in patients treated with amiodarone. In some cases, visual impairment has progressed to permanent blindness. Optic neuropathy or neuritis may occur at any time following initiation of therapy. A causal relationship to the drug has not been clearly established. If symptoms of visual impairment appear, prompt ophthalmic examination is recommended. The presence of optic neuropathy or neuritis calls for reevaluation of therapy. Regular ophthalmic examination, including fundoscopy and slit lamp examination, is recommended during administration of amiodarone. Amiodarone can also cause a distinctive keratopathy early in the course of treatment. The onset may be as early as 6 days following initiation of treatment, but it more commonly appears after 1 to 3 months of therapy. Virtually all patients will demonstrate corneal changes after 3 months of treatment. The corneal deposits are bilateral and are initially similar to the horizontal configuration of a Hudson-Stahli line, but eventually assume the configuration of a whorl-like opacity in the corneal epithelium. Once amiodarone therapy is discontinued, the keratopathy gradually resolves within 6 to 18 months. Lenticular opacities generally cause no visual symptoms, but moderate-to-severe keratopathy can lead to complaints of blurred vision, glare, and halos around lights or light sensitivity. Visual acuity is usually normal.

DRUGS AFFECTING THE CONJUNCTIVA AND LIDS

Isotretinoin

Ocular complications of isotretinoin (*Accutane*) include blepharoconjunctivitis, dry eye symptoms, contact lens intolerance, and subepithelial corneal opacities. There appears to be a dose-dependent relationship between isotretinoin therapy and blepharoconjunctivitis.

Chlorpromazine

Discoloration of the conjunctiva, sclera, and exposed skin has been reported with phenothiazine therapy. The discoloration is usually slate blue. Melanin-like granules have been observed in the superficial dermis.

Minocycline

Reports of blue, blue-gray, dark blue, or brownish sclera have been associated with minocycline therapy. This is an indication to stop the drug because these have been associated with irreversible papilledema, possibly more frequently than tetracycline because of minocycline's greater lipid solubility. This drug may aggravate keratitis sicca or cause irritation in contact lens wearers.

Tetracyclines

Conjunctival deposits similar to those seen in epinephrine-treated glaucoma patients have been reported in patients treated with oral tetracycline. These deposits appear as dark-brown to black granules in the palpebral conjunctiva. When observed under ultraviolet light, the brown pigment concentrations give a yellow fluorescence characteristic of tetracycline.

DRUGS THAT DECREASE AQUEOUS TEAR SECRETION

Anticholinergics

Dryness of mucous membranes is a common side effect of anticholinergic drugs because atropine and related agents inhibit glandular secretion in a dose-dependent manner.

Antihistamines

H_1 antihistamines have varying degrees of atropine-like actions, including the ability to alter tear film integrity. Both aqueous and mucin production may decrease with use of systemic antihistamines.

Isotretinoin

Dry eye symptoms are commonly reported with use of isotretinoin. The incidence has been estimated to be as high as 20%, and approximately 8% of patients experience contact lens intolerance.

Beta-Blockers

Reduced tear secretion is a reported side effect of oral beta-blockers. Most of the reported cases have occurred with practolol (not available in the US), but other beta-blockers also have been implicated in patients with dry eye syndrome.

DRUGS AFFECTING THE IRIS

Tamsulosin

Tamsulosin (*Flomax*), an alpha-adrenergic receptor antagonist, is used routinely to treat signs and symptoms of benign prostatic hypertrophy (BPH). This drug has been associated with intraoperative floppy iris syndrome (IFIS) during cataract surgery, characterized by the following:

- Billowing of the iris with normal intraocular irrigation currents
- Prolapse of the iris to the phacoemulsification probe and incision sites
- Progressive miosis during cataract surgery

These characteristics can increase surgical complications. Surgical precautions eg, (iris hooks, iris dilator rings) may be required. Discontinuation of the medication 2 to 14 days prior to surgery may also be helpful.

DRUGS CAUSING MYDRIASIS

The iris is an excellent indicator of autonomic activity because of the delicate balance between adrenergic and cholinergic innervation to the iris dilator and sphincter muscles, respectively. Adrenergic and cholinergic agents can thus easily influence pupil size and activity.

Anticholinergics

Drugs with pronounced anticholinergic action, such as atropine or related compounds, can cause significant mydriasis. Systemic administration of atropine 2 mg or more can cause pupillary dilation and cycloplegia. Both mydriasis and reduced pupillary light response can occur when transdermal scopolamine (*Transderm Scōp*) is used for 3 or more days. This usually occurs through direct contamination of the eye by rubbing with fingers following application of the patch.

Central Nervous System Stimulants

CNS stimulants, such as amphetamines, methylphenidate, and cocaine, can cause mydriasis. Likewise, CNS depressants, such as phenobarbital and antianxiety agents, can dilate the pupil through their action on the adrenergic division of the autonomic nervous system.

DRUGS CAUSING MIOSIS

Opiates (eg, heroin, morphine, codeine) characteristically constrict the pupil. Systemically administered anticholinesterase agents also can cause miosis.

DRUGS AFFECTING EXTRAOCULAR MUSCLES

Drugs that affect the autonomic nervous system or central vestibular system or cause extrapyramidal effects may cause nystagmus, diplopia, extraocular muscle palsy, or oculogyric crisis. Nystagmus can be caused by intoxication with salicylates, phenytoin, antihistamines, gold salts, and barbiturates. Diplopia has been associated with phenothiazines, antianxiety agents, and antidepressants. Alcohol can impair both smooth pursuits and saccades.

DRUGS CAUSING MYOPIA

Systemically administered sulfonamides can induce transient myopia. The myopia is acute in onset and subsides within days or weeks following withdrawal of the medication. Diuretics and carbonic anhydrase inhibitors also may cause myopia. Topiramate therapy has been associated with both myopia and angle-closure glaucoma.

DRUGS CAUSING CYCLOPLEGIA

Drugs with mild anticholinergic properties (eg, antianxiety agents, antihistamines, tricyclic antidepressants) and agents with strong anticholinergic effects (eg, atropine, scopolamine), can dilate the pupil and cause dry eye symptoms, but the cycloplegic effects are less commonly encountered in clinical practice.

DRUGS AFFECTING INTRAOCULAR PRESSURE

Drugs known to be capable of dilating the pupil can cause acute or subacute angle-closure glaucoma if the anterior chamber angle is narrow. Steroids are widely known to elevate intraocular pressure in the presence of open angles. Other drugs, such as beta-blockers, can reduce intraocular pressure.

DRUGS AFFECTING THE RETINA

Denileukin Difitox

Denileukin difitox (*Ontak*) is indicated for treatment of patients with persistent or recurrent cutaneous T-cell lymphoma whose malignant cells express the CD_{25} component of the IL-2 receptor. It has been reported to cause visual acuity loss with loss of color vision with or without retinal pigment mottling. Some patients report persistent visual impairment.

Glitazones

Glitazones are oral agents including rosiglitazone and pioglitazone used to reduce insulin resistance in type 2 diabetes. Macular edema has been associated with drugs in this class.

Hydroxychloroquine

Hydroxychloroquine maculopathy consists of a granular hyperpigmentation surrounded by a zone of depigmentation, which is surrounded by another ring of pigment. This clinical picture can vary in intensity, but is characteristic of chloroquine retinopathy and is referred to as a "bull's eye" lesion. Variations of pigmentary disturbances can occur, and some patients may show retinal changes resembling retinitis pigmentosa.

Thioridazine

Thioridazine can cause significant retinal toxicity, leading to reduced visual acuity, color vision changes, and disturbances of dark adaptation. These symptoms usually occur 30 to 90 days after initiation of treatment. Fundus appearance is often normal during the early stages, but within several weeks or months a pigmentary retinopathy develops, characterized by clumps of pigment developing first in the periphery and then progressing toward the posterior pole.

Quinine

Acute vision loss is common in quinine toxicity (eg, overdose due to attempted suicide) and frequently consists of a clinical presentation of no light perception along with dilated and nonreactive pupils. In the early stages, visual fields usually demonstrate concentric contraction. Improvement of the visual fields may require days or months, but the field loss can sometimes become permanent.

Talc

Medication tablets intended for oral use contain inert filler materials, such as talc (magnesium silicate), cornstarch, cotton fibers, and other substances. Chronic drug abusers may prepare a suspension of medication for injection by dissolving a crushed tablet of cocaine, methylphenidate, codeine, or other narcotic in water. The solution is then boiled and filtered through a crude cigarette or cotton filter prior to injection. The talc particles eventually embolize to the retinal circulation and produce a characteristic form of retinopathy. Multiple, tiny, yellow-white, glistening particles are scattered throughout the posterior pole and are more numerous in the capillary bed and small arterioles of the perimacular area. Retinal neovascularization also can occur.

Cardiac glycosides

Digitoxin and digoxin can cause changes in color vision and impairment of vision. Various visual phenomena often precede cardiac abnormalities as the earliest symptoms of digitoxin intoxication. A common symptom is snowy vision, wherein objects appear to be covered with frost or snow.

Indomethacin

Indomethacin can induce pigmentary changes of the macula and other areas of the retina. The lesions usually consist of discrete pigment scattering and fine areas of depigmentation around the macula.

Tamoxifen

Tamoxifen can cause white or yellow refractile opacities in the macular and paramacular area, with or without macular edema. The patient can experience reduced visual acuity associated with the macular lesions, and the visual fields can demonstrate abnormalities.

Isotretinoin

Isotretinoin therapy in dosages of 1 mg/kg body weight daily can impair dark adaptation, with or without excessive glare sensitivity. Once therapy is discontinued, both the abnormal dark adaptation and abnormal electroretinogram (ERG) usually resolve within several months.

Sildenafil

Sildenafil (*Viagra*) can cause retinal dysfunction and affect vision function for more than 5 hours. Visual disturbances include bluish color tinge, light sensitivity, and blurred vision. There is no safety information on the administration of sildenafil to patients with retinitis pigmentosa; administer with caution to these patients.

Vigabatrin

Vigabatrin can cause symptomatic or asymptomatic field loss, mainly bilateral concentric peripheral constriction with variable degree of visual field defects. Cases of tunnel vision have occurred.

DRUGS AFFECTING THE OPTIC NERVE

Amiodarone

Optic neuropathy occurs in about 2% of patients taking this drug. The optic nerve appearance is characterized by disc swelling with or without parapapillary disc hemorrhages.

Ethambutol

Ethambutol can cause ocular symptoms of reduced visual acuity, color vision changes, and visual field loss. Signs of ocular toxicity can appear several weeks following initial therapy, but the onset of ocular complications usually occurs several months after treatment is begun. The primary ocular manifestation of ethambutol toxicity is retrobulbar neuritis.

Chloramphenicol

Chloramphenicol causes both optic neuritis and retrobulbar neuritis. There is severe bilateral reduction of visual acuity accompanied by dense central scotomas. The optic discs are usually edematous and hyperemic, the retinal veins are engorged and tortuous, and hemorrhages are often seen. Optic atrophy is a late complication.

For More Information

Bartlett JD. Ophthalmic toxicity by systemic drugs. In: Chiou GC, ed. *Ophthalmic Toxicology*. 2nd ed. Philadelphia, PA: Taylor and Francis, Inc; 1999.

Chang DF, Campbell JR. Intraoperative floppy iris syndrome associated with tamsulosin. *J Cataract Refract Surg*. 2005;31:664-673.

Craig JE, Ong TJ, Louis DL, et al. Mechanism of topiramate-induced acute-onset myopia and angle-closure glaucoma. *Am J Ophthalmol*. 2004;137:193-195.

Flomax [package insert]. Ridgefield, CT; Boerhringer Ingelheim; 2006.

Fraunfelder FT, Fraunfelder FW. *Drug Induced Ocular Side Effects and Drug Interactions*. 5th ed. Boston, MA: Butterworth-Heinemann; 2001.

Fraunfelder FW, Fraunfelder FT, Keates EU. Topiramate-associated acute, bilateral, secondary angle-closure glaucoma. *Ophthalmology*. 2004;111:109-111.

Grant WM, Schuman JS. *Toxicology of the Eye*. 4th ed. Springfield, IL: Charles C. Thomas; 1993.

Koneru PB, Lien EJ, Koda RT. Oculotoxicities of systemically administered drugs. *J Ocul Pharmacol*. 1986;2:385-404.

Prokopich L, Bartlett JD, Jaanus SD. Ocular effects of systemic drugs. In: Bartlett JD, Jaanus SD, eds. *Clinical Ocular Pharmacology*. 5th ed. St. Louis, MO: Elsevier; 2008.

Ryan EH, Han DP, Ramsay RC, et al. Diabetic macular edema associated with glitazone use. *Retina*. 2006;26:562-570.

SYSTEMIC MEDICATIONS USED FOR OCULAR CONDITIONS

Topical, peribulbar, or intraocular drug administration may not be effective routes of administration for treatment of all eye diseases. Systemic medication is often required to achieve effective concentrations of drug in and around the ocular tissues. Included in this chapter are the more common indications and systemic medications employed for the treatment of these ocular conditions. Dosages may vary depending upon patient response, new recommendations, and guidelines. Some conditions require concurrent treatment by other routes of administration (eg, topical drops, subconjunctival or intravitreal injections).

ANTIMICROBIAL AGENTS

Antimicrobial agents may be given by topical, intraocular, peribulbar, and systemic routes of administration. Systemic antimicrobial agents are used for anterior segment, posterior segment or orbital infections, often in conjunction with topical treatment. Duration of treatment may vary, although generally 7 to 14 days is adequate in most cases. The etiology of the various conditions may vary, but the more prevalent causes are listed.

Antibacterials				
Condition	**Etiology**	**Antibiotic**	**Dose**	**Comment**
Blepharitis/ meibomian gland/ acne rosacea	*Staphylococcal* species	Tetracycline	250 to 500 mg orally every 6 hours. May be reduced to 250 mg daily in some cases.	Not for antibacterial effect. Reduces free fatty acid by-products. Tetracycline is contraindicated in pregnancy and in children < 10 years of age. Treat for ≥ 1 month for meibomian gland dysfunction.
		Doxycycline	50 to 100 mg 1 to 2 times/day	
Internal hordeolum	*Staphylococcal* species	Dicloxacillin	250 mg orally every 6 hours	Use with caution in penicillin allergy.
		Cephalexin	250 to 500 mg orally every 6 hours	Use with caution in penicillin allergy.
Acute dacryocystitis	*Staphylococcal* sp., *pneumoniae Haemophilus influenzae*	Dicloxacillin	250 mg orally every 6 hours	Use with caution in penicillin allergy.
		Cephalexin	250 to 500 mg orally every 6 hours	Use with caution in penicillin allergy.
		Amoxicillin/ Clavulanate (*Augmentin*)	125 to 250 mg orally every 8 hours	Amoxicillin/clavulanate is recommended in children to treat *H. influenzae*.

Antibacterials				
Condition	**Etiology**	**Antibiotic**	**Dose**	**Comment**
Conjunctivitis	*Gonococcal*[1] (ophthalmic)	Ceftriaxone		
		neonatal	25 to 50 mg/kg, up to 125 mg IV or IM	AAO practice standards require daily injections for 7 days.
		adult	1 g IV or IM daily	May treat up to 5 days.
		Cefixime (*Suprax*)	400 mg orally for 1 dose	Ciprofloxacin 500 mg or ofloxacin 400 mg is also indicated as single-dose treatment.
	Chlamydial[1] (adult inclusion)	Doxycycline	100 mg orally twice daily	Treat for ≥ 3 weeks.
		Tetracycline	500 mg orally 3 times daily	Treat for ≥ 3 weeks.
		Erythro-mycin	500 mg orally 4 times daily	Treat for ≥ 3 weeks.
		Ofloxacin (*Floxin*)	300 mg orally twice daily	Treat for 7 days.
		Azithro-mycin (*Zithromax*)	1 g orally once daily	Azithromycin may require only single dose.
	(neonatal inclusion)	Erythro-mycin	50 mg/kg/day orally in 4 divided doses	Treat for 14 days.
	H. influenzae	Amoxicillin	125 to 250 mg orally every 8 hours	Often used in conjunction with topical therapy.
Keratitis	*Pseudomonas* (various others possible)	Gentamicin	3 mg/kg every 8 hours (request peak & trough serum levels)	Use if pending scleral involvement. Antibiotic selection depends upon organism isolated.
Lid trauma/ oculoplastics procedures	*Staphylococcus*, *Streptococcus*, *H. influenzae*, etc.	Cephalexin	250 to 500 mg orally every 6 hours	Prophylaxis
		Dicloxacillin	250 to 500 mg orally every 6 hours	
		Amoxicillin/ Clavulanate (*Augmentin*)	125 to 500 mg orally every 8 hours	Suggest amoxicillin/ clavulanate if *H. influenzae* is suspected (more often in children).
Preseptal cellulitis	*Streptococcus*, *H. influenzae*, *Staphylococcus*, etc.	Amoxicillin/ Clavulanate	250 to 875 mg orally 2 to 3 times daily	Oral antibiotics may be sufficient.
Orbital cellulitis	*Streptococcus*, *H. influenzae*, *Staphylococcus*, etc.	Ceftriaxone and antistaphy-lococcal penicillins (*Nafcillin*)	1 g IV every 12 hours 1 to 2 g IV every 4 to 6 hours	IV therapy is required.
Endophthalmitis/ penetrating eye injury prophylaxis	*Staphylococcus*, *Streptococcus* *Bacillus*, etc.	Aminogly-coside and cefa-zolin (IV); moxifloxa-cin or levofloxacin (oral)	Gentamicin 3 mg/kg every 8 hours and cefazolin 1 g every 8 hours; moxifloxacin 400 mg daily or levofloxacin 500 mg daily	Not all clinicians use systemic therapy. Oral fluoroquinolones have been used systemically because of good aqueous and vitreous penetration, although study data is lacking.
Retinitis	*Toxoplasmosis*	Sulfadiazine and	1 g orally every 6 hours	Watch for sulfa hypersensitivity. Treat for 3 to 6 weeks.
		Pyrimeth-amine (*Daraprim*) and	25 mg orally 1 to 2 times/day (loading dose 75 mg)	May need folinic acid to prevent bone marrow depression; treat for 3 to 6 weeks.
		Clindamycin (optional)	300 mg orally every 6 hours	Treat for 3 to 6 weeks; pseudomembranous colitis is a risk.

Antibacterials				
Condition	**Etiology**	**Antibiotic**	**Dose**	**Comment**
Neurosyphilis	*Treponema pallidum*	Aqueous crystalline penicillin G	12 MU/day IV for 10 days	Caution if allergies; in HIV up to 24 MU/day for 14 to 21 days. CNS toxicity in doses > 20 MU/day.
		Ceftriaxone	1 g daily IV or IM for 14 days	

[1] Recommend concurrent treatment for gonorrhea and chlamydia.

Antivirals				
Condition	**Etiology**	**Antiviral**	**Dose**	**Comment**
Keratitis/ keratoconjunctivitis	Herpes zoster	Acyclovir (*Zovirax*)	600 to 800 orally 5 times daily for 7 to 10 days	Best if used within 72 hours of onset.
		Valacyclovir (*Valtrex*)	1,000 mg orally 3 times daily for 7 days	Best if used within 72 hours of onset.
		Famciclovir (*Famvir*)	500 mg orally 3 times daily for 7 days	Best if used within 72 hours of onset.
Cytomegalovirus (CMV) Retinitis		Ganciclovir	IV-induction - 5 mg/kg every 12 hours for 14 to 21 days; maintenance 5 mg/kg every day or 6 mg/kg 5 days/week	Bone marrow suppression; granulocytopenia, thrombocytopenia. Dosing may vary with renal impairment.
			Oral capsule - 1,000 mg 3 times daily	Maintenance
		Foscarnet (*Foscavir*)	IV-induction - 60 mg/kg every day, maintenance - 90 to 120 mg/kg every day	Renal toxicity, adjust for dose. Other side effects include headache, nausea, vomiting.
		Cidofovir (*Vistide*)	IV-5 mg/kg once per week for 2 weeks then 5 mg/kg every 2 weeks	IV saline and oral probenecid given before and after each dose; dosage reduction required with increased serum creatinine.
Varicella or Herpes Simplex (ARN; PORN)		Acyclovir (*Zovirax*)	IV - 14 mg/kg every 8 hours (or 1,500 mg/m^2)	Adequate hydration is essential.
		Famcyclovir or valacyclovir	PO - 500 mg 3 times daily (famciclovir) or 1 g 3 times daily (valacyclovir)	Pilot study resulted in regression of ARN.

Antifungals[1]				
Condition	**Etiology**	**Antifungals[1]**	**Dose**	**Comment**
Endophthalmitis	*Candida, Aspergillus, Fusarium,* etc.	Itraconazole (*Sporanox*)	200 to 400 mg orally twice a day	Monitor liver function tests (LFTs).
		Ketoconazole (*Nizoral*)	200 mg orally every 6 to 8 hours	Monitor LFTs.
		Amphotericin B	0.5 to 0.8 mg/kg/day IV	More effective in endogenous type. Systemic toxicity (eg, hypokalemia, chills, nausea, vomiting) Liposomal preparation causes fewer side effects.
		Fluconazole (*Diflucan*)	100 to 200 mg orally 1 to 2 times/day (or IV)	Well tolerated, minimal side effects. Antifungal spectrum limited.
		Flucytosine (*Ancobon*)	50 to 150 mg/kg/day orally in 4 doses	Not used alone because of potential resistance.
		Voriconazole (*Vfend*)	200 mg twice daily	Data from case reports only, but broader spectrum than fluconazole.

[1] Rifampin 600 mg/day has been added to regimen to supplement antifungal activity. Various protocols and combinations have been used. Most have not been studied adequately to recommend one regimen or antifungal agent over another. Some clinicians may add systemic antifungal agents to supplement treatment of fungal keratitis.

ANALGESICS

Various types of systemic analgesics may be used for pain. Nonnarcotic analgesics may be sufficient for minor eye pain. Acetaminophen and nonsteroidal anti-inflammatory drugs (NSAIDs) (eg, ibuprofen, aspirin, naproxen) commonly are used, also. Narcotic-containing medications such as acetaminophen with codeine (*Tylenol #3*) or acetaminophen with hydrocodone (*Vicodin*) may be required for more severe pain. Pain will vary significantly among individuals. Therefore, careful assessment is required by the clinician to determine the appropriate amount of pain relief the patient may require.

Narcotic Analgesics				
Condition	**Etiology**	**Analgesic**	**Dose**	**Comment**
Keratitis	PRK/RK Corneal abrasions	Acetaminophen with codeine 30 mg (narcotic)	1 to 2 tablets every 4 to 6 hours	Short-term control of severe eye pain. May cause drowsiness, nausea, or constipation.
		Acetaminophen with hydrocodone 5 to 7.5 mg	1 to 2 tablets every 4 to 6 hours	Short-term control of severe eye pain. May cause drowsiness, nausea, or constipation.

Nonnarcotic Analgesics				
Condition	**Etiology**	**Analgesic**	**Dose**	**Comment**
Keratitis	Epithelial defect General eye pain	Acetaminophen 500 mg	1 to 2 tablets every 4 to 6 hours	For mild eye pain
		Ketorolac (*Toradol*) 10 mg	1 tablet every 4 to 6 hours (40 mg/day maximum)	Not to exceed 5 days combined IM/IV and PO GI bleeding.
		Ibuprofen 200 mg (otc)	1 to 2 tablets every 4 to 6 hours	Take with food. Some bleeding risk.
		Tramadol (*Ultram*) 50 mg	1 to 2 tablets every 6 hours (400 mg/day maximum)	Drowsiness; potential for abuse.

ANTIHISTAMINES

The systemic administration of antihistamines for signs or symptoms of seasonal allergies may benefit patients with ocular symptoms. Patients may not require topical medication for treatment of conjunctivitis if systemic antihistamines control or alleviate systemic and ocular symptoms. Some patients do not wish to take systemic antihistamines; therefore, local treatment with various topical agents may be preferred. Other patients receiving systemic antihistamines may require supplemental therapy with topical medication to achieve adequate control of ocular symptoms.

Nonsedating Antihistamines			
Condition	**Etiology**	**Antihistamine**	**Dose**
Conjunctivitis	Seasonal allergic	Loratadine (*Claritin*) Cetirizine (*Zyrtec*) Fexofenadine (*Allegra*)[1]	10 mg every day 10 mg every day 60 mg twice daily

[1] Nonsedating antihistamines may interact with erythromycin, antifungals, phenytoin, or cyclosporine. May cause cardiac toxicity (torsades de pointes).

Sedating Antihistamines				
Condition	**Etiology**	**Antihistamine**	**Dose**	**Comment**
Conjunctivitis	Seasonal allergic	Chlorpheniramine Diphenhydramine Many others	4 to 12 mg every 4 to 12 hours 25 to 50 mg every 4 to 6 hours	Sedation may be a problem.

ANTI-INFLAMMATORY AGENTS

Systemic corticosteroids have been used in many ocular conditions, and their use is not limited to the conditions below because systemic NSAIDs probably do not penetrate the eye in sufficient levels to provide good intraocular anti-inflammatory effect and have somewhat limited application. However, generally, immunosuppressive agents are reserved for more severe or unresponsive conditions.

Corticosteroids				
Condition	**Etiology**	**Corticosteroid**	**Dose**	**Comment**
Scleritis	Autoimmune vascular-collagen disease (eg, arthritis, SLE, Wegener) Other etiologies include infectious, metabolic, or granulomatous diseases	Prednisone	Variable - 20 to 100 mg/day	Watch for side effects, including rebound inflammation, psychosis, electrolyte disturbance, peptic ulcer aggravation, hyperglycemia, aseptic necrosis, hypertension, pancreatitis. Informed consent requires review with patient.
Hyphema	Trauma Red blood cells	Prednisone	20 mg twice daily (adult)	Decreasing dose in children.
Keratitis	Viral/bacterial	Prednisone	20 to 60 mg/day	If infection is not under control or if topical steroids cannot be used (ie, with an epithelial defect).
Vitritis	Post-op membrane	Prednisone	20 to 100 mg/day	Short course under 2 weeks; taper dose to prevent rebound inflammation.

Corticosteroids				
Condition	**Etiology**	**Corticosteroid**	**Dose**	**Comment**
Retinitis	Toxoplasmosis	Prednisone	20 to 100 mg/day	Used if impending macular involvement or severe posterior segment inflammation.
Optic neuropathy	Traumatic	Methylprednisolone	30 mg/kg loading dose then, starting 2 hours later, 15 mg/kg every 6 hours, usually for a maximum of 3 to 5 days	Megadose steroid Watch for side effects (hyperglycemia, steroid sycosis, aggravation of peptic ulcer, rebound inflammation, electrolyte imbalance).
Neuritis	Demyelinizing Optic	Methylprednisolone	250 mg every 6 hours for 3 days IV followed by oral prednisone 1 mg/kg/day for 11 days	Same as megadose.

Nonsteroidal Anti-inflammatory Drugs (NSAIDs)				
Condition	**Etiology**	**NSAID**	**Dose**	**Comment**
Conjunctivitis	Vernal	Aspirin 325 mg	650 mg 3 times daily	May give additional relief with topical mast cell stabilizers or steroids.
Scleritis	Diffuse or nodular; necrotizing	Indomethacin	75 to 150 mg/day	Take with food; combination with prednisone 60 to 80 mg/day is more effective than either alone.
		Ibuprofen	400 to 800 mg/day 3 to 4 times per day (2400 mg max)	Take with food.
		Naproxen	250 to 500 mg 2 to 3 times per day	Take with food.
Myositis	Idiopathic orbital	Indomethacin	25 to 50 mg 3 times/day	Not used often.

IMMUNOSUPPRESSIVE AGENTS

Many of the immunosuppressive agents listed below have been used in treating other autoimmune-related diseases in addition to those listed. Most are reserved for cases unresponsive to initial therapy because of concerns for increased systemic toxicity and vigilant monitoring that is required. Doses may vary because extensive clinical studies are lacking.

Immunosuppressive Agents				
Condition	**Etiology**	**Agent**	**Dose**	**Comment**
Uveitis	Unknown Autoimmune	Azathioprine[1]	1 to 2.5 mg/kg/day orally (50 mg 3 times daily)	Bone marrow depression, nausea, vomiting.
		Bromocriptine	Variable	Headache, nausea, vomiting, fatigue, dizziness.
		Cyclosporine A[1] (eg, *Neoral*)	4 to 5 mg/kg/day orally (variable)	Nephrotoxicity, hypertension, gingival hyperplasia, hypertrichosis, etc.
		Methotrexate	12.5 to 15 mg/week	Watch for bone marrow depression, nausea, vomiting, pneumonitis.
Cicatricia pemphigoid	Unknown	Dapsone	25 mg/day orally for week 1, increase to 50 mg/day variable dosing	Hemolytic anemia, nausea, vomiting, anorexia, methemoglobinemia.
		Azathioprine (*Imuran*)	1 to 2 mg/kg/day orally	Bone marrow depression, nausea, vomiting. Often combined with corticosteroids.
		Cyclophosphamide[1] (eg, *Cytoxan*)	2 to 3 mg/kg/day orally	Hemorrhagic cystitis, nausea, vomiting, alopecia, thrombocytopenia.
Behçet syndrome	Unknown	Chlorambucil (*Leukeran*)	Up to 2.5 mg orally 4 times daily	Bone marrow depression, mutagenicity; start with low dose, increase slowly.
		Colchicine	1 to 1.5 mg/day orally	Nausea, vomiting, diarrhea.

[1] Also used in Behçet syndrome.

AMINOCAPROIC ACID

Aminocaproic acid (*Amicar*) is an antifibrinolytic agent used orally for the prevention of secondary rebleeds in traumatic hyphemas. Corticosteroids may also be effective, cost less, and exhibit fewer side effects than aminocaproic acid.

Aminocaproic Acid				
Condition	**Etiology**	**Drug**	**Dose**	**Comment**
Hyphema	Traumatic	Aminocaproic acid (*Amicar*)	50 mg/kg orally every 4 hours for 5 days; not to exceed 5 g every 4 hours (max 30 g/day)	Treat for 5 days. Nausea, vomiting, hypotension.

OCULAR HYPOTENSIVE AGENTS

Systemic ocular hypotensive agents are some of the most effective agents for decreasing intraocular pressure (IOP). Carbonic anhydrase inhibitors effectively decrease IOP, but are associated with various systemic side effects. Hyperosmotic agents are especially effective in reducing very elevated IOPs, although the underlying cause must be corrected to prevent rebound increase in IOP. Hyperosmotic agents are generally indicated for short-term control of IOP because their effects last for 6 to 8 hours.

Carbonic Anhydrase Inhibitors				
Condition	**Etiology**	**CAI**	**Dose**	**Comment**
Glaucoma	Open-angle	Acetazolamide	125 to 500 mg orally every 6 to 12 hours	Systemic side effects include GI intolerance, paresthesias, hypokalemia, CNS (drowsiness, lethargy, depression), renal stones, sulfa hypersensitivity, etc.
		Methazolamide	25 to 50 mg orally 2 to 3 times daily	Same as acetazolamide, more CNS, fewer GI effects.
	Acute	Acetazolamide	500 mg injectable IV	Systemic side effects include GI intolerance, paresthesias, hypokalemia, CNS (drowsiness, lethargy, depression), renal stones, sulfa hypersensitivity, etc.

Hyperosmotic Agents				
Condition	**Etiology**	**Osmotic Agent**	**Dose**	**Comment**
Glaucoma	Acute Preoperative (to lower IOP)	Mannitol IV 15 to 25% (*Osmitrol*)	1.5 to 2 g/kg IV	Watch crystal formation; use with in-line IV filter, keep warm. Infuse over 30 minutes. Watch for electrolyte disturbances, thirst, diuresis, potential cardiovascular overload.

VITAMINS/MINERALS

Various vitamins and minerals have established roles in the treatment of ophthalmic conditions. Others are not well documented.

Vitamin/Minerals				
Condition	**Etiology**	**Vitamin/Mineral**	**Dose**	**Comment**
Dry eye/ keratitis	Vitamin A deficiency	Vitamin A	50,000 U every day	Fat soluble vitamin, toxicity includes dry mucous membranes, increased eye irritation.
Optic neuritis	Nutritional or toxic	Vitamin B_{12} hydroxocobalamin	1,000 U IM daily, reduce dose to weekly then monthly	Cyanocobalamin may not be as effective.
	Drug toxicity (INH)	Pyridoxine (B_6)	50 mg/day	Often given concurrently with INH.
Macular degeneration	Deficiency of antioxidant vitamins (eg, E, C, A) Zinc Selenium Copper	*Ocuvite*, *Icaps Plus*- various mfr.	1 tablet 1 to 2 times daily	Causative agent not well established; recent evidence has suggested beta-carotene may not be beneficial.
		Ocuvite PreserVision	2 tablets, 2 times daily or as directed	

For More Information

Aizman A, Johnson MW, Elner SG. Treatment of acute retinal necrosis syndrome with oral antiviral medications. *Ophthalmology*. 2007:114:307-312.

Bartlett JD, Jaanus SD, eds. *Clinical Ocular Pharmacology*. 5th ed. St. Louis, MO: Elsevier; 2008.

Breit SM, Hariprasad SM, Mieler WF, et al. Management of endogenous fungal endophthalmitis with voriconazole and caspofungin. *Am J Ophthalmol*. 2005;139:135-140.

Optometric Clinical Practice Guidelines, American Optometric Association, St. Louis MO.

Preferred Practice Pattern Series, American Academy of Ophthalmology, San Francisco CA.

Sanford JP, Gilbert DN, Sande MA, eds. *Guide to Antimicrobial Therapy*. Dallas, TX: Antimicrobial Therapy Inc.; 1995.

Tabbara KF, Hyyndiuk RA, eds. *Infections of the Eye*, 2nd ed. Boston, MA: Little, Brown and Company; 1996.

Wickersham RM, Novak KK, managing eds. *Drug Facts and Comparisons*. St. Louis, MO: Wolters Kluwer Health, Inc.; 2008.

Zimmerman TJ, ed. *Textbook of Ocular Pharmacology*. New York, NY: Lippincott-Raven Press; 1997.

Appendix

Orphan Drugs

In addition to the Food and Drug Administration (FDA) approved drugs and the drugs with unlabeled ophthalmic uses (see the Drugs with Off-labeled Ophthalmic Uses chapter), two other groups of drugs are of interest to eye care practitioners: Investigational New Drugs (INDs) and Orphan Drugs. INDs are drugs that are not approved by the FDA, but are being investigated by a pharmaceutical company or sponsor. Orphan drugs are drugs made available by manufacturers for the treatment of rare diseases.

The term "orphan drug" first appeared in the medical literature in a 1968 editorial. It was used to disclaim nonapproved substances as drugs and included compounds such as lithium carbonate, d-xylose, and sodium fluoride. These products were frequently labeled "for chemical purposes, not for drug use," "for research use only, not for clinical use," and "for manufacturing use only." The term "orphan drug" has since been applied to drugs and devices used in the treatment or diagnosis of rare diseases.

The Orphan Drug Act has provided an environment for the development of products for rare diseases and should continue to facilitate this process. In 1984, the Orphan Drug Act was amended to define a rare disease or condition as that which (a) affects less than 200,000 people or (b) affects greater than 200,000 people and for which the manufacturing company has no reasonable prospect of recovering research and development costs from sales within the US. Occasionally, a drug that is already commercially available may achieve orphan status for an indication that does not involve a large patient population. The incentives provided by both the Orphan Drug Act and other federal initiatives make it possible for commercial manufacturers to produce drugs for FDA approval at minimal costs. Individuals with rare diseases can be assured that efforts will continue to be made to find treatments.

The FDA established the Office of Orphan Products Development in 1982. These products consist of drugs, biologicals (eg, vaccines), medical devices, and foods for the diagnosis, treatment, or prevention of rare diseases.

Government Incentives To Assist In Orphan Drug Development[1]
♦ Developers of orphan drugs have 7 years of exclusive licensing, during which time the product may not be marketed by another company in the US without the sponsor's permission.
♦ Developers may claim up to 63% of the cost of clinical investigations as a tax credit.
♦ The FDA can grant up to $200,000 in support of a sponsor's orphan drug clinical research. The Orphan Drug Act authorizes $12,000,000 per year for these research grants.
♦ The FDA can assist sponsors of orphan drugs in the development of investigational guidelines and protocols.
♦ When appropriate, the FDA can modify approval requirements for specific orphan drugs (eg, modify the size of study populations).
♦ The FDA can assign to orphan drugs a high review priority. The review phase (time from a new drug application submission to approval) for 9 orphan drugs receiving approval in 1985 and 1986 was 2.7 years.

[1] Tatro, DS. Orphan drugs. *Drug Newsletter.* 1988 Apr;7(4):26.

Ophthalmic drugs established by the FDA as Orphan Drugs are listed in the following table.

Orphan Drugs		
Drug generic (*Trade*)	**Indication**	**Manufacturer/Sponsor**
AI-RSA	Autoimmune uveitis	AutoImmune
Allogeneic retinal epithelial cells transfected with plasmid vector expressing ciliary neurotrophic growth factor	Retinitis pigmentosa	Neurotech USA
Aminocaproic acid (*Caprogel*)	Topical treatment of traumatic hyphema of the eye	Eastern Virginia Medical School
Botulinum toxin type A (*Botox*)	Blepharospasm or strabismus associated w/dystonia in adults (12 years of age and older)[1]	Allergan
	Synkinetic closure of the eyelid associated with VII cranial nerve aberrant regeneration	Botulinum Toxic Research
Botulinum toxin type F	Essential blepharospasm	Ipsen
Brimonidine (*Alphagan*)	Anterior ischemic optic neuropathy	Allergan
Bromhexine (*Bisolvon*)	Mild to moderate keratoconjunctivitis sicca in patients with Sjogren syndrome	Boehringer Ingelheim
Chondroitinase	Patients undergoing vitrectomy	Bausch & Lomb
Cromolyn sodium 4% ophthalmic solution (*Opticrom 4% Ophthalmic Solution*)	Vernal keratoconjunctivitis[1]	Fisons
Cyclosporine 2% ophthalmic ointment	Patients at high risk of graft rejection following penetrating keratoplasty; corneal melting syndromes of known or presumed immunologic etiopathogenesis, including Mooren ulcer	Allergan
Cyclosporine ophthalmic (*Optimmune*)	Severe keratoconjunctivitis sicca associated with Sjogren syndrome	University of Georgia
Cysteamine Hydrochloride	Corneal cystine crystal accumulation in cystinosis patients	Sigma-Tau
Dexamethasone (*Posurdex*)	In posterior segment drug delivery system in idiopathic intermediate uveitis	Allergan
Dextran 70 (*Dehydrex*)	Recurrent corneal erosion unresponsive to conventional therapy	Holles Labs
Epidermal growth Factor (human)	Acceleration of corneal epithelial regeneration and the healing of stromal tissue in nonhealing corneal defects	Chiron Vision
Fibronectin (human plasma-derived)	Nonhealing corneal ulcers or epithelial defects that have been unresponsive to conventional therapy and the underlying cause has been eliminated	Melville Biologics
Fibronectin (plasma-derived)	Nonhealing corneal ulcers or epithelial defects that are unresponsive to conventional therapy and for which any infectious cause of the defect has been eliminated	Chiron Vision
Fluocinolone (*Retisert*)	Uveitis involving the posterior segment of the eye[1]	Bausch & Lomb
Ganciclovir intravitreal implant (*Vitrasert Implant*)	Cytomegalovirus retinitis[1]	Bausch & Lomb, Chiron Vision
Ganciclovir sodium (*Cytovene*)	Cytomegalovirus retinitis in immunocompromised patients with AIDS[1]	Syntex
Gangliosides as sodium salts (*Cronassial*)	Retinitis pigmentosa	Fidia

Orphan Drugs		
Drug generic (*Trade*)	**Indication**	**Manufacturer/Sponsor**
Human umbilical tissue-derived cells	Retinitis pigmentosa	Centocor
Levocabastine hydrochloride ophthalmic suspension 0.05%	Vernal keratoconjunctivitis	Iolab
Lodoxamide tromethamine (*Alomide Ophthalmic Solution*)	Vernal keratoconjunctivitis[1]	Alcon
Matrix metalloproteinase inhibitor (*Galardin*)	Corneal ulcers	Glycomed
Mitomycin-C	Refractory glaucoma as an adjunct to ab externo glaucoma surgery	IOP
Monoclonal antibody to cytomegalovirus (human)	Cytomegalovirus retinitis in AIDS	Protein Design Labs
Myo-inositol	Prevent retinopathy of prematurity in preterm infants at risk of developing the condition	Ross Products Division
Ofloxacin (*Ocuflox Ophthalmic Solution*)	Bacterial corneal ulcers[1]	Allergan
Pilocarpine hydrochloride (*Salagen*)	Xerostomia and keratoconjunctivitis sicca in Sjorgren syndrome[1]	MGI Pharma
Transforming growth factor-beta 2	Full thickness macular holes	Celtrix
Tretinoin	Squamous metaplasia of the ocular surface epithelia (conjunctiva and/or cornea) with mucous deficiency and keratinization	Hannan Ophthalmic
Urea for intravitreal injection (*Neurosolve*)	Retinitis pigmentosa	Vitreo Retinal Technologies
Urogastrone	Accelerate corneal epithelial regeneration and healing of stromal incisions from corneal transplant surgery	Chiron Vision

[1] Approved for marketing.

Published information about orphan drugs is made available by various agencies. These sources can be contacted to obtain information about the acquisition or availability of an orphan drug product.

Information Sources For Rare Diseases And Orphan Drug Treatment[1]			
Organization	**Information**	**Telephone**	**Web site**
National Organization for Rare Disorders (NORD) PO Box 8923 New Fairfield, CT 06812-8923	Information on rare diseases and their treatment.	(203) 744-0100	http://www.rarediseases.org
Federal Register: Dockets Management Branch (HFA-305) FDA Room 1061 5630 Fishers Lane Rockville, MD 20852	List of orphan drugs and biologicals, designated uses, sponsor's name and address. Available under Docket #84N-0102.	Not available	http://www.fda.gov/ohrms/dockets
Office of Orphan Products Development (HF-35) FDA 5600 Fishers Lane Rockville, MD 20857	Technical information on orphan drug development, product availability, research grants, and drug sponsorship.	(301) 827-3666 (800) 300-7469	http://www.fda.gov/orphan

[1] Tatro, DS. Orphan Drugs. *Drug Newsletter*. 1988 Apr;7(4):26.

MANUFACTURERS AND DISTRIBUTORS INDEX

00074
Abbott Laboratories
200 Abbott Park Rd.
Abbott Park IL 60064-6400
800-633-9110
http://www.abbott.com

Advanced Medical Optics
1700 East St. Andrew Pl.
P.O. Box 25162
Santa Ana CA 92799-5162
714-247-8200
http://www.amo-inc.com

Advanced Vision Research
12 Alfred St., Ste. 200
Woburn MA 01801
781-932-8327
800-579-8327
http://www.theratears.com

17478
Akorn, Inc.
2500 Millbrook Dr.
Buffalo Grove IL 60089
800-535-7155
888-519-8384
http://www.akorn.com

00065, 00998
Alcon Laboratories, Inc.
6201 S. Freeway
Fort Worth TX 76134-2009
800-451-3937
800-862-5266
http://www.alconlabs.com

00023, 11980
Allergan, Inc.
2525 DuPont Dr.
Irvine CA 92623-9534
714-246-4500
800-433-8871
http://www.allergan.com

Alliance Pharm. Corp.
6175 Lusk Blvd.
San Diego CA 92121
858-410-5200
http://www.allp.com

54569
Allscripts, Inc.
2401 Commerce Dr.
Libertyville IL 60048-4464
847-680-3515
800-654-0889
http://www.allscripts.com

Altaire Pharmaceuticals, Inc.
311 West Lane
P.O. Box 849
Aquebogue NY 11931
800-258-2471

17314
Alza Corp.
1900 Charleston Rd.
Mt. View CA 94039
650-564-5000
http://www.alza.com

89709, 90605
Amcon Laboratories
40 N. Rock Hill Rd.
St. Louis MO 63119
314-961-5758
800-255-6161
http://www.amconlabs.com

00517
American Regent (Luitpold Pharmaceuticals, Inc.)
1 Luitpold Dr.
Shirley NY 11967
800-645-1706
631-924-4000
http://www.luitpold.com

00003, 00015
Apothecon, Inc.
See Bristol-Myers Squibb

00186
AstraZeneca LP
1800 Concord Pike
Wilmington DE 19850
800-842-9920
800-237-8898
800-456-3669
http://www.astrazeneca-us.com

Aton Pharma
3150 Brunswick Pike
Lawrenceville NJ 08648
877–286–6549

AutoImmune, Inc.
1199 Madia St.
Pasadena CA 91103
626-792-1235
http://www.autoimmuneinc.com

00264
B. Braun Medical Inc.
1601 Wallace Dr., Ste. 150
Carrollton TX 75006
800-627-7867
800-854-6551
http://www.bbraunusa.com

10119
Bausch & Lomb North American Vision Care
1400 N. Goodman St.
P.O. Box 450
Rochester NY 14603-0450
585-338-6000
800-344-8815
800-553-5340
http://www.bausch.com

24208, 57782
Bausch & Lomb Pharmaceuticals
8500 Hidden River Pkwy.
Tampa FL 33637
813-975-7770
800-323-0000
http://www.bausch.com

Bausch & Lomb Surgical
180 Via Verde
San Dimas CA 91773
800-338-2020
http://www.blsurgical.com

Baxter Healthcare Corp.
1 Baxter Pkwy.
Deerfield IL 60015
888-229-0001
800-422-9837
http://www.baxter.com

12843, 16500
Bayer Consumer Care Division
36 Columbia Rd.
P.O. Box 1910
Morristown NJ 07962
800-800-4793
800-331-4536
http://www.bayercare.com

31280
BD (Becton Dickinson & Co.)
1 Becton Dr.
Franklin Lakes NJ 07417
201-847-6800
888-237-2762
http://www.bd.com

55390
Bedford Laboratories
300 Northfield Rd.
Bedford OH 44146
440-232-3320
800-562-4797
http://www.bedfordlabs.com

50486
Blairex Labs, Inc.
1600 Brian Dr.
Columbus IN 47202
812-378-1864
800-252-4739
http://www.blairex.com

Boehringer Ingelheim Pharmaceuticals, Inc.
900 Ridgebury Rd.
Ridgefield CT 06877-0368
203-798-9988
800-542-6257
http://www.boehringer-ingelheim.com

Burroughs Wellcome Co.
See GlaxoSmithKline

Celltech Pharmaceutical Co.
755 Jefferson Rd.
Rochester NY 14623
800-234-5535
585-475-9000
http://www.celltechgroup.com

Celtrix Pharmaceuticals, Inc.
2033 Gateway Pl., Ste. 600
San Jose CA 95110
408-988-2500
http://www.bioportfolio.com

Centocor, Inc.
200 Great Valley Pkwy.
Malvern PA 19355
610-651-6000
800-457-6399
http://www.centocor.com

00436
Century Pharmaceuticals, Inc.
10377 Hague Rd.
Indianapolis IN 46256-3399
317-849-4210
866-343-2576

Chiron Vision
See Bausch & Lomb Surgical

00346
Ciba Vision Corporation
11460 Johns Creek Pkwy.
Duluth GA 30097
770-476-3937
800-845-6585
http://www.cibavision.com

Clintec Nutrition
See Baxter Healthcare

54799
Cynacon/OCuSOFT
P.O. Box 429
Richmond TX 77406-0429
800-233-5469
http://www.ocusoft.com

10310
Del Pharmaceuticals
565 Broad Hollow Rd.
Farmingdale NY 11735
516-844-2020
800-645-9888
http://www.dellabs.com

00777
Dista Products Co.
See Eli Lilly and Co.

00168
E. Fougera Co.
60 Baylis Rd.
Melville NY 11747
800-432-6673
http://www.fougera.com

Eagle Vision, Inc.
8500 Wolf Lake Drive; Ste. 110
P.O. Box 34877
Memphis TN 38184
901-380-7000
800-222-7584
http://www.eaglevis.com

00002, 59075
Eli Lilly and Co.
Lilly Corp. Center
Indianapolis IN 46285
317-276-2000
800-545-5979
http://www.lilly.com

00641
Elkins-Sinn, Inc.
See Wyeth-Ayerst

Escalon Medical Corp.
2440 South 179th St.
New Berlin WI 53146
262-821-9182
800-433-8197
http://www.escalonmed.com

Falcon Ophthalmics, Inc.
6201 S. Freeway
Fort Worth TX 76134
817-551-8710
800-343-2133
http://www.falconpharma.com

Fidia Pharmaceutical Corp.
2000 K St. N.W., # 700
Washington DC 20006

Fisons Corp.
See Celltech Pharmaceutcal Co.

Focus Laboratories, Inc.
North Little Rock AK 72113

00258, 00456, 00535
Forest Pharmaceuticals, Inc.
13600 Shoreline Dr.
St. Louis MO 63045
314-493-7000
800-678-1605
http://www.forestpharm.com

Fougera & Co.
See E. Fougera Co.

10432
Freeda Vitamins, Inc.
36 E. 41st St.
New York NY 10017-6203
212-685-4980
800-777-3737
http://www.freedavitamins.com

00469, 57317
Fujisawa Healthcare, Inc.
3 Pkwy. North
Deerfield IL 60015-2548
800-727-7003
800-888-7704
http://www.fujisawa.com

00781
Geneva Pharmaceuticals, Inc.
See Sandoz Inc.

GlaxoSmithKline
1 Franklin Plaza
Philadelphia PA 19102
215-751-4000
888-825-5249
http://www.gsk.com

GlaxoSmithKline Consumer Healthcare, L.P.
100 Beecham Dr.
Pittsburgh PA 15205
800-245-1040
http://www.gsk.com

00081, 00173
GlaxoWellcome, Inc.
See GlaxoSmithKline

00182
Goldline Laboratories, Inc.
See Ivax Pharmaceuticals

Hannan Ophthalmic Marketing Services, Inc.
34 Sherrill Rd.
Nashville MA 02050
781-834-8111

Henry Schein, Inc.
135 Duryea Rd.
Melville NY 11747
631-843-5500
800-472-4346
http://www.henryschein.com

H.L. Bouton
11 Kendrick Rd.
Wareham MA 02571
508-295-3300
800-426-1881
http://www.hlbouton.com

00839
H.L. Moore Drug Exchange, Inc.
See Moore Medical Corp.

00004, 00033, 00140, 18393, 42987
Hoffmann-La Roche Inc.
See Roche Laboratories

47992
Holles Laboratories, Inc.
30 Forest Notch
Cohasset MA 02025-1198
781-383-0005
800-356-4015

00548
I.M.S., Ltd.
See Celltech Pharmaceutical Co.

00814
Interstate Drug Exchange
See Henry Schein, Inc.

Iolab Pharmaceuticals
See Ciba Vision Corporation

IOP, Inc.
3151 Airway Ave., Ste. I-1
Costa Mesa CA 92626
714-549-1185
800-535-3545
http://www.iopinc.com

ISTA Pharmaceuticals
15279 Alton Parkway
Irvine CA 92618
949-788-6000
http://www.istavision.com

Ivax Pharmaceuticals, Inc.
4400 Biscayne Blvd.
Miami FL 33137
305-575-6000
800-327-4114
http://www.ivaxpharmaceuticals.com

00137
Johnson & Johnson
1 Johnson & Johnson Plz.
New Brunswick NJ 08933
732-524-0400
http://www.jnj.com

KabiVitrum, Inc.
See Pharmacia Corp.

00588
Keene Pharmaceuticals, Inc.
303 S. Mockingbird
P.O. Box 7
Keene TX 76059-0007
817-645-8083
800-541-0530

La Haye Laboratories, Inc.
See US Nutraceuticals, LLC

Lacrimedics, Inc.
P.O. Box 1209
Eastbound WA 98245
360-376-7095
800-367-8327
http://www.lacrimedics.com

10651
Lavoptik Co., Inc.
661 Western Ave.
St. Paul MN 55103

00005, 53124
Lederle Pharmaceuticals Division
See Wyeth-Ayerst Labs

23558
Lee Pharmaceuticals
1434 Santa Anita Ave.
South Elmonte CA 91733
800-950-5337
http://www.leepharmaceuticals.com

00619
Luyties
P.O. Box 8080
Richford VT 05476
800-466-3672
http://www.1800homeopathy.com

00904
Major Pharmaceuticals
31778 Enterprise Dr.
Livonia MI 48150
734-525-8700
800-688-9696
http://www.harvarddrugs.com

Marlin Industries
P.O. Box 560
Grover City CA 93483-0560
805-473-2743
800-423-5926

00259
Mayrand, Inc.
See Merz Pharmaceuticals

00264
McGaw, Inc.
See B. Braun Medical Inc.

Med Pointe Healthcare, Inc.
265 Davidson Ave., Ste. 300
Somerset NJ 08873-4120
732-564-2200
http://www.medpointeinc.com

00585
Medeva Pharmaceuticals
See Celltech Pharmaceutical Co.

00348, 75137
Medtech Laboratories, Inc.
3510 N. Lake Creek
Jackson WY 83001-1108
914-524-6810
800-443-4908
800-803-4471
http://www.medtechinc.com

Melville Biologics

(Precision Pharma Services)
155 Duryea Rd.
Melville NY 11747
631-752-7320
http://www.precisionpharma.com

Menicon America
1840 Gateway Dr., Second Floor
San Mateo CA 94404
650-378-1424
800-636-4266
http://www.menicon.com

00006
Merck & Co., Inc.
1 Merck Drive
Whitehouse Station NJ 08889-1000
908-423-1000
800-672-6372
http://www.merck.com

Merz Pharmaceuticals
4215 Tudor Lane
Greensboro NC 27410
888-637-9872
336-856-2003
800-335-0514
http://www.merzusa.com

MGI Pharma, Inc.
5775 W. Old Shakopee Rd., Ste. 100
Bloomington MN 55437-3714
952-346-4700
800-562-5580
http://www.mgipharma.com

00682, 46672
Mikart, Inc.
1750 Chattahoochee Ave.
Atlanta GA 30318
404-351-4510
888–4MIKART
http://www.mikart.com

Moore Medical Corp.
389 John Downey Dr.
P.O. Box 2740
New Britain CT 06050-1500
800-234-1464
http://www.mooremedical.com

53489
Mutual Pharmaceutical Co., Inc.
(United Research Laboratories)
1100 Orthodox St.
Philadelphia PA 19124
800-523-3684
215-288-6500
http://www.urlmutual.com

Novartis Consumer Health
200 Kimball Dr.
Parsippany NJ 07054-0622
973-503-8000
http://www.novartis.com

Novartis Ophthalmics, Inc.
11695 Johns Creek Pkwy.
Duluth GA 30097-1556
866-393-6336
http://www.novartisophthalmics.com

00028, 00067, 00083, 58887
Novartis Pharmaceuticals Corp.
59 Route 10
East Hanover NJ 04936
973-781-8300
888-669-6682
http://www.pharma.us.novartis.com

00362
Novocol
See Septodont, Inc.

NutraMax Laboratories, Inc.
2208 Lakeside Blvd.
Edgewood MD 21040
410-776-4000
800-925-5187
http://www.nutramaxlabs.com

51944
Ocumed, Inc.
119 Harrison Ave.
Roseland NJ 07068
973-226-2330
http://www.ocumedgroupinc.com

OCuSOFT
See Cynacon/OCuSOFT

Optikem International
2172 S. Jason St.
Denver CO 80223
303-936-1137
800-525-1752

59148
Otsuka America Pharmaceutical, Inc.
2440 Research Blvd., Ste. 250
Rockville MD 20850
301-990-0030
800-562-3974
http://www.otsuka.com

60758
Pacific Pharma
See Allergan

00071
Parke-Davis
A Pfizer Company
235 E. 42nd St.
New York NY 10017
800-438-1985

00349
ParMed Pharmaceuticals
4220 Hyde Park Blvd.
Niagara Falls NY 14305
800-727-6331
http://www.parmed.com

00418
Pasadena Research Labs
See Taylor Pharmaceuticals

00927
Pfeiffer Co.
71 University Ave. SW
Atlanta GA 30315
404-614-0255
800-342-6450
http://pfeifferpharmaceuticals.com

00069, 00663, 74300
Pfizer US Pharmaceutical Group
235 E. 42nd St.
New York NY 10017
800-438-1985
http://www.pfizer.com

00013, 00016
Pharmacia Corp.
A Division of Pfizer
235 E. 42nd St.
New York NY 10017
800-323-4204
http://www.pnu.com

Pharmafair
See Bausch & Lomb Pharmaceuticals

Pharmics, Inc.
2702 South 3600 West, Suite H
Salt Lake City UT 84119
801-966-4138
800-456-4138
http://www.pharmics.com

47144
Polymer Technology Corp.
100 Research Dr.
Wilmington MA 01887
978-658-6111

Protein Design Labs, Inc.
34801 Campus Dr.
Fremont CA 94555
510-574-1400
http://www.pdl.com

00603
Qualitest Pharmaceuticals
130 Vintage Dr.
Huntsville AL 35811
256-859-4011
800-444-4011

54092
Roberts Pharmaceutical Corp.
See Shire

Roche Laboratories
340 Kingsland St.
Nutley NJ 07110-1199
973-235-5000
800-526-6367
http://www.rocheusa.com

00049
Roerig
See Pfizer US Pharmaceutical Group

00074
Ross Products Division, Abbott Labs
625 Cleveland
Columbus OH 43215
800-986-8510
http://www.ross.com

00536
Rugby Labs, Inc.
See Watson Pharmaceuticals

Sandoz, Inc.
506 Carnegie Center Dr.
Suite 400
Princeton NJ 08540
609-627-8500
800-525-8747
http://www.us.sandoz.com

00024
Sanofi-Synthelabo, Inc.
90 Park Ave.
New York NY 10016
212-551-4000
800-223-1062
http://en.sanofi-aventis.com

65086
Santen, Inc.
555 Gateway Rd.
Napa CA 94558
707-254-1750
800-611-2011
http://www.santeninc.com

00364, 00591
Schein Pharmaceutical, Inc.
See Watson Pharmaceuticals

00274, 00032
Scherer Laboratories, Inc.
84 Church St., Ste. C
Marietta GA 30060
770-514-1333
800-310-5357

00085, 11017, 41000, 41100
Schering-Plough Corp.
2000 Galloping Hill Rd.
Kenilworth NJ 07033-0530
908-298-4000
800-842-4090
http://www.sch-plough.com

Septodent, Inc.
245 C Quigley Blvd.
New Castle DE 19720
302-328-1102
800-872-8305
http://www.septodentinc.com

Shire US Inc.
1 Riverfront Place
Newport KY 41071
859-669-8000
800-828-2088
http://www.shire.com

Sigma-Tau Pharmaceuticals
800 S. Frederick Ave., Ste. 300
Gaithersburg MD 20877-4150
301-948-1041
800-447-0169
http://www.sigmatau.com

00766
SmithKline Beecham Consumer Healthcare
1500 Littleton Rd.
Parsippany NJ 07084
973-889-2100
http://www.sb.com

51318
Star Pharmaceuticals, Inc.
1990 N.W. 44th St.
Pompano Beach FL 33064-8712
954-971-9704
800-845-7827
http://www.starpharm.com

Stellar Pharmacal Corp.
1881 W. State Road 84, Ste. 101
Ft. Lauderdale FL 33309
954-759-3436
800-845-7827

00402
Steris Corp.
5960 Heisley Rd.
Mentor OH 44060-1834

57706
Storz Ophthalmics
See Bausch & Lomb Surgical

00033, 18393, 42987
Syntex Laboratories
See Roche Pharmaceuticals

00418
Taylor Pharmaceuticals (Akorn)
2500 Millbrook Dr.
Buffalo Grove IL 60089
847-279-6100
800-223-9851

00677
United Research Laboratories
See Mutual Pharmaceutical Co.

00009
Upjohn Co.
See Pfizer

US Nutraceuticals, LLC
2751 Nutra Lane
Eustis FL 32726
352-357-2004
877-729-7256
http://www.usnutra.com

54891
Vision Pharmaceuticals, Inc.
1022 N. Main St.
Mitchell SD 57301-0400
605-996-3356
800-325-6789
http://www.visionpharm.com

00047, 52544, 51875, 55515
Watson Pharmaceuticals
311 Bonnie Circle Dr.
Corona CA 92880
951-493-5300
800-272-5525
http://www.watsonpharm.com

00008, 00031
Wyeth-Ayerst
5 Giralda Farms
Madison NJ 07940
800-934-5556
610-688-4400
http://www.wyeth.com

00172, 00182
Zenith Goldline Pharmaceuticals
See Ivax Pharmaceuticals

Chapter Summaries

The following tables are provided as a quick-look product guide. The tables cover Chapter 2 (Ophthalmic Dyes) through Chapter 12 (Agents For Retinal Disease) and Chapter 14 (Miscellaneous Products) and contain a summary of product information including: generic name, trade name, manufacturer(s), ingredient(s), strength(s), doseform(s), and how supplied. For complete information about a particular product, please consult the index for the appropriate page number.

Ophthalmic Dyes

Generic Name *Trade Name*	**Doseform/ Strength**	**How Supplied**
Fluorescein Sodium *Ak-Fluor, Rx* (Akorn)	**Injection**: 10%	In 5 mL amps and vials.
Angiofluor, Rx (OcuSoft)	**Injection**: 10%	In 5 mL single-dose vials and boxes of 12 vials.
Angiofluor Lite, Rx (OcuSoft)	**Injection**: 10%	In 5 mL single-dose vials and boxes of 12 vials.
Fluorescite, Rx (Alcon)	**Injection**: 10%	In 5 mL amps with syringes.
AK-Fluor, Rx (Akorn)	**Injection**: 25%	In 2 mL amps and vials.
Angiofluor, Rx (OcuSoft)	**Injection**: 25%	In 2 mL single-dose vials and boxes of 12 vials.
Angiofluor Lite, Rx (Alliance Pharm.)	**Injection**: 25%	In 2 mL single-dose vials and boxes of 12 vials.
Ful-Glo, Rx (Akorn)	**Strips**: 0.6 mg	In 300s.
Fluorexon *Fluoresoft, otc* (Various, eg, Holles)	**Solution**: 0.35%	In 0.3 mL ampules (20s).
Indocyanine Green *IC-Green, Rx* (Akorn)	**Powder for Injection**: 25 mg	In 10 mL amps of aqueous solvent (6s).
Lissamine Green *Lissamine Green, otc* (Cyanacon/Ocusoft)	**Strips**: 1.5 mg	100 sterile strips per carton.
Rose Bengal *Rose Bengal, otc* (Akorn)	**Strips**: 1.3 mg/strip	In 100s.

Local Anesthetics, Injectable

Generic Name *Trade Name*	Doseform/ Strength	How Supplied
Lidocaine Hydrochloride and Lidocaine Combinations		
Xylocaine MPF, Rx (Astra Zeneca)	**Injection**: 4%	In 5 mL amps and 5 mL disp. syringe with laryngotracheal cannula.
Xylocaine, Rx (Astra Zeneca)	**Injection**: 0.5% with 1:200,000 epinephrine	In 50 mL multiple-dose vials.[1]
Xylocaine, Rx (Astra Zeneca)	**Injection**: 1% with 1:100,000 epinephrine	In 10, 20, and 50 mL multiple-dose vials.[1]
Xylocaine MPF, Rx (Astra Zeneca)	**Injection**: 1% with 1:200,000 epinephrine	In 30 mL ampules, and 10 and 30 mL single-dose vials.[2]
Xylocaine MPF, Rx (Astra Zeneca)	**Injection**: 1.5% with 1:200,000 epinephrine	In 5 and 30 mL ampules, 10 and 30 mL single-dose vials.[2]
Xylocaine, Rx (Astra Zeneca)	**Injection**: 2% with 1:100,000 epinephrine	In 20 and 50 mL multiple-dose vials.[1]
Xylocaine MPF, Rx (Astra Zeneca)	**Injection**: 2% with 1:200,000 epinephrine	In 20 mL ampules, and 10 and 20 mL single-dose vials.[2]
Mepivacaine Hydrochloride		
Polocaine, Rx (Astra Zeneca)	**Injection**: 1%	In 50 mL vials.
Polocaine MPF, Rx (Astra Zeneca)	**Injection**: 1%	In 30 mL vials.
Polocaine MPF, Rx (Astra Zeneca)	**Injection**: 1.5%	In 30 mL vials.
Polocaine, Rx (Astra Zeneca)	**Injection**: 2%	In 50 mL vials.
Polocaine MPF, Rx (Astra Zeneca)	**Injection**: 2%	In 20 mL vials.
Bupivacaine Hydrochloride and Bupivacaine Combinations		
Bupivacaine Hydrochloride, Rx (Abbott)	**Injection**: 0.75%	In 20 mL amps.
Sensorcaine MPF, Rx (Astra Zeneca)	**Injection**: 0.75%	In 30 mL vials.
Sensorcaine MPF, Rx (Astra Zeneca)	**Injection**: 0.75% with 1:200,000 epinephrine	In 30 mL amps and 10 and 30 mL vials.[2]

[1] With methylparaben.
[2] With sodium metabisulfite.

Local Anesthetics, Topical

Generic Name *Trade Name*	**Doseform/ Strength**	**How Supplied**
Tetracaine Hydrochloride *Tetracaine Hydrochloride, Rx* (Various, eg, Bausch & Lomb)	**Solution**: 0.5%	In 2 and 15 mL.
Tetcaine, Rx (OCuSOFT)	**Solution**: 0.5%	In 15 mL.
Proparacaine Hydrochloride *Proparacaine Hydrochloride, Rx* (Various, eg, Bausch & Lomb, Falcon)	**Solution**: 0.5%	In 15 mL.
AK-TAINE, Rx (Akorn)	**Solution**: 0.5%	In 15 mL.[1,2]
Alcaine, Rx (Various, eg, Alcon)	**Solution**: 0.5%	In 15 mL *Drop-Tainers*.[3,4]
Ophthetic, Rx (Various, eg, Allergan)	**Solution**: 0.5%	In 15 mL.[1,2]
Paracaine, Rx (OCuSOFT)	**Solution**: 0.5%	In 15 mL.[1,3]
Miscellaneous Local Anesthetic Combinations *Flucaine, Rx* (OCuSOFT)	**Solution**: 0.5% proparacaine hydrochloride and 0.25% fluorescein sodium	In 5 mL.[1,5]
Altafluor, Rx (Altaire)	**Solution**: 0.4% benoxinate hydrochloride and 0.25% fluorescein sodium	In 5 mL with dropper.[1,6]
Flurox, Rx (OCuSOFT)	**Solution**: 0.4% benoxinate hydrochloride and 0.25% fluorescein sodium	In 5 mL with dropper.[1,6]
Fluress, Rx (Various, eg, Akorn)	**Solution**: 0.4% benoxinate hydrochloride and 0.25% fluorescein sodium	In 5 mL with dropper.[6]
FluraSafe, Rx (Altaire)	**Solution**: 0.4% benoxinate hydrochloride and 0.35% fluorexon disodium	In 6 mL with dropper.[1,7]

[1] Refrigerate.
[2] With benzalkonium Cl 0.01%, glycerin, and sodium Cl.
[3] With glycerin and benzalkonium Cl 0.01%.
[4] Refrigerate after opening.
[5] With glycerin, povidone, polysorbate 80, and thimerosal 0.01%.
[6] With povidone, boric acid, and chlorobutanol 1%.
[7] With povidone, boric acid, and chlorobutanol 0.5%.

Mydriatics

Generic Name *Trade Name*	Doseform/ Strength	How Supplied
Phenylephrine Hydrochloride *Phenylephrine Hydrochloride, Rx* (Various, eg, Bausch & Lomb)	**Solution**: 2.5%	In 2, 5, and 15 mL.
AK-Dilate, Rx (Akorn)	**Solution**: 2.5%	In 2 and 15 mL.[1]
Mydfrin 2.5%, Rx (Alcon)	**Solution**: 2.5%	In 3 and 5 mL *Drop-Tainers*.[2]
Neofrin 2.5%, Rx (OCuSOFT)	**Solution**: 2.5%	In 2, 5, and 15 mL.[2]
Phenylephrine Hydrochloride, Rx (Various, eg, Novartis Ophthalmic)	**Solution**: 10%	In 1, 2, and 5 mL.
AK-Dilate, Rx (Akorn)	**Solution**: 10%	In 2 and 5 mL.[1]
Neofrin 10%, Rx (OCuSOFT)	**Solution**: 10%	In 5 and 15 mL.[1]

[1] With benzalkonium chloride.
[2] With benzalkonium chloride 0.01%, EDTA, and sodium bisulfite.

Cycloplegic Mydriatics

Generic Name *Trade Name*	Doseform/ Strength	How Supplied
Atropine Sulfate *Atropine Sulfate Ophthalmic, Rx* (Various, eg, Bausch & Lomb)	**Ointment**: 1%	In 3.5 g.
Atropine Sulfate, Rx (Various, eg, Alcon, Bausch & Lomb, Fougera)	**Solution**: 1%	In 2, 5, and 15 mL.
Homatropine HBr *Isopto Homatropine, Rx* (Alcon)	**Solution**: 2%	In 5 mL *Drop-Tainers*.[1]
Homatropine HBr, Rx (Various, eg, OCuSOFT	**Solution**: 5%	In 2 and 5 mL.
AK-Homatropine, Rx (Akorn)	**Solution**: 5%	In 5 mL.
Isopto Homatropine, Rx (Alcon)	**Solution**: 5%	In 5 and 15 mL *Drop-Tainers*.[2]
Scopolamine HBr (Hyoscine HBr) *Isopto Hyoscine, Rx* (Alcon)	**Solution**: 0.25%	In 5 and 15 mL *Drop-Tainers*.[3]
Cyclopentolate Hydrochloride *Cyclogyl, Rx* (Alcon)	**Solution**: 0.5%	In 15 mL *Drop-Tainers*.[4]
Cyclopentolate Hydrochloride, Rx (Various, eg, Bausch & Lomb)	**Solution**: 1%	In 2 and 15 mL.

Cycloplegic Mydriatics

Generic Name *Trade Name*	**Doseform/ Strength**	**How Supplied**
AK-Pentolate, Rx (Akorn)	**Solution**: 1%	In 2, 5, and 15 mL.[4]
Cylate, Rx (OCuSOFT)	**Solution**: 1%	In 2 and 15 mL.[4]
Cyclogyl, Rx (Alcon)	**Solution**: 1%	In 2, 5, and 15 mL.[4]
Cyclogyl, Rx (Alcon)	**Solution**: 2%	In 2, 5, and 15 mL *Drop-Tainers*.[4]
Tropicamide		
Tropicamide, Rx (Various, eg, Bausch & Lomb, Falcon)	**Solution**: 0.5%	In 15 mL.
Mydral, Rx (OCuSOFT)	**Solution**: 0.5%	In 15 mL.[5]
Tropicacyl, Rx (Akorn)	**Solution**: 0.5%	In 2 and 15 mL.
Tropicamide, Rx (Various, eg, Falcon)	**Solution**: 1%	In 3 and 15 mL.
Mydriacyl, Rx (Alcon)	**Solution**: 1%	In 3 and 15 mL *Drop-Tainers*.[5]
Mydral, Rx (OCuSOFT)	**Solution**: 1%	In 2 and 15 mL.[5]
Tropicacyl, Rx (Akorn)	**Solution**: 1%	In 2 and 15 mL.[6]

[1] With benzalkonium chloride 0.01%, hydroxypropyl methylcellulose 0.5%, and polysorbate 80.
[2] With benzethonium chloride 0.005% and hydroxypropyl methylcellulose 0.5%.
[3] With benzalkonium chloride 0.01% and hydroxypropyl methylcellulose 0.5%.
[4] With benzalkonium chloride, EDTA, and boric acid.
[5] With benzalkonium chloride 0.01% and EDTA.
[6] With benzalkonium chloride 0.1% and EDTA.

Mydriatic Combinations

Trade Name	Doseform/Strength	How Supplied
Cyclomydril, Rx (Alcon)	**Solution**: 0.2% cyclopentolate hydrochloride and 1% phenylephrine hydrochloride	In 2 and 5 mL *Drop-Tainers*.[1]
Paremyd, Rx (Akorn)	**Solution**: 0.25% tropicamide and 1% hydroxyamphetamine HBr	In 15 mL.[2]
Murocoll-2, Rx (Bausch & Lomb)	**Drops**: 0.3% scopolamine HBr and 10% phenylephrine hydrochloride	In 5 mL.[3]

[1] With benzalkonium chloride 0.01%, EDTA, and boric acid.
[2] With benzalkonium chloride 0.005%, EDTA 0.015%, and NaCl.
[3] With benzalkonium chloride 0.01%, sodium metabisulfite, and EDTA.

Antiallergy and Decongestants

Generic Name *Trade Name*	Doseform/ Strength	How Supplied
Naphazoline Hydrochloride		
20/20 Eye Drops, otc (S.S.S.)	**Solution**: 0.012%	In 15 mL.[1]
Clear Eyes, otc (Allscripts)	**Solution**: 0.012%	In 15 mL.[2]
Naphcon, otc (Alcon)	**Solution**: 0.012%	In 15 mL.[3]
Naphazoline Hydrochloride, Rx (Various, eg, S.S.S.)	**Solution**: 0.1%	In 15 mL.
AK-Con, Rx (Various, eg, Akorn)	**Solution**: 0.1%	In 15 mL.[3]
Albalon, Rx (Allergan)	**Solution**: 0.1%	In 15 mL.[4]
Vasocon Regular, Rx (Novartis Ophthalmics)	**Solution**: 0.1%	In 15 mL.[5]
Oxymetazoline		
Visine L.R., otc (Pfizer)	**Solution**: 0.025%	In 15 and 30 mL.[6]
Phenylephrine Hydrochloride		
Relief, otc (Allergan)	**Solution**: 0.12%	Preservative free. In 15 mL.[7]
Tetrahydrozoline Hydrochloride		
Tetrahydrozoline Hydrochloride, otc (Rugby)	**Solution**: 0.05%	In 15 and 30 mL.
Collyrium Fresh, otc (Wyeth-Ayerst)	**Solution**: 0.05%	In 15 mL.[8]
Altazine Irritation Relief, otc (Altaire)	**Solution**: 0.05%	In 15 mL.[9]
Altazine Moisturizing Relief, otc (Altaire)	**Solution**: 0.05%	In 15 mL.[10]

Antiallergy and Decongestants

Generic Name *Trade Name*	Doseform/ Strength	How Supplied
Eyesine, otc (Akorn)	**Solution:** 0.05%	In 15 mL.[3]
Geneyes, otc (Ivax)	**Solution:** 0.05%	In 15 and 22.5 mL.[3]
Murine Tears Plus, otc (Prestige/ Medtech)	**Solution:** 0.05%	In 15 mL.[11]
Optigene 3, otc (Pfeiffer)	**Solution:** 0.05%	In 15 mL.[3]
Visine, otc (Various, eg, Pfizer)	**Solution:** 0.05%	In 15 and 30 mL.[3]
Visine A.C., otc (Pfizer)	**Solution:** 0.05%	In 15 mL.[12]
Visine Advanced Relief, otc (Pfizer)	**Solution:** 0.05%	In 15 and 30 mL.[13]

[1] With benzalkonium chloride 0.01%, glycerin 0.4%, zinc sulfate 0.25%, and EDTA.
[2] With benzalkonium chloride, EDTA, glycerin 0.2%, and boric acid.
[3] With benzalkonium chloride 0.01% and EDTA.
[4] With benzalkonium chloride 0.004%, EDTA, and polyvinyl alcohol 1.4%.
[5] With benzalkonium chloride, polyvinyl alcohol, EDTA, and PEG-800.
[6] With benzalkonium chloride 0.01% and EDTA 0.1%.
[7] With polyvinyl alcohol 1.4, EDTA.
[8] With benzalkonium chloride 0.01%, EDTA 0.1%, and glycerin 1%.
[9] With benzalkonium chloride and zinc sulfate 0.25%.
[10] With benzalkonium chloride, dextran 70 (1%), polyethylene glycol 400 (1%), povidone 1%.
[11] With benzalkonium chloride, EDTA, polyvinyl alcohol 1.4%, and povidone 0.6%.
[12] With benzalkonium chloride 0.01%, EDTA, and zinc sulfate 0.25%.
[13] With benzalkonium chloride, polyethylene glycol 400 1%, povidone 1%, dextran 70 (0.1%), and EDTA.

Antihistamines

Generic Name *Trade Name*	Doseform/ Strength	How Supplied
Azelastine Hydrochloride *Optivar, Rx* (MedPointe)	**Solution:** 0.05%	In 6 mL.[1]
Emedastine Difumarate *Emadine, Rx* (Alcon)	**Ophthalmic suspension:** 0.05%	In 5 mL *Drop-Tainers.*[2]
Epinastine Hydrochloride *Elestat, Rx* (Allergan)	**Solution:** 0.05%	In 5 mL opaque, white plastic bottles with dropper tips and caps.[3]
Ketotifen Fumarate *Zaditor, Rx* (Novartis)	**Solution:** 0.25 mg/mL (ketotifen fumarate 0.345 mg/mL)	In 5 mL.[4]

Antihistamines

Generic Name *Trade Name*	Doseform/ Strength	How Supplied
Olopatadine Hydrochloride		
Patanol, Rx (Alcon)	**Ophthalmic solution:** 0.1%	In 5 mL *Drop-Tainers.*[5]
Olopatadine Hydrochloride, Rx (Alcon)	**Ophthalmic solution:** 0.2%	In 2.5 mL fill in 4 mL bottle.[6]
Pataday, Rx (Alcon)	**Ophthalmic solution:** 0.2%	In 2.5 mL *Drop-Tainer.*[5]

[1] With benzalkonium chloride 0.125 mg, disodium edetate dihydrate, hydroxypropylmethylcellulose, sorbitol solution, and sodium hydroxide.
[2] With benzalkonium 0.01%, tromethamine, sodium chloride, hydroxypropylmethylcellulose, and hydrochloric acid/sodium hydroxide.
[3] With benzalkonium chloride 0.01%, EDTA, sodium chloride, sodium phosphate monobasic, hydrochloric acid/sodium hydroxide.
[4] With benzalkonium chloride 0.01%, glycerol, and sodium hydroxide/hydrochloric acid.
[5] With benzalkonium chloride 0.01%.
[6] With benzalkonium chloride 0.01%, EDTA, povidone, dibasic sodium phosphate, sodium chloride, hydrochloric acid/sodium hydroxide.

Mast Cell Inhibitors

Generic Name *Trade Name*	Doseform/ Strength	How Supplied
Cromolyn Sodium		
Cromolyn Sodium, Rx (Various, eg, Akorn)	**Solution**: 4%	In 10 and 15 mL.
Crolom, Rx (Bausch & Lomb)	**Solution**: 4%	In 10 mL bottles with controlled drop tip.[1]
Opticrom, Rx (Allergan)	**Solution**: 4%	In 10 mL opaque polyethylene eye drop bottles.[2]
Lodoxamide Tromethamine		
Alomide, Rx (Alcon)	**Solution**: 0.1%	In 10 mL *Drop-Tainers.*
Nedocromil Sodium		
Alocril, Rx (Allergan)	**Solution**: 2%	In 5 mL bottle with a controlled dropper tip.[3]
Pemirolast Potassium		
Alamast, Rx (Johnson & Johnson Vision Care)	**Solution**: 0.1%	In 10 mL bottles with a controlled dropper tip.[4]

[1] With benzalkonium chloride 0.01%, EDTA 0.1%, hydrochloric acid and/or sodium hydroxide.
[2] With benzalkonium chloride 0.01% and EDTA 0.1%.
[3] With benzalkonium chloride 0.01%, sodium chloride 0.5%, and EDTA 0.05%.
[4] With lauralkonium chloride 0.005%, glycerin, dibasic sodium phosphate, monobasic sodium phosphate, phosphoric acid, and sodium hydroxide.

Decongestants and Antihistamines

Trade Name	Decongestant	Antihistamine	How Supplied
Naphcon-A Solution, otc (Alcon)	naphazoline hydrochloride 0.025%	pheniramine maleate 0.3%	In 15 mL *Drop-Tainers.*[1]
Opcon-A Solution, otc (Bausch & Lomb)	naphazoline hydrochloride 0.027%	pheniramine maleate 0.315%	In 15 mL.[2]
Vasocon-A Solution, otc (Novartis)	naphazoline hydrochloride 0.05%	antazoline phosphate 0.5%	In 15 mL.[3]
Visine•A, otc (Visine)	naphazoline hydrochloride 0.025%	pheniramine maleate 0.3%	In 15 mL.[4]

[1] With benzalkonium chloride 0.01%, and EDTA.
[2] With hydroxypropyl methylcellulose 0.5%, benzalkonium chloride 0.01%, EDTA 0.1%, and boric acid.
[3] With benzalkonium chloride 0.01%, PEG 8000, polyvinyl alcohol, and EDTA.
[4] With benzalkonium chloride 0.01%, EDTA 0.1%, boric acid, sodium borate.

Corticosteroids

Generic Name *Trade Name*	Doseform/ Strength	How Supplied
Dexamethasone		
Dexamethasone Sodium Phosphate, Rx (Various, eg, Bausch & Lomb)	**Solution**: dexamethasone phosphate 0.01% (as sodium phosphate)	In 5 mL.
AK-Dex, Rx (Various, eg, Akorn)	**Solution**: dexamethasone phosphate 0.01% (as sodium phosphate)	In 5 mL.[1]
Maxidex, Rx (Alcon)	**Suspension**: dexamethasone 0.1%	In 5 and 15 mL *Drop-Tainers.*[2]
Fluorometholone		
FML, Rx (Allergan)	**Suspension**: fluorometholone alcohol 0.1%	In 1, 5, 10, and 15 mL.[3]
Flarex, Rx (Alcon)	**Suspension**: fluorometholone acetate 0.1%	In 5 mL *Drop-Tainers.*[4]
eFLone, Rx (Novartis)	**Suspension**: fluorometholone acetate 0.1%	In 5 and 10 mL.[4]
FML Forte, Rx (Various, eg, Allergan)	**Suspension**: fluorometholone alcohol 0.25%	In 5, 10, and 15 mL.[5]
FML S.O.P., Rx (Various, eg, Allergan)	**Ointment**: 0.1%	In 3.5 g.[6]

Corticosteroids

Generic Name *Trade Name*	**Doseform/ Strength**	**How Supplied**
Loteprednol Etabonate		
Alrex, Rx (Bausch & Lomb)	**Suspension**: 0.2%	In 5 and 10 mL.[7]
Lotemax, Rx (Bausch & Lomb)	**Suspension**: 0.5%	In 2.5, 5, 10, and 15 mL.[7]
Prednisolone		
Pred Mild, Rx (Allergan)	**Suspension**: prednisolone acetate 0.12%	In 5 and 10 mL.[8]
Econopred Plus, Rx (Alcon)	**Suspension**: prednisolone acetate 1%	In 5 and 10 mL *Drop-Tainers*.[9]
Pred Forte, Rx (Allergan)	**Suspension**: prednisolone acetate 1%	In 1, 5, 10, and 15 mL.[8]
Prednisolone Acetate Ophthalmic, Rx (Falcon)	**Suspension**: prednisolone acetate 1%	In 5 and 10 mL.[9]
Prednisolone Sodium Phosphate, Rx (Various, eg, Bausch & Lomb)	**Solution**: prednisolone sodium phosphate 1%	In 5, 10, and 15 mL.
Rimexolone		
Vexol, Rx (Alcon)	**Suspension**: 1%	In 5 and 10 mL *Drop-Tainers*.

[1] With benzalkonium chloride 0.01%, EDTA, and hydroxyethylcellulose.
[2] With benzalkonium chloride 0.01%, EDTA, hydroxypropyl methylcellulose 0.5%, and polysorbate 80.
[3] With benzalkonium chloride 0.004%, EDTA, polysorbate 80, and polyvinyl alcohol 1.4%.
[4] With benzalkonium chloride 0.01%, EDTA, hydroxyethylcellulose, and tyloxapol.
[5] With benzalkonium chloride 0.005%, EDTA, polysorbate 80, and polyvinyl alcohol 1.4%.
[6] With phenylmercuric acetate 0.0008%, white petrolatum, mineral oil, petrolatum, and lanolin alcohol.
[7] With EDTA, glycerin, povidone, and tyloxapol.
[8] With benzalkonium chloride 0.01%, EDTA, polysorbate 80, hydroxypropyl methylcellulose, and glycerin.
[9] With benzalkonium chloride 0.01%, EDTA, hydroxypropyl methylcellulose, and sodium bisulfite.

Nonsteroidal Anti-Inflammatory Agents (NSAIDs)

Generic Name *Trade Name*	**Doseform/ Strength**	**How Supplied**
Bromfenac		
Xibrom, Rx (Bausch & Lomb)	**Solution**: 0.09%	In 5 mL dropper bottles.[1]
Diclofenac Sodium		
Voltaren, Rx (Novartis)	**Solution**: 0.1%	In 2.5 and 5 mL dropper bottles.[2]
Flurbiprofen Sodium		
Ocufen, Rx (Allergan)	**Solution**: 0.03%	In 2.5 mL dropper bottles.[3]
Flurbiprofen Sodium Ophthalmic, Rx (Various, eg, Bausch & Lomb)	**Solution**: 0.03%	In 2.5 mL.[3]

Nonsteroidal Anti-Inflammatory Agents (NSAIDs)

Generic Name *Trade Name*	Doseform/ Strength	How Supplied
Ketorolac Tromethamine		
Acular LS, Rx (Allergan)	**Solution**: 0.4%	In 5 mL dropper bottles.[4]
Acular, Rx (Allergan)	**Solution**: 0.5%	In 5 mL dropper bottles.[5]
Acular PF, Rx (Allergan)	**Solution**: 0.5%	In 12 single-use 0.4 mL vials.[6]
Nepafenac		
Nevanac, Rx (Alcon)	**Solution**: 0.1%	In 3 mL.

[1] With benzalkonium chloride 0.05 mg/mL, EDTA 0.2 mg/mL, povidone 20 mg/mL, and sodium hydroxide.
[2] With EDTA 1 mg/mL, boric acid, polyoxyl 35 castor oil, sorbic acid 2 mg/mL, and tromethamine.
[3] With polyvinyl alcohol 1.4%, thimerosal 0.005%, and EDTA.
[4] With benzalkonium chloride 0.006%, EDTA 0.015%, octoxynol 40.
[5] With benzalkonium chloride 0.01%, EDTA 0.1%, and octoxynol 40.
[6] With ketorolac tromethamine 0.5%.

Immunomodulators

Generic Name *Trade Name*	Doseform/ Strength	How Supplied
Cyclosporine *Restasis, Rx* (Allergan)	**Emulsion**: 0.05%	In 0.4 mL fill in a 0.9 mL single-use vial. In 32s.[1]

[1] With glycerin and polysorbate 80.

Artificial Tear Solutions

Trade Name	Doseform/Strength	How Supplied
20/20 Tears, otc (S.S.S.)	**Solution**: PVA 1.4%, benzalkonium Cl 0.01%, EDTA 0.05%, KCl, NaCl	Thimerosal free. In 15 mL.
Akwa Tears, otc (Akorn)	**Solution**: PVA 1.4%, benzalkonium Cl 0.005%, EDTA, NaCl, sodium phosphate	In 15 mL.
Artificial Tears, otc (Various, eg, Rugby, United)	**Solution**: PVA 1.4%, benzalkonium Cl 0.01%, EDTA, NaCl, KCl	In 15 mL.
Bion Tears, otc (Alcon)	**Solution**: dextran 70 (0.1%), hydroxypropyl methylcellulose 2910 (0.3%), sodium hydroxide, carbon dioxide, hydrochloric acid	Preservative free. In 0.45 mL (UD 28s).
Celluvisc, otc (Allergan)	**Solution**: carboxymethylcellulose 1%, calcium chloride, NaCl, KCl, sodium lactate	Preservative free. In 0.1 mL (UD 30s).
Dry Eye Therapy, otc (Bausch & Lomb)	**Solution**: glycerin 0.3%, NaCl, KCl, sodium citrate, sodium phosphate	Preservative free. In 3 mL.

Artificial Tear Solutions

Trade Name	Doseform/Strength	How Supplied
FreshKote, otc (Focus Laboratories)	**Solution**: PVP 2%, PVA 0.9% and 1.8%, Amisol clear, NaCl, KCl, boric acid, EDTA, polixetonium	In 3.5 and 15 mL.
GenTeal Mild, otc (Novartis)	**Solution**: hydroxypropyl methylcellulose 0.2%, boric acid, NaCl, KCl, phosphoric acid, sodium perborate, calcium chloride dihydrate	In 15 and 25 mL.
HypoTears, otc (Novartis)	**Solution**: PVA 1%, PEG-400 1%, benzalkonium Cl 0.01%, dextrose, EDTA	In 15 and 30 mL.
Isopto Tears, otc (Alcon)	**Solution**: hydroxypropyl methylcellulose 2910 (0.5%), benzalkonium C 0.01%l, NaCl, sodium phosphate, sodium citrate	In 15 mL.
Moisture Eyes, otc (Bausch & Lomb)	**Solution**: propylene glycol 1%, glycerin 0.3%, benzalkonium Cl 0.01%, boric acid, NaCl, KCl, sodium borate, EDTA	In 10 mL.
Moisture Eyes Preservative Free, otc (Bausch & Lomb)	**Solution**: propylene glycol 1%	In 0.6 mL (UD 32s).
Moisture Eyes Liquid Gel, otc (Bausch & Lomb)	**Solution**: dextran 70 (0.1%), hypromellos 0.8%	In 15 and 30 mL.
Moisture Eyes Liquid Gel Preservative Free, otc (Bausch & Lomb)	**Solution**: dextran 70 (0.1%), hypromellos 0.8%	In 0.5 mL (UD 28s).
Murine Tears For Dry Eyes, otc (Prestige/ Medtech)	**Solution**: PVP 0.6%, PVA 0.5%, benzalkonium Cl, dextrose, EDTA, NaCl, sodium bicarbonate, sodium phosphate, KCl, sodium citrate	In 15 and 30 mL.
Murocel, otc (Bausch & Lomb)	**Solution**: methylcellulose, propylene glycol 1%, NaCl, methylparaben 0.028%, propylparaben 0.012%, boric acid, sodium borate	In 15 mL.
Optive, otc (Allergan)	**Solution**: CMC 0.5%, glycerin 0.9%, in *Purite*	In 15 and 30 mL.
Puralube Tears, otc (Fougera)	**Solution**: PVA 1%, PEG-400 1%, EDTA, benzalkonium Cl	In 15 mL.
Refresh, otc (Allergan)	**Solution**: PVA 1.4%, PVP 0.6%, NaCl	Preservative free. In 0.3 mL (UD 30s and 50s).

Artificial Tear Solutions

Trade Name	Doseform/Strength	How Supplied
Refresh Endura, otc (Allergan)	**Solution**: glycerin 1%, polysorbate 80 (1%)	Preservative free. In 0.4 mL single-use containers (20s).
Refresh Plus, otc (Allergan)	**Solution**: carboxymethylcellulose sodium 0.5%, KCl, NaCl, calcium chloride, magnesium chloride, sodium lactate	Preservative free. In 0.3 mL (UD 30s, 50s, and 70s).
Refresh Tears, otc (Allergan)	**Solution**: carboxymethylcellulose sodium 0.5%, boric acid, calcium chloride, magnesium chloride, KCl, NaCl, stabilized oxychloro complex	*Purite* preservative. In 3, 15, and 30 mL and 30 mL twin pack.
Soothe, otc (Alimera Sciences)	**Solution**: *Testoryl* (*Drakeol-15* and *Drakeol-35* 4.5%), polysorbate 80 (0.4%), octoxynol 40, NaCl, sodium phosphate, EDTA, polyhexamethylene biguanide preservative	In 15 mL.
Systane, otc (Alcon)	**Solution**: PEG-400 (0.4%), propylene glycol 0.3%, boric acid, calcium chloride, hydroxypropyl guar, magnesium chloride, polyquaternium preservative, KCl, NaCl, zinc chloride	In 15 and 30 mL.
Teargen II, otc (Zenith-Goldline)	**Solution**: hydroxypropyl methylcellulose 2910 (0.4%), benzalkonium Cl 0.01%, sodium phosphate, EDTA, KCl, NaCl	In 15 mL.
Tears Again Eye Drops, otc (OCuSOFT)	**Solution**: polyvinyl alcohol 1.4%, benzalkonium chloride 0.01%, sodium phosphate, EDTA, NaCl, phosphoric acid	In 15 mL.
Tears Again Gel Drops, otc (OCuSOFT)	**Solution**: carboxymethyl cellulose 0.7%, boric acid, phosphoric acid, NaCl, potassium chloride, carbopol 940, dissipate preservative (stabilized peroxy-complex)	In 15 mL.
Tears Again MC, otc (OCuSOFT)	**Solution**: hydroxypropyl methylcellulose 0.3%, boric acid, phosphoric acid, KCl	Preservative free. In 15 mL.
Tears Naturale II, otc (Alcon)	**Solution**: hydroxypropyl methylcellulose 2910 (0.3%), dextran 70 (0.1%), polyquarternium-1 (0.001%), NaCl, KCl, sodium borate	In 15 and 30 mL *Drop-Tainers*.
Tears Naturale Forte, otc (Alcon)	**Solution**: dextran 70 (0.1%), hydroxypropyl methylcellulose 0.3%, glycerin 0.2%, polyquaternium-1 (0.001%), NaCl, KCl, sodium borate	In 15 and 30 mL.

Artificial Tear Solutions

Trade Name	Doseform/Strength	How Supplied
Tears Naturale Free, otc (Alcon)	**Solution**: hydroxypropyl methylcellulose 2910 (0.3%), dextran 70 (0.1%)	Preservative free. In 0.6 mL (UD 36s and 60s).
Tears Plus, otc (Allergan)	**Solution**: PVA 1.4%, PVP 0.6%, chlorobutanol 0.5%, NaCl	In 15 and 30 mL.
Tears Renewed, otc (Akorn)	**Solution**: hydroxypropyl methylcellulose 2906 (0.3%), benzalkonium Cl 0.01%, EDTA, dextran 70 (0.1%), NaCl, hydrochloric acid, KCl, NaCl, sodium hydroxide	In 15 mL.
TheraTears, otc (Advanced Vision)	**Gel**: sodium carboxymethylcellulose 1%, borate buffers, calcium chloride, magnesium chloride, KCl, sodium bicarbonate, NaCl, sodium phosphate	In 17 mL.
TheraTears, otc (Advanced Vision)	**Solution**: sodium carboxymethylcellulose 0.25%, borate buffers, calcium chloride, KCl, magnesium chloride, NaCl, sodium bicarbonate, sodium phosphate	Preservative free. In 15 and 30 mL.
Visine Tears, otc (Pfizer)	**Solution**: PEG-400 (1%), hydroxypropyl methylcellulose 0.2%, glycerin 0.2%, ascorbic acid, benzalkonium Cl, boric acid, dextrose, disodium phosphate, glycine, KCl, magnesium chloride, NaCl, sodium borate, sodium citrate, sodium lactate	In 15 mL.
Visine Pure Tears, otc (Pfizer)	**Solution**: PEG-400 (1%), hypromellose 0.2%, glycerin 0.2%	In 9.5 mL single-drop dispenser.
Viva-Drops, otc (Vision Pharm)	**Solution**: Polysorbate 80, citric acid, NaCl, EDTA, retinyl palmitate, mannitol, sodium citrate, pyruvate	Preservative free. In 10 and 15 mL.
Zi, otc (Rohto)	**Solution**: PVP 1.8%, alcohol 0.1%, benzalkonium chloride, boric acid, NaCl, KCl, poloxamer 407, polysorbate 80, sodium borate	In 13 mL.

Ocular Lubricants, Ointments and Gels

Trade Name	Doseform/Strength	How Supplied
GenTeal Gel, otc (Novartis)	**Gel**: hydroxypropyl methylcellulose 0.3%, sodium perborate 0.028%, carbopol 980, phosphoric acid, sorbitol	In 10 mL.
Refresh Liquigel, otc (Allergan)	**Gel**: carboxymethylcellulose 1%, *Purite* (stabilized oxychloro complex)	In 15 and 30 mL.
Tears Again Night & Day, otc (OCuSOFT)	**Gel**: carboxymethylcellulose sodium 1.5%, povidone 0.1%(polyvinylpyrrolidone)	In 3.5 g.
Tears Again Preservative Free, otc (OCuSOFT)	**Gel**: carboxymethyl cellulose 1.5%	Preservative free. In 3.5 g
Akwa Tears, otc (Akorn)	**Ointment**: white petrolatum, mineral oil, lanolin	Preservative free. In 3.5 g.
Artificial Tears, otc (Rugby)	**Ointment**: white petrolatum 83%, mineral oil 15%, lanolin oil	In 3.5 g.
Lacri-Lube S.O.P., otc (Allergan)	**Ointment**: white petrolatum 56.8%, mineral oil 42.5%, chlorobutanol, lanolin alcohols	In 3.5, and 7 g.
Moisture Eyes PM, otc (Bausch & Lomb)	**Ointment**: white petrolatum 80%, mineral oil 20%	Preservative free. In 3.5 g.
Puralube, otc (Fougera)	**Ointment**: white petrolatum, light mineral oil	In 3.5 g.
Refresh PM, otc (Allergen)	**Ointment**: white petrolatum 56.8%, mineral oil 41.5%, lanolin alcohols, NaCl	Preservative free. In 3.5 g.
Stye, otc (Del Pharm)	**Ointment**: white petrolatum 57.7%, mineral oil 31.9%, stearic acid, wheat germ oil, microcrystalline wax	In 3.5 g.
Tears Again Ointment, otc (OCuSOFT)	**Ointment**: white petrolatum, mineral oil	In 3.5 g.
Tears Naturale P.M., otc (Alcon)	**Ointment**: white petrolatum, anhydrous liquid lanolin, mineral oil	Preservative free. In 3.5 g.
Tears Renewed, otc (Akorn)	**Ointment**: white petrolatum, light mineral oil	Preservative free. In 3.5 g.
Tears Again Liposome Spray, otc (OCuSOFT)	**Spray**: purified water, lecithin, ethanol 1%, vitamin A, vitamin E, NaCl, phenoxyethanol 0.5%	In 10 mL.

Artificial Tear Insert

Trade Name	Doseform/Strength	How Supplied
Lacrisert, Rx (Merck & Co.)	**Insert**: hydroxypropyl cellulose 5 mg	Preservative free. In 60s with applicator.

Collagen Implants

Trade Name	Doseform/Strength	How Supplied
Collagen Implant, Rx (Lacrimedics)	**Implant**: collagen implant	In 0.3, 0.4, and 0.5 mm sizes.
TearSaver, Rx (Ciba Vision)	**Implant**: collagen implant	In 0.2, 0.3, and 0.4 mm sizes.
Temporary Punctal/ Canalicular Collagen Implant, Rx (Eagle Vision)	**Implant**: collagen implant	In 0.2, 0.3, and 0.4 mm sizes (60s).

Cleaning/Lubricant for Artificial Eyes

Generic Name *Trade Name*	Doseform/ Strength	How Supplied
Tyloxapol		
Enuclene, otc (Alcon)	**Solution**: 0.25%[1]	In 15 mL *Drop-Tainers*.

[1] With benzalkonium Cl 0.02.

Antibiotics

Generic Name *Trade Name*	Doseform/ Strength	How Supplied
Bacitracin		
Bacitracin, Rx (Various, eg, Fougera)	**Ointment**: 500 units/g	In 3.5 and 3.75 g.
Erythromycin		
Erythromycin, Rx (Various, eg, Akorn)	**Ointment**: 5 mg/g	In 3.5 g.
Romycin, Rx (OCuSOFT)	**Ointment**: 5 mg/g	In 3.5 g.[1]
Gentamicin Sulfate		
Gentamicin Ophthalmic, Rx (Various, eg, Akorn)	**Solution**: 3 mg/mL	In 5 and 15 mL.
Gentak, Rx (Akorn)	**Solution**: 0.3%	In 5 mL dropper bottles.[2]
Gentamicin Ophthalmic, Rx (Various, eg, Akorn)	**Ointment**: 0.3%	In 3.5 g.
Gentak, Rx (Akorn)	**Ointment**: 3 mg/g	In 3.5 g.[3]

Antibiotics

Generic Name *Trade Name*	**Doseform/ Strength**	**How Supplied**
Tobramycin		
Tobramycin, Rx (Various, eg, Bausch & Lomb)	**Solution**: 0.3%	In 5 mL bottle.
AKTob, Rx (Akorn)	**Solution**: 0.3%	In 5 mL.[4]
Tobrasol, Rx (OCuSOFT)	**Solution**: 0.3%	In 5 mL.[4]
Tobrex, Rx (Alcon)	**Solution**: 0.3%	In 5 mL *Drop-Tainers*.[5]
Tobrex, Rx (Alcon)	**Ointment**: 3 mg/g	In 3.5 g.[6]
Ciprofloxacin		
Ciprofloxacin, Rx, (Various, eg, Falcon)	**Solution**: 0.3% (equivalent to 3 mg base)	In 2.5, 5, and 10 mL bottles.
Ciloxan, Rx (Alcon)		In 5 and 10 mL *Drop-Tainers*.[7]
Ciloxan, Rx (Alcon)	**Ointment**: 0.3% (equivalent to 3 mg base)	In 3.5 g tube.[1]
Ofloxacin		
Ofloxacin, Rx (Various, eg, Bausch & Lomb, Falcon, Pacific Pharma)	**Solution**: 0.3%	In 5 and 10 mL.
Ocuflox, Rx (Allergan)	**Solution**: 0.3%	In 5 mL.[8]
Levofloxacin		
Quixin, Rx (Santen/J&J Vista-kon)	**Solution**: 0.5%	In 5 mL.[8]
Moxifloxacin Hydrochloride		
Vigamox, Rx (Alcon)	**Solution**: 0.5%	Preservative free. In 3 mL *Drop-Tainers*.[9]
Gatifloxacin		
Zymar, Rx (Allergan)	**Solution**: 0.3%	In 5 mL bottles.[10]

[1] With white petrolatum and mineral oil.
[2] With benzalkonium chloride 0.1 mg/mL, disodium phosphate 1.4%, NaCl, monosodium phosphate.
[3] With white petrolatum.
[4] With benzalkonium chloride 0.01%, boric acid, and sodium sulfate.
[5] With benzalkonium chloride, tyloxapol, boric acid, and NaCl.
[6] With white petrolatum, mineral oil, and chlorobutanol 0.5%.
[7] With benzalkonium chloride 0.006%, mannitol 4.6%, and EDTA 0.05%.
[8] With benzalkonium chloride 0.005% and NaCl.
[9] With boric acid, NaCl, and purified water.
[10] With benzalkonium chloride 0.005%, EDTA, and NaCl. May contain hydrochloric acid and/or sodium hydroxide.

Combination Antibiotics

Trade Name	Antibiotics	How Supplied
Bacitracin Zinc-Neomycin-Polymyxin B Ointment, Rx (Various, eg, Bausch and Lomb)	Polymyxin B Sulfate (units/g or mL): 10,000 Neomycin Sulfate (mg/g or mL): 3.5 Bacitracin Zinc (units/g): 400	In 3.5 g.
Neomycin Sulfate-Polymyxin B Sulfate-Gramicidin Solution, Rx (Various, eg, Bausch and Lomb, URL)	Polymyxin B Sulfate (units/g or mL): 10,000 Neomycin Sulfate (mg/g or mL): 1.75 Gramicidin: 0.025 mg/mL	In 2 and 10 mL.
Neosporin Ophthalmic Solution, Rx (Monarch)	Polymyxin B Sulfate (units/g or mL): 10,000 Neomycin Sulfate (mg/g or mL): 1.75 Gramicidin: 0.025 mg/mL	In 10 mL *Drop Dose.*[1]
Bacitracin Zinc and Polymyxin B Ointment, Rx (Bausch & Lomb)	Polymyxin B Sulfate (units/g or mL): 10,000 Bacitracin Zinc (units/g): 500	White petrolatum and mineral oil. In 3.5 g.
AK-Poly-Bac Ointment, Rx (Akorn)	Polymyxin B Sulfate (units/g or mL): 10,000 Bacitracin Zinc (units/g): 500	Preservative free. White petrolatum, mineral oil. In 3.5 g.
Terramycin w/Polymyxin B Ointment, Rx (Roerig)	Polymyxin B Sulfate (units/g or mL): 10,000 Oxytetracycline hydrochloride: 5 mg/g	White and liquid petrolatum. In 3.5 g.
Trimethoprim Sulfate and Polymyxin B Sulfate Ophthalmic Solution, Rx (Various, eg, Falcon)	Polymyxin B Sulfate (units/g or mL): 10,000 Trimethoprim: 1 mg/mL	In 10 mL.[2]
Polytrim Ophthalmic Solution, Rx (Allergan)	Polymyxin B Sulfate (units/g or mL): 10,000 Trimethoprim: 1 mg/mL	In 10 mL.[2]

[1] With thimerosal 0.001%, alcohol 0.5%, propylene glycol, and NaCl
[2] With benzalkonium chloride 0.004%, sodium hydroxide, and NaCl.

Sulfonamides

Generic Name *Trade Name*	**Doseform/ Strength**	**How Supplied**
Sulfacetamide Sodium *Sulster, Rx* (Akorn)	**Solution**: 1%	In 5 and 10 mL.
Sulfacetamide Sodium, Rx (Various, eg, Bausch & Lomb)	**Solution**: 10%	In 15 mL.
AK-Sulf, Rx (Akorn)	**Solution**: 10%	In 2, 5, and 15 mL.[1]
Bleph-10, Rx (Allergan)	**Solution**: 10%	In 5 mL.[2]

Sulfonamides

Generic Name *Trade Name*	**Doseform/ Strength**	**How Supplied**
Sulf-10, Rx (Novartis)	**Solution:** 10%	In 1 mL *Dropperettes.*[3]
Sulfacetamide Sodium, Rx (Various, eg, Fougera)	**Ointment:** 10%	In 3.5 g.
AK-Sulf, Rx (Akorn)	**Ointment:** 10%	In 3.5 g.[4]
Bleph-10, Rx (Allergan)	**Ointment:** 10%	In 3.5 g.[5]

[1] With sodium thiosulfate pentahydrate 3.1 mg, methylcellulose 5 mg, methylparaben 0.5 mg, and propylparaben 0.1 mg per mL.
[2] With polyvinyl alcohol 1.4%, benzalkonium chloride 0.005%, polysorbate 80, sodium thiosulfate, and EDTA.
[3] With sodium thiosulfate, thimerosal 0.005%, and boric acid.
[4] With methylparaben 0.5 mg, propylparaben 0.1 mg, benzalkonium chloride 0.25 mg, and petrolatum base per g.
[5] With phenylmercuric acetate 0.0008%, white petrolatum, mineral oil, petrolatum, and lanolin alcohol.

Steroid and Sulfonamide Combinations, Suspensions and Solutions

Trade Name	**Steroid**	**Sulfonamide**	**How Supplied**
FML-S Suspension, Rx (Allergan)	fluorometholone 0.1%	sodium sulfacetamide 10%	In 5 and 10 mL.[1]
Blephamide Suspension, Rx (Allergan)	prednisolone acetate 0.2%	sodium sulfacetamide 10%	In 5 and 10 mL.[2]
AK-Cide Suspension, Rx (Akorn)	prednisolone acetate 0.5%	sodium sulfacetamide 10%	In 5 mL dropper bottle.[3]
Sulfacetamide Sodium and Prednisolone Sodium Phosphate Solution, Rx (Various, eg, Falcon)	prednisolone sodium phosphate 0.25%	sodium sulfacetamide 10%	In 5 and 10 mL.[4]
Sulster Solution, Rx (Akorn)			In 5 and 10 mL.[5]

[1] With EDTA, polyvinyl alcohol 1.4%, benzalkonium chloride 0.006%, polysorbate 80, povidone, sodium thiosulfate, and sodium chloride.
[2] With EDTA, polyvinyl alcohol 1.4%, polysorbate 80, sodium thiosulfate, and benzalkonium chloride.
[3] With phenethyl alcohol 5 mg, tyloxapol, sodium thiosulfate, benzalkonium chloride 0.25 mg, and EDTA per mL.
[4] With phenylethyl alcohol 0.5%, benzalkonium chloride 0.025%, sodium thiosulfate, EDTA, and tyloxapol.
[5] With thimerosal 0.01% mg and EDTA.

Steroid and Sulfonamide Combinations, Ointments

Trade Name	Steroid	Sulfonamide	How Supplied
Blephamide S.O.P., Rx (Allergan)	prednisolone acetate 0.2%	sodium sulfacetamide 10%	In 3.5 g.[1]
AK-Cide, Rx (Akorn)	prednisolone acetate 0.5%	sodium sulfacetamide 10%	In 3.5 g applicator tube.[2]
Vasocine, Rx (Novartis)			In 3.5 g.[3]

[1] With phenylmercuric acetate 0.0008%, mineral oil, white petrolatum, and lanolin alcohol.
[2] With methylparaben 0.5 mg, propylparaben 0.1 mg per g, mineral oil, and white petrolatum.
[3] With mineral oil and white petrolatum.

Steroid and Antibiotic Ointments

Trade Name	Steroid (per g)	Antibiotic (per g)	How Supplied
Bacitracin Zinc/ Neomycin Sulfate/ Polymyxin B Sulfate/ Hydrocortisone, Rx (Various, eg, Fougera)	hydrocortisone 1%	Neomycin sulfate equivalent to neomycin base 0.35%, bacitracin zinc 400 units, polymyxin B sulfate 10,000 units	In 3.5 g.
Cortisporin, Rx (Monarch)			In 3.5 g.[1]
Pred-G S.O.P., Rx (Allergan)	prednisolone acetate 0.6%	Gentamicin sulfate equivalent to gentamicin base 0.3%	In 3.5 g.[2]
Neomycin/Polymyxin B Sulfate/ Dexamethasone, Rx (Various, eg, Bausch & Lomb)	dexamethasone 0.1%	Neomycin sulfate equivalent to neomycin base 0.35%, polymyxin B sulfate 10,000 units.	In 3.5 g.
AK-Trol, Rx (Akorn)			In 3.5 g.[3]

[1] With white petrolatum.
[2] With chlorobutanol 0.5%, white petrolatum, mineral oil, petrolatum, and lanolin alcohol.
[3] With white petrolatum, lanolin oil, mineral oil, and parabens.

Steroid and Antibiotic Solutions and Suspensions

Trade Name	Steroid (per mL)	Antibiotic (per mL)	How Supplied
Neomycin/Polymyxin B Sulfate/Hydrocortisone, Rx (Various, eg, Falcon)	hydrocortisone 1%	Neomycin sulfate equivalent to neomycin base 0.35%, polymyxin B sulfate 10,000 units	In 10 mL.

Steroid and Antibiotic Solutions and Suspensions

Trade Name	Steroid (per mL)	Antibiotic (per mL)	How Supplied
AK-Spore H.C. Ophthalmic Suspension, Rx (Akorn)			In 7.5 mL.[1]
Cortisporin Suspension, Rx (Monarch)			In 7.5 mL *Drop Dose.*[2]
Poly-Pred Suspension, Rx (Allergan)	prednisolone acetate 0.5%	Neomycin sulfate equivalent to neomycin base 0.35%, polymyxin B sulfate 10,000 units	In 5 mL.[3]
Pred-G Suspension, Rx (Allergan)	prednisolone acetate 1%	Gentamicin sulfate equivalent to gentamicin base 0.3%	In 5 and 10 mL.[1]
Neomycin Sulfate/ Dexamethasone Sodium Phosphate Solution, Rx (Various)	dexamethasone phosphate 0.1% (as sodium phosphate)	Neomycin sulfate equivalent to neomycin base 0.35%	In 5 mL.
TobraDex Suspension, Rx (Alcon)	dexamethasone 0.1%	tobramycin 0.3%	In 2.5, 5, and 10 mL *Drop-Tainers.*[4]
Neomycin/Polymyxin B Sulfate/ Dexamethasone Suspension, Rx (Various, eg, Falcon, Fougera, Major)	dexamethasone 0.1%	neomycin sulfate equivalent to neomycin base 0.35%, polymyxin B sulfate 10,000 units	In 5 mL.
AK-Trol Suspension, Rx (Akorn)			In 5 mL.[5]
Maxitrol Suspension, Rx (Alcon)			In 5 mL *Drop-Tainers.*[6]
Poly-Dex Suspension, Rx (OCuSOFT)			In 5 mL *Drop-Tainers.*[7]
Zylet Suspension, Rx (Bausch and Lomb)	loteprednol etabonate 0.5%	tobramycin 0.3%	In 2.5, 5, and 10 mL.[8]

[1] With polyvinyl alcohol 1.4%, benzalkonium chloride 0.005%, EDTA, hydroxypropyl methylcellulose, polysorbate 80, and NaCl.
[2] With thimerosal 0.001%, cetyl alcohol, glyceryl monostearate, polyoxyl 40 stearate, propylene glycol, mineral oil, and NaCl.
[3] With polyvinyl alcohol 1.4%, thimerosal 0.001%, polysorbate 80, and propylene glycol.
[4] With benzalkonium chloride 0.01%, tyloxapol, EDTA, hydroxyethylcellulose, sodium sulfate, and NaCl.
[5] With benzalkonium chloride 0.004%, polysorbate 20, hydroxypropyl methylcellulose 0.5%, and NaCl.
[6] With hydroxypropyl methylcellulose 0.5%, polysorbate 20, benzalkonium chloride 0.004%.
[7] With hydroxypropyl methylcellulose, benzalkonium chloride 0.004%.
[8] With edetate disodium, glycerin, povidone, tyloxapol, benzalkonium chloride 0.01%.

Antiviral and Antifungal Agents

Generic Name *Trade Name*	Doseform/ Strength	How Supplied
Natamycin *Natacyn, Rx* (Alcon)	**Suspension**: 5%	With 0.02% benzalkonium. In 15 mL.
Trifluridine (Trifluorothymidine) *Viroptic, Rx* (Monarch)	**Solution**: 1%	In aqueous solution with NaCl and 0.001% thimerosal. In 7.5 mL *Drop-Dose.*

Anti-infective Agents

Generic Name *Trade Name*	Doseform/ Strength	How Supplied
Zinc Sulfate Solution *20/20 Eye Drops, otc* (S. S. S.)	**Solution**: 0.25%	In 15 mL.[1]
Clear Eyes ACR Eye Drops, otc (Prestige/Medtech)	**Solution**: 0.25%	In 15 and 30 mL.[2]
Visine A.C., otc (Pfizer)	**Solution**: 0.25%	In 15 mL.[3]

[1] With glycerin 0.4%, naphazoline hydrochloride 0.12%, EDTA, KCl, and camphor.
[2] With glycerin 0.2%, naphazoline hydrochloride 0.12%, benzalkonium chloride, boric acid, EDTA, NaCl, and sodium citrate.
[3] With tetrahydrozoline hydrochloride 0.05%, EDTA, boric acid, and NaCl.

Epinephrines

Generic Name *Trade Name*	Doseform/ Strength	How Supplied
Dipivefrin Hydrochloride (Dipivalyl epinephrine) *Dipivefrin Hydrochloride, Rx* (Falcon)	**Solution**: 0.1%	In 5, 10, and 15 mL.
Propine, Rx (Allergan)	**Solution**: 0.1%	In 10 and 15 mL.[1]

[1] With benzalkonium chloride 0.005%, sodium chloride, EDTA, and hydrochloric acid.

Alpha-2 Adrenergic Agonists

Generic Name *Trade Name*	Doseform/ Strength	How Supplied
Apraclonidine Hydrochloride *Iopidine, Rx* (Alcon)	**Solution**: 0.5%	With 0.01% benzalkonium chloride. In 5 and 10 mL *Drop-Tainers.*
Iopidine, Rx (Alcon)	**Solution**: 1%	With 0.01% benzalkonium chloride. In 0.1 mL.

Alpha-2 Adrenergic Agonists

Generic Name *Trade Name*	**Doseform/ Strength**	**How Supplied**
Brimonidine Tartrate		
Brimonidine Tartrate, Rx (Bausch & Lomb)	**Solution:** 0.2%	With citric acid, polyvinyl alcohol, NaCl, sodium citrate. In 5, 10, and 15 mL bottles.
Alphagan P, Rx (Allergan)	**Solution:** 0.15%	With sodium borate, boric acid, NaCl, KCl. In 5, 10, and 15 mL dropper bottles.

Beta-Adrenergic Blocking Agents

Generic Name *Trade Name*	**Doseform/ Strength**	**How Supplied**
Betaxolol Hydrochloride		
Betoptic S, Rx (Alcon)	**Suspension:** 2.8 mg (equivalent to 2.5 mg base) per mL (0.25%)	In 2.5, 5, 10, and 15 mL *Drop-Tainers.*[1]
Carteolol Hydrochloride		
Ocupress, Rx (Novartis)	**Solution:** 1%	In 5, 10 and 15 mL dropper bottles.[2]
Levobunolol Hydrochloride		
Levobunolol, Rx (Various, eg, Bausch & Lomb)	**Solution:** 0.25%	In 5 and 10 mL.
Betagan Liquifilm, Rx (Allergan)	**Solution:** 0.25%	In 5 and 10 mL dropper bottles with *B.I.D. C Cap.*[3]
Levobunolol, Rx (Various, eg, Bausch & Lomb)	**Solution:** 0.5%	In 5, 10, and 15 mL.
Betagan Liquifilm, Rx (Allergan)	**Solution:** 0.5%	In 2, 5, 10, and 15 mL bottles with *B.I.D.* and *Q.D. C Cap.*[3]
Metipranolol Hydrochloride		
OptiPranolol, Rx (Bausch & Lomb)	**Solution:** 0.3%	In 5 or 10 mL dropper bottles.[4]
Timolol Hemihydrate		
Betimol, Rx (Johnson & Johnson Vision Care)	**Solution:** 0.25%	In 2.5, 5, 10, and 15 mL.[5]
Betimol, Rx (Johnson & Johnson Vision Care)	**Solution:** 0.5%	In 2.5, 5, 10, and 15 mL.[5]
Timolol Maleate		
Timolol Maleate, Rx (Various, eg, Falcon)	**Solution:** 0.25%	In 5, 10, and 15 mL.
Timoptic, Rx (Merck)	**Solution:** 0.25%	In 2.5, 5, 10, and 15 mL *Ocumeters.*[6]

Beta-Adrenergic Blocking Agents

Generic Name *Trade Name*	**Doseform/ Strength**	**How Supplied**
Timolol Maleate, Rx (Various, eg, Falcon)	**Solution**: 0.5%	In 5, 10, and 15 mL.
Timoptic, Rx (Merck)	**Solution**: 0.5%	Preservative free. In UD 60s *Ocudose.*[7]
Timoptic, Rx (Merck)	**Solution**: 0.5%	In 2.5 mL *Ocumeters.*[6]
Istalol, Rx (IstaPharma)	**Solution**: 0.5%	In 2.5 and 5 mL.
Timolol Maleate Ophthalmic, Rx (Falcon)	**Solution, gel-forming**: 0.25%	In 5 mL.[6]
Timoptic-XE, Rx (Merck)	**Solution, gel-forming**: 0.25%	In 2.5 and 5 mL *Ocumeters.*[8]
Timolol Maleate Ophthalmic, Rx (Falcon)	**Solution, gel-forming**: 0.5%	In 5 mL.[6]
Timoptic-XE, Rx (Merck)	**Solution, gel-forming**: 0.5%	In 2.5 and 5 mL *Ocumeters.*[8]

[1] With benzalkonium chloride 0.01%, mannitol, poly sulfonic acid, carbomer 934P, hydrochloric acid or sodium hydroxide, and EDTA.
[2] With benzalkonium chloride 0.005%, NaCl, and sodium phosphate.
[3] With polyvinyl alcohol 1.4%, benzalkonium chloride 0.004%, sodium metabisulfite, and EDTA.
[4] With benzalkonium chloride 0.004% and EDTA.
[5] With benzalkonium chloride 0.01%, and monosodium and disodium phosphate dihydrate.
[6] With benzalkonium chloride 0.01%, sodium hydroxide, and monobasic and dibasic sodium phosphate.
[7] Use immediately after opening; discard remaining contents. With monobasic and dibasic sodium phosphate and sodium hydroxide.
[8] With benzododecinium bromide 0.012%.

Miotics, Direct-Acting

Generic Name *Trade Name*	**Doseform/ Strength**	**How Supplied**
Carbachol, Topical		
Isopto Carbachol, Rx (Alcon)	**Solution**: 1.5%	In 15 mL *Drop-Tainers.*[1]
Isopto Carbachol, Rx (Alcon)	**Solution**: 3%	In 15 and 30 mL *Drop-Tainers.*[1]
Pilocarpine Hydrochloride		
Pilocarpine Hydrochloride, Rx (Various, eg, Bausch % Lomb)	**Solution**: 0.5%	In 15 mL.
Isopto Carpine, Rx (PolyMedica)	**Solution**: 0.5%	In 15 and 30 mL.[2]
Pilocarpine Hydrochloride, Rx (Various, eg, Alcon)	**Solution**: 1%	In 2 and 15 mL.
Akarpine, Rx (Akorn)	**Solution**: 1%	In 15 mL.
Isopto Carpine, Rx (Alcon)	**Solution**: 1%	In 15 mL.[2]

Miotics, Direct-Acting

Generic Name *Trade Name*	**Doseform/ Strength**	**How Supplied**
Pilocarpine Hydrochloride, Rx (Various, eg, Alcon)	**Solution**: 2%	In 2 and 15 mL.
Akarpine, Rx (Akorn)	**Solution**: 2%	In 15 mL dropper bottles.
Isopto Carpine, Rx (Alcon)	**Solution**: 2%	In 15 mL.[2]
Pilostat, Rx (Bausch & Lomb)	**Solution**: 2%	In 15 mL and twin-pack (2 × 15 mL).[3]
Pilocar, Rx (Novartis)	**Solution**: 3%	In 15 mL, twin-pack (2 × 15 mL).[4]
Pilocarpine Hydrochloride, Rx (Various, eg, Alcon)	**Solution**: 4%	In 2 and 15 mL.
Akarpine, Rx (Akorn)	**Solution**: 4%	In 15 mL dropper bottles.
Isopto Carpine, Rx (Alcon)	**Solution**: 4%	In 15 mL.[2]
Pilocarpine Hydrochloride, Rx (Various, eg, Bauch & Lomb)	**Solution**: 6%	In 15 mL.
Isopto Carpine, Rx (PolyMedica)	**Solution**: 10%	In 15 mL.[2]
Pilopine HS, Rx (Alcon)	**Gel**: 4%	In 4 g.[5]
Miochol-E, Rx (Novartis)	**Solution**: 1:100 acetylcholine chloride when reconstituted.	In 2 mL dual chamber univial (lower chamber 20 mg lyophilized acetylcholine chloride and 56 mg mannitol; upper chamber 2 mL electrolyte diluent and sterile water[6] for injection).

[1] With benzalkonium chloride 0.005%, hydroxypropyl methylcellulose 1%, sodium chloride, boric acid, and sodium borate.
[2] With hydroxypropyl methylcellulose 0.5% and benzalkonium chloride 0.01%.
[3] With hydroxypropyl methylcellulose, benzalkonium chloride 0.01%, and EDTA.
[4] With hydroxypropyl methylcellulose, benzalkonium chloride, and EDTA.
[5] With benzalkonium chloride 0.008%, carbopol 940, and EDTA.
[6] Sodium chloride, potassium chloride, magnesium chloride hexahydrate, calcium chloride dihydrate.

Cholinesterase Inhibitors

Generic Name *Trade Name*	**Doseform/ Strength**	**How Supplied**
Echothiophate Iodide *Phospholine Iodide, Rx* (Wyeth)	**Powder for reconstitution:** 6.25 mg to make 0.125%	With 5 mL diluent.[1]

[1] With potassium acetate, chlorobutanol 0.55%, and mannitol 1.2%.

Carbonic Anhydrase Inhibitors

Generic Name *Trade Name*	**Doseform/ Strength**	**How Supplied**
Acetazolamide *Acetazolamide, Rx* (Various, eg, Mutual, URL)	**Tablets**: 125 mg	In 50s, 100s, 250s, 500s, and 1000s.
Diamox, Rx	**Tablets**: 125 mg	In 100s.
Diamox Sequels, Rx (Barr)	**Capsules, sustained-release**: 500 mg	In 100s.
Acetazolamide, Rx (Various, eg, Bedford)	**Powder for injection, lyophilized**: 500 mg (as sodium)	In 10 mL vials.
Diamox, Rx (Barr)	**Powder for injection, lyophilized**: 500 mg (as sodium)	In vials.
Methazolamide *Methazolamide, Rx* (Various, eg, Teva)	**Tablets**: 25 mg	In 100s and 1000s.
GlaucTabs, Rx (Akorn)	**Tablets**: 25 mg	In 100s.
Methazolamide, Rx (Various, eg, Teva)	**Tablets**: 50 mg	In 100s and 1000s.
GlaucTabs, Rx (Akorn)	**Tablets**: 50 mg	In 100s.
Dorzolamide Hydrochloride *Trusopt, Rx* (Merck)	**Solution**: 2%	In 5 and 10 mL.[1]
Brinzolamide *Azopt, Rx* (Alcon)	**Suspension**: 1%	In 2.5, 5, 10, and 15 mL *Drop-Tainers.*

[1] 0.0075% benzalkonium chloride.

Carbonic Anhydrase Inhibitor/Beta-Adrenergic Blocking Agent

Generic Name *Trade Name*	**Doseform/ Strength**	**How Supplied**
Dorzolamide/Timolol Maleate *Cosopt, Rx* (Merck)	**Solution**: 20 mg dorzolamide, 5 mg timolol maleate	In 5 and 10 mL dispenser with controlled tip.[1]

[1] With sodium citrate, hydroxyethyl cellulose, sodium hydroxide, and mannitol. Benzalkonium chloride 0.0075% is added as a preservative.

Prostaglandins

Generic Name *Trade Name*	**Doseform/ Strength**	**How Supplied**
Latanoprost *Xalatan, Rx* (Pharmacia)	**Solution**: 0.005%	In 2.5 mL plastic ophthalmic dispenser bottle with dropper tip.[1]
Travoprost *Travatan, Rx* (Alcon)	**Solution**: 0.004%	In 2.5 mL *Drop-Tainers* and twin-pack (5 mL).[2]
Travatan Z, Rx (Alcon)	**Solution**: 0.004%	In 2.5 and 5 mL *Drop-Tainers*.[3]
Bimatoprost *Lumigan, Rx* (Allergan)	**Solution**: 0.03%	In 2.5, 5, and 7.5 mL.[4]
Unoprostone Isopropyl *Rescula, Rx* (Novartis)	**Solution**: 0.15%	In 5 mL.[5]

[1] With benzalkonium chloride 0.2%, sodium chloride, sodium dihydrogen phosphate monohydrate, and disodium hydrogen phosphate anhydrous.
[2] With benzalkonium chloride 0.015%, EDTA.
[3] Polyoxyl 40 hydrogenated castor oil, *sofZia* (boric acid, propylene glycol, sorbitol, zinc chloride) as a preservative.
[4] With benzalkonium chloride 0.05 mg/mL.
[5] With benzalkonium chloride 0.015%, EDTA, sodium hydroxide, hydrochloric acid.

Hyperosmotic Agents

Generic Name *Trade Name*	**Doseform/ Strength**	**How Supplied**
Sodium Chloride, Hypertonic *Muro 128, Rx* (Bausch & Lomb)	**Solution**: 2%	In 15 mL.[1]
AK-NaCl, Rx (Akorn)	**Solution**: 5%	In 15 mL.[2]
Muro 128, Rx (Bausch & Lomb)	**Solution**: 5%	In 15 and 30 mL.[3]
Sochlor Solution, Rx (OCuSOFT)	**Solution**: 5%	In 15 mL.[2]
AK-NaCl, Rx (Akorn)	**Ointment**: 5%	Preservative free. In 3.5 g.[4]
Muro 128, Rx (Bausch & Lomb)	**Ointment**: 5%	In 3.5 g single and twin packs.[5]
Sochlor Ointment, Rx (OCu-SOFT)	**Ointment**: 5%	In 3.5 g.
Mannitol *Osmitrol Viaflex, Rx* (Clintec)	**Injection**: 5%	In 1,000 mL.
Osmitrol Viaflex, Rx (Clintec)	**Injection**: 10%	In 500 and 1,000 mL.
Osmitrol Viaflex, Rx (Clintec)	**Injection**: 15%	In 500 mL.

Hyperosmotic Agents

Generic Name *Trade Name*	**Doseform/ Strength**	**How Supplied**
Mannitol, Rx (Various, eg, Astra)	**Injection**: 20%	In 250 and 500 mL.
Osmitrol Viaflex, Rx (Clintec)	**Injection**: 20%	In 250 and 500 mL.

[1] With hydroxypropyl methylcellulose 2910, methylparaben 0.028%, propylparaben 0.01%, propylene glycol, and boric acid.
[2] With hydroxypropyl methylcellulose 2906, propylene glycol, methylparaben 0.023%, propylparaben 0.01%, and boric acid.
[3] With boric acid, hydroxypropyl methylcellulose 2910, propylene glycol, methylparaben 0.023%, and propylparaben 0.01%.
[4] With mineral oil, white petrolatum, and lanolin oil.
[5] With mineral oil, white petrolatum, and lanolin.

Surgical Adjuncts

Generic Name *Trade Name*	**Doseform/ Strength**	**How Supplied**
Intraocular Irrigating Solutions		
Balanced Salt Solution, Rx (B. Braun)	**Solution**: 0.64% NaCl, 0.075% KCl, 0.03% magnesium chloride, 0.048% calcium chloride, 0.39% sodium acetate, 0.17% sodium citrate and sodium hydroxide acid or hydrochloric acid	In 500 mL.
BSS, Rx (Alcon)	**Solution**: 0.64% NaCl, 0.075% KCl, 0.03% magnesium chloride, 0.048% calcium chloride, 0.39% sodium acetate, 0.17% sodium citrate and sodium hydroxide or hydrochloric acid	Preservative free. In 15, 30, 250, and 500 mL.
BSS Plus, Rx (Alcon)	**Solution**: Part 1: 7.44 mg NaCl, 0.395 mg KCl, 0.433 mg dibasic sodium phosphate, 2.19 mg sodium bicarbonate, hydrochloric acid or sodium hydroxide/mL *Mix aseptically just prior to use.*	Preservative free. In 250 and 500 mL.
	Solution: Part 2: 3.85 mg calcium chloride dihydrate, 5 mg magnesium chloride hexahydrate, 23 mg dextrose, 4.6 mg glutathione disulfide/mL *Mix aseptically just prior to use.*	Preservative free. In 10 mL.

Surgical Adjuncts		
Generic Name *Trade Name*	**Doseform/ Strength**	**How Supplied**
B-Salt Forte, Rx (Akorn)	**Solution**: Part 1: 7.14 mg NaCl, 0.38 mg KCl, 0.154 mg calcium chloride dihydrate, 0.2 mg magnesium chloride hexahydrate, 0.92 mg dextrose, hydrochloric acid or sodium hydroxide/mL	Preservative free. In 515 mL.
	Solution: Part 2: 1081 mg sodium bicarbonate, 216 mg dibasic sodium phosphate (anhydrous), 95 mg glutathione disulfide (oxidized glutathione)/vial	Preservative free. In 60 mL.
Povidone Iodine		
Betadine 5% Sterile Ophthalmic Prep Solution, Rx (Alcon)	**Solution**: 5%	In 30 mL.[1]
Sodium Hyaluronate		
Healon, Rx (AMO)	**Injection**: 10 mg/mL[2]	In 0.4, 0.55, 0.85, and 2 mL disp. syringes.
ProVisc, Rx (Alcon)	**Injection**: 10 mg/mL[2]	In 0.4, 0.55, and 0.85 mL disp. glass syringes.
Amvisc, Rx (Chiron)	**Injection**: 12 mg/mL[3]	In 0.5 or 0.8 mL disp. syringes.
Coease, Rx (Advanced Medical Optics)	**Injection**: 12 mg/mL[3]	In 0.5 or 0.8 mL disp. syringes.
Shellgel, Rx (Cyotosol Ophthalmics)	**Injection**: 12 mg/mL[3]	In 0.8 mL disp. syringes.
Healon GV, Rx (AMO)	**Injection**: 14 mg/mL[2]	In 0.85 mL disp. syringes.
Amvisc Plus, Rx (Chiron)	**Injection**: 16 mg/mL[3]	In 0.5 or 8 mL disp. syringes.
Healon5, Rx (AMO)	**Injection**: 23 mg/mL[4]	In 0.6 mL disp. syringes.
Sodium Hyaluronate and Chondroitin Sulfate		
Viscoat, Rx (Alcon)	**Solution**: ≤ 40 mg sodium chondroitin sulfate, 30 mg sodium hyaluronate per mL	In 0.5 and 0.75 mL disp. syringes.
Hyaluronidase		
Vitrase, Rx (Ista)	**Injection**: 6,200 units lyophilized ovine hyaluronidase nonpreserved	In single-use 5 mL vial, one 1 mL syringe, one 5 mcm filter needle.

Surgical Adjuncts

Generic Name *Trade Name*	**Doseform/ Strength**	**How Supplied**
Hydroxypropyl Methylcellulose		
Gonak, Rx (Akorn)	**Solution**: 2.5%	In 15 mL.[5]
Goniosoft, Rx (Akorn)	**Solution**: 2.5%	In 15 mL.
Goniosol, Rx (Novartis)	**Solution**: 2.5%	In 15 mL.[6]
Absorbable Gelatin Film, Sterile		
Gelfilm, Rx (Pharmacia)	**Film**: 100 mm × 125 mm	In 1s.
Gelfilm Ophthalmic, Rx (Pharmacia)	**Film**: 25 mm × 50 mm	In 6s.
Miotics, Direct-Acting Acetylcholine Chloride, Intraocular		
Miochol-E, Rx (Novartis)	**Solution**: 1:100 acetylcholine chloride when reconstituted	In 2 mL dual chamber univial (lower chamber 20 mg lyophilized acetylcholine chloride and 56 mg mannitol; upper chamber 2 mL electrolyte diluent[7] and sterile water for injection).
Miotics, Direct-Acting Carbachol, Intraocular		
Carbastat, Rx (Novartis)	**Solution**: 0.01%	In 1.5 mL vials.[8]
Miostat, Rx (Alcon)	**Solution**: 0.01%	In 1.5 mL vials.[8]
Polydimethylsiloxane (Silicone Oil)		
AdatoSil 5000, Rx (Bausch & Lomb)	**Injection**: Polydimethysiloxane oil	In single-use 10 and 15 mL vials.
Botulinum Toxin Type A		
Botox, Rx (Allergan)	**Powder for injection, lyophilized**: 100 units of lyophilized *Clostridium botulinum* toxin type A.[9]	Preservative free. 0.05 mg albumin (human), 0.9 mg sodium chloride. In vials.

[1] With glycerin, sodium chloride, sodium hydroxide, and sodium phosphate.
[2] With NaCl 8.5 mg per mL.
[3] With 9 mg NaCl per mL.
[4] With NaCl 8.5 mg, 0.28 mg disodium hydrogen phosphate dihydrate, 0.04 mg sodium dihydrogen phosphate monohydrate per mL.
[5] With benzalkonium chloride 0.01%, EDTA, boric acid, KCl, sodium borate, hydrochloric acid or sodium hydroxide.
[6] With benzalkonium chloride 0.01%, boric acid, KCl, and EDTA.
[7] With sodium chloride, potassium chloride, magnesium chloride hexahydrate, and calcium chloride dihydrate.
[8] With sodium chloride 0.64%, potassium chloride 0.075%, calcium chloride dihydrate 0.048%, magnesium chloride hexahydrate 0.03%, sodium acetate trihydrate 0.39%, sodium citrate dihydrate 0.17%, sodium hydroxide, and hydrochloric acid.
[9] One unit corresponds to the calculated median lethal intraperitoneal dose (LD_{50}) in mice of the reconstituted drug injected.

Agents For Retinal Disease

Generic Name *Trade Name*	**Doseform/** **Strength**	**How Supplied**
Ganciclovir (DHPG) *Ganciclovir, Rx* (Various, eg, Ranbaxy)	**Capsules**: 250 mg	In 180s.
Cytovene, Rx (Roche)	**Capsules**: 250 mg	In 180s.
Ganciclovir, Rx (Various, eg, Ranbaxy)	**Capsules**: 500 mg	In 60s, 180s, and 1,000s.
Cytovene, Rx (Roche)	**Powder for injection, lyophilized**: 500 mg/vial ganciclovir (as sodium)	In 10 mL vials.
Ganciclovir Intravitreal Implant *Vitrasert, Rx* (Bausch & Lomb Surgical)	**Implant**: Minimum 4.5 mg	In individual unit boxes in a sterile *Tyvek* package.
Foscarnet Sodium (Phosphonoformic Acid) *Foscavir, Rx* (Astra)	**Injection**: 24 mg/mL	In 500 mL bottles.
Cidofovir *Vistide, Rx* (Gilead Sciences)	**Injection**: 75 mg/mL	5 mL amps.
Valganciclovir Hydrochloride *Valcyte, Rx* (Roche)	**Tablets, film-coated**: 450 mg	In 60s.
Verteporfin *Visudyne, Rx* (Novartis)	**Lyophilized cake**: 15 mg (reconstituted to 2 mg/mL)[1]	In single-use vials.
Pegaptanib Sodium *Macugen, Rx* (Eyetech)	**Injection**: 0.3 mg[2]	In 1 mL glass syringe. With 27∞gauge needle and shield.
Ranibizumab *Lucentis, Rx* (Genentech)	**Injection**: 10 mg/mL[3]	Preservative-free. In single-use glass vials.

[1] Egg phosphatidylglycerol.
[2] Equivalent to 1.6 mg pegaptanib sodium (pegylated oligonucleotide) or 3.2 mg when expressed as the sodium salt form of the oligonucleotide moiety.
[3] 10% alpha, alpha-trehalose dihydrate, 0.01% polysorbate 20, 10 mM histidine. Designed to deliver 0.05 mL.

Nonsurgical Adjuncts

Generic Name *Trade Name*	**Doseform/ Strength**	**How Supplied**
Dapiprazole Hydrochloride		
Rēv-Eyes, otc (Lederle)	**Powder, lyophilized**: 25 mg (0.5% solution when reconstituted)	In vial with 5 mL diluent and dropper.[1]
Extraocular Irrigating Solutions		
Collyrium for Fresh Eyes Wash, otc (Bausch & Lomb)	**Solution**: Boric acid, sodium borate, benzalkonium chloride	In 120 mL.
Eye Stream, otc (Alcon)	**Solution**: 0.64% NaCl, 0.075% KCl, 0.03% magnesium chloride hexahydrate, 0.048% calcium chloride dihydrate, 0.39% sodium acetate trihydrate, 0.17% sodium citrate dihydrate, 0.013% benzalkonium chloride	In 30 and 120 mL.
Eye Wash, otc (Bausch & Lomb)	**Solution**: Boric acid, KCl, EDTA, sodium carbonate, 0.01% benzalkonium chloride	In 118 mL.
Eye Wash, otc (Zenith-Goldline)	**Solution**: Boric acid, KCl, EDTA, anhydrous sodium carbonate, 0.01% benzalkonium chloride	In 118 mL.
Eye Wash, otc (Altaire)	**Solution**: Edetate disodium, potassium Cl, sodium Cl, sodium phosphate dibasic, sodium phosphate monobasic, benzalkonium Cl	In 118 mL.
Eye Irrigating Solution, otc (Rugby)	**Solution**: Sodium borate, NaCl, boric acid, sorbic acid, EDTA	In 180 mL with eyecup.
OCuSOFT Eye Wash, otc (OCuSOFT)	**Solution**: Benzalkonium chloride, edetate disodium, NaCl, sodium phosphate dibasic, sodium phosphate monobasic	In 30 mL.
Lid Scrubs		
Eye-Scrub, otc (Ciba Vision)	**Solution**: PEG-200 glyceryl tallowate, disodium laureth sulfosuccinate, cocoamidopropylamine oxide, PEG-78 glyceryl cocoate, benzyl alcohol, EDTA	In UD 30s (pads) and kit (120 mL and 60 pads).
Eye-Scrub, otc (Novartis)	**Solution**: PEG-200 hydrogenated glyceryl palmate, disodium laureth sulfosuccinate, cocoamidopropylamine oxide, PEG-80 glyceryl cocoate, benzyl alcohol, EDTA	In UD 30s (pads).

Nonsurgical Adjuncts

Generic Name *Trade Name*	**Doseform/ Strength**	**How Supplied**
Lid Wipes-SPF, otc (Akorn)	**Solution:** PEG-200 glyceryl tallowate, PEG-80 glyceryl cocoate, laureth-23, cocoamidopropylamine oxide, NaCl, glycerin, sodium phosphate, sodium hydroxide	Preservative free. In UD 30s (pads).
OCuSOFT, otc (OCuSOFT)	**Solution:** PEG-80 sorbitan laurate, sodium trideceth sulfate, PEG-150 distearate, cocoamidopropyl hydroxysultaine, lauroamphacarboxyglycinate, sodium laureth-13 carboxylate, PEG-15 tallow polyamine, quarternium-15	Alcohol and dye free. In UD 30s (pads), 30, 100, 120, and 240 mL and compliance kit (120 mL and 100 pads).
Tear Test Strips		
Sno-Strips, otc (Akorn)	**Strips:** Sterile tear flow test strips	In 100s.
Schirmer Tear Test, otc (Alcon)	**Strips:** Sterile test strips	In 250s.
Zone-Quick, otc (Menicon USA)	**Threads:** Phenol red threads (PRT)	In 50 Aluminum package sets (100 threads).
Zinc Sulfate Solution		
Eye-Sed, otc (Scherer)	**Solution:** 0.25%	In 15 mL.[2]
Vitamins and Minerals		
Vitamin A Palmitate, otc (Freeda)	**Tablets:** 10,000 IU	In 100s and 250s.
Vitamin A Palmitate, otc (Freeda)	**Tablets:** 15,000 IU	In 100s and 250s.
Beta Carotene, otc (Freeda)	**Tablets:** 10,000 IU	In 100s, 250s, and 500s.
Palmitate-A, otc (Akorn)	**Tablets:** 15,000 IU vitamin A palmitate	In 100s.
Palmitate-A 5000, otc (Akorn)	**Tablets:** 5000 IU vitamin A	In 100s.
Icaps Plus, otc (Alcon)	**Tablets:** 6000 IU vitamin A,[3] 200 mg C, 20 mg B_2, 60 IU E, 40 mg Zn,[4] 2 mg Cu, 5 mg Mn, 20 mcg Se	In 60s and 120s.
Icaps Time Release, otc (Alcon)	**Tablets:** 7000 IU vitamin A,[3] 200 mg C, 20 mg B_2, 100 IU E, 40 mg Zn,[4] 2 mg Cu, 20 mcg Se	In 60s and 120s.

Nonsurgical Adjuncts

Generic Name *Trade Name*	Doseform/ Strength	How Supplied
AntiOxidants, otc (Akorn)	**Caplets:** 5000 IU vitamin A,[3] 400 mg C,[5] 200 IU E,[6] 40 mg Zn,[7] 5 mg L-glutathione, 3 mg sodium pyruvate, 2 mg Cu,[8] 40 mcg Se[9]	In 60s.
Oxi-Freeda, otc (Freeda)	**Tablets:** 5000 IU beta carotene, 150 IU E, 20 mg B_1, 20 mg B_2, 20 mg B_6, 10 mcg B_{12}, 15 mg elemental Zn, 50 mcg Se, 20 mg calcium pantothenate, 40 mg glutathione, 40 mg B_3, 100 mg C, 75 mg L-cysteine	In 100s and 250s.
OCuSOFT VMS, otc (OCuSOFT)	**Tablets:** 5000 IU vitamin A, 30 IU E, 60 mg C, 40 mg Zn, 2 mg Cu, 40 mcg Se	Film coated. In 60s.
Ocuvite, otc (Bausch & Lomb)	**Tablets:** 40 mg elemental Zn,[10] 2 mg elemental Cu,[11] 40 mcg elemental Se,[12] 5000 IU vitamin A,[3] 30 IU E,[5] 60 mg C[6]	In 60s and 120s.
Ocuvite Extra, otc (Bausch & Lomb)	**Tablets:** 40 mg elemental Zn,[10] 2 mg elemental Cu,[11] 200 mg C, 50 IU E, 6000 IU vitamin A,[3] 40 mcg elemental Se, 3 mg B_2, 40 mg B_3, 5 mg elemental Mn, 5 mg L-glutathione	In 50s.
Ocuvite PreserVision, otc (Bausch & Lomb)	**Tablets:** 7,160 IU vitamin A[3,] 100 mg E, 113 mg C, 17.4 mg Zn, 0.4 mg Cu, lactose	In 120s.

[1] With mannitol 2%, hydroxypropyl methycellulose 0.4%, EDTA 0.01%, benzalkonium chloride 0.01%, and sodium chloride.
[2] With tetrahydrozoline hydrochloride 0.05%, EDTA, benzalkonium chloride, and sodium chloride.
[3] As beta carotene.
[4] As zinc acetate.
[5] As ascorbic acid.
[6] As dl-alpha tocopheryl acetate.
[7] As zinc ascorbate.
[8] As copper ascorbate.
[9] As L-selenomethionine.
[10] As zinc oxide.
[11] As cupric oxide.
[12] As sodium selenate.

Index

INDEX

The Index lists all generic names, brand names *(italics)*, and group names included in *Ophthalmic Drug Facts*. Additionally, many drug tables, synonyms, pharmacological actions, and therapeutic uses for the agents listed are included.

Index entries may refer to more than one form of a product (eg, tablets, solutions, suspensions, ointments) when all forms are included on the single page. Separate index entries are included when multiple forms of a product appear on different pages or when products are listed in more than one therapeutic group.